# History and Health Policy
# in the United States

**Critical Issues in Health and Medicine**

Edited by Rima Apple, University of Wisconsin–Madison,
and Janet A. Golden, Rutgers University, Camden

Growing criticism of the U.S. healthcare system is coming from consumers, politicians, the media, activists, and healthcare professionals. Critical Issues in Health and Medicine is a collection of books that explores these contemporary dilemmas from a variety of perspectives, among them political, legal, historical, sociological, and comparative, and with attention to crucial dimensions such as race, gender, ethnicity, sexuality, and culture.

# History and Health Policy in the United States

## in the United States

## Putting the Past Back In

**Edited by**
**Rosemary A. Stevens, Charles E. Rosenberg, and Lawton R. Burns**

**Rutgers University Press**

New Brunswick, New Jersey, and London

Library of Congress Cataloging-in-Publication Data

History and health policy in the United States : putting the past back in / edited by
Rosemary A. Stevens, Charles E. Rosenberg, and Lawton R. Burns.
    p. ;   cm. — (Critical issues in health and medicine)
  Includes bibliographical references and index.
  ISBN-13: 978-0-8135-3837-2 (cloth : alk. paper)
  ISBN-13: 978-0-8135-3838-9 (pbk : alk. paper)
    1. Medical policy—United States—History.   I. Stevens, Rosemary, 1935–  .
  II. Rosenberg, Charles E.   III. Burns, Lawton R.   IV. Series.
  RA395.A3H57   2006
  362.1'0973—dc22                           2005023051

A British Cataloging-in-Publication record for this book is available from the British Library.

Manufactured in the United States of America

# Contents

## Part III    Priorities and Politics

## Part IV    Policy Management and Results

# Foreword

Henry Ford may have told us that history is bunk, but the fact remains that much of what goes on in our social and political lives is an outgrowth of happenings in the past, the social institutions and arrangements we have developed over time, and the existing physical and social infrastructure on which we build. Scientific discovery, technical innovations, and social revolutions may bring large changes, but most of our policies and processes evolve from preexisting patterns. Some get comfort from thinking we are avant garde and that we are on the threshold of new ways of thinking and doing, but legacies carry great weight. Many so-called innovations are, when investigated further, little more than a recasting of earlier ideas and arrangements.

Some might think that health and medicine are different, reflected in the dramatic expansion of knowledge and technological innovation in the past fifty years—the unraveling of the genome and fantastic new developments in the pipeline such as new biomaterials (artificial skin and blood) and treatments fitted to individuals' genes. Some may even believe that in this dynamic scientific arena an understanding of history is more avocation than necessity. But these beliefs lead us to reinvent the wheel and repeat mistakes that could be avoided with a broader cultural, social, and historical perspective. Many think that HMOs are new organizational inventions, but similar entities in a great variety of forms have been around for more than a century; others may believe that new forms of payment such as capitation, prospective reimbursement of institutions, and blended reimbursement systems are innovative payment arrangements to deal with modern changes in health care, but these arrangements, too, are older than most of us. Under the British National Insurance Act of 1911, for example, capitation was established as a way of paying general practitioners. Few if any of the problems we have faced in paying professionals in the past twenty years would have been in any way surprising with even minimal attention to the past, in the United States and elsewhere. And even a cursory examination of the history of anti-smoking efforts would provide useful guidance about future challenges in preventing not only smoking but also obesity.

This volume on history and social policy is a product of The Robert Wood Johnson Foundation's Investigator Awards in Health Policy Research program. Initiated in 1992, this competitive program provides awards each year to a select group of investigators with innovative ideas and interdisciplinary projects that promise to contribute meaningfully to our understanding of significant health and health-care issues and to improve policy formulation. Since 1992 we have supported a broad range of approximately 150 scholars from medicine, public health, economics, political science, sociology, law, journalism, and history. The program is tied to no individual discipline or orientation. It seeks to support scholars with ambitious perspectives and ideas whose broad investigations would not ordinarily be supported by research organizations like the National Institutes of Health, the National Science Foundation, or other funding organizations.

The program is more than just a collection of individuals and a portfolio of research projects. We also bring together scholars and researchers from different disciplines and areas of research, and with varying perspectives, to think about and work on important cross-cutting issues. This is a voluntary activity, building on the enthusiasm and interest of our investigators in cross-disciplinary understanding and collaboration. The book's authors are associated with The RWJF Investigators' Awards program and have participated in an ongoing group seeking to better illuminate how the lessons of history can enhance our understanding of how to deal with emerging and future policy challenges. The contributors come from different disciplines and points of view and there is no "party line" here. This work is based on the belief that exploring the historical basis of health-care events will contribute to overall understanding of the health-care system and more discerning policy making.

As director of the program I want to especially thank Rosemary Stevens, an investigator awardee and member of our National Advisory Committee, who led this group effort with her usual sagacity and thoughtfulness and her co-editors Charles Rosenberg and Lawton Burns. Lynn Rogut, deputy director of the program, provided administrative support and guidance, and the contributors enthusiastically and often passionately participated in this effort. Special thanks are due to David Colby and James Knickman of the Robert Wood Johnson Foundation and Risa Lavizzo-Mourey, the foundation's president, for their understanding and support of the importance of a broad approach to policy making in health and health care.

**David Mechanic**
National Program Director
Robert Wood Johnson Foundation

# Acknowledgments

This book was made possible through the support of the Robert Wood Johnson Foundation Investigator Awards program in health-policy research. We thank the foundation, and particularly the program's leaders, David Mechanic and Lynn Rogut. Enthusiastic support and keen criticism came from Marlie Wasserman, the director, and Audra Wolfe, science editor, at Rutgers University Press. Kennie Lyman, our editor, worked long hours with the authors on style and readability. Students at the University of Pennsylvania also provided useful critiques of each chapter.

# History and Health Policy in the United States

# Introduction

History matters. Shared perceptions of history can move audiences, offer powerful explanatory narratives for the present, suggest intriguing analogies with past events, and help build consensus around policy and management goals. When visible at all, however, policy history is often tailored to specific aims, interests, and agendas. Policy-making is strewn with dubious historical analogies and powerful myths.[1]

One reason for studying the history of health policy is to avoid the pitfalls of thinking too narrowly about the present; in other words, to let one's imagination rove beyond the seductions of convenient but outdated partisan history. Among the pitfalls: assuming that past trends and/or current beliefs, as presented by advocates, will continue; uncritically accepting common or group belief in a new strategy in reaction to a perceived past; and neglecting the possibility that there may be promising alternative futures.

A second reason is that history is particularly important when policy directions seem unclear, as they are for health policy in most countries today, though perhaps most evidently in the United States. Without history, how are we to think about health policy in the twenty-first century? There are no ruling paradigms or canned solutions for health services in the United States (or for that matter in most other countries), save for rhetorical commitments to market and consumer principles and to providing care to every member of the population (while an estimated sixty percent of all health-care expenditures are incurred through the public sector and forty-five million Americans are uninsured). The lack of preconceived solutions may be good, allowing diverse, creative approaches to the organization, distribution, resource development, and evaluation of health care for the future. But good intentions are not enough. All of us—policy makers, employers, workers, investors, taxpayers, and patients, Republicans and Democrats—seek better ways to resolve the confusion and understand the complexities of our particular present. The essays in this book are designed to take a longer view of the present, and thus to open up the future, by looking at the history of health care through new prisms.

A third reason—and opportunity—for advancing historical policy work today is the breadth and depth of historical analysis and interpretations, across a range of subjects and from a variety of perspectives, now being produced by historians of medicine and health care. Though we do not confine ourselves here to card-carrying historians of medicine (that is, those who claim history of medicine as their primary discipline) the field has become more open to policy studies in recent years, including recent policy history.[2] At the same time, sociologists, political scientists, and others have brought their disciplinary interests to bear on historical themes. There is now a critical mass of historical scholarship, characterized by diversity of goals, purposes, and ideas.

We present here the work of seventeen scholars to illustrate the vitality of the work being done, the range of styles and points of view, and the relevance of history as a policy field. The essayists come from ten universities, two policy research centers outside of universities, and one private legal practice and represent ten scholarly and professional disciplines (history, history of science, medicine, public health, organizational theory and practice, bioethics, health policy, law, sociology, and social service administration). The writers bring their own questions to history and policy.

The resulting diversity of purposes and points of view is a major strength of this collection. We want to suggest, collectively, that there is no single definition of policy nor, therefore, of policy history; nor should there be. We hope that you, like us, will find this concept liberating.

Health policy is more than politics as we commonly understand that term; that is, more than an accretion of written policies inscribed in legislation after battles waged and compromises made among politicians and private interests. Policies reflect more general perceptions about what is important or fair or doable (or all three) in a particular culture, at a particular time, in a particular place. Hence the United States has consistently rejected universal health insurance for the whole population, though in 1965 the Congress voted for Medicare and Medicaid as proactive and self-protective actions. Policies rest on the evolution of culturally crafted institutions, such as hospitals, nursing homes, and organized health professions; on shared language (a commitment to equality of opportunity, for example); and on the prevalence of historical myths (that equality of opportunity can actually be achieved). Belief in the power of the market as a prime social tool, to be preferred where possible over government initiative, is also an expression of a nation's cultural—and thus policy—preferences. American health policy, to be understood in its rich complexity, expresses who we are, what we believe, the institutions we have created, and how we think.

What assumptions about health policy inform the health-care system of today—and thus may shape what we as a society find necessary tomorrow? Why have both private and governmental initiatives often failed? Are the "new" questions—such as reliance on information technology or on consumer-centered health care—really new? How (and why) do Americans accept deficiencies in major parts of the health-care system and deflect intractable problems from one set of institutions to another? Examples from the essays include: patients seeking primary care flocking to emergency rooms, leading to a perceived crisis in emergency medicine; otherwise middle-class nursing home residents embedded in major welfare programs designed for the poor (Medicaid); and many individuals with severe behavioral problems receiving their medical care in prisons. The politics of deflection have become policies of convenience. Why do leaders in both major political parties express their belief in smaller government yet expand government services and expenditures during their administrations? These and many other questions in this volume are historical questions; indeed, they are the very stuff of history.

This book has three goals. We hope, first, to stimulate debate over such questions and thus to demonstrate the importance of history in evaluating health-care policy, past and present, and in imagining new paths for the future. These essays are written by an outstanding group of health-care historians and others who use history as a fundamental policy skill. We write for a general audience rather than for any one academic field and have included explanatory language and descriptive materials for those without a health-care background (for example, in recounting the history of health maintenance organizations, or HMOs). Though health care is replete with acronyms such as HMO and DRG, we have done our best to keep the reader on-course and engaged.

Our second goal is to reconceptualize health policy problems by looking at their historical roots—including the often unexamined values and assumptions that infuse them—and thus energize and sometimes polarize political policy in the United States. Targeted historical studies illuminate an array of policies, programs, institutions, and fields, ranging from the policy issues involved in biomedical research, public health, and medical specialization through the dynamics and perils of different health organizations, policies, and programs. While the chapters cover a variety of subjects, most of the focus is on health-care history and policy since the 1960s. The essayists provide a historical overview of major systems of health-care delivery, including hospitals, emergency rooms, managed care, insurance, nursing homes, and mental health. We also examine important institutional actors and longer themes, such as the National Institutes of Health, consumers, privacy, and public health. We do not address every aspect of the U.S. health-care system, nor could we without writing a vast and/or tendentious synthesis. What we do provide is a tapestry of essays based on the shared assumption that thinking historically is essential for understanding the characteristics and idiosyncrasies of health services in the United States.

Our third goal is to demonstrate the role of social scientists (historians in particular) in framing and imagining policy for the future, that is, to confirm the place of history as a fundamental policy science. We are not arguing for a new historical discipline: quite the reverse. As we have noted, the essays here draw on the research of scholars in many disciplines, and we see this as a strength. What we seek is greater historical awareness among participants in health-care management and health policy and greater awareness among historians (whatever their training) of the contributions they can make. And we hope as well to make historians more generally aware that health-care history and policy history are rich sources for research and analysis. Historians of health care still do not communicate well with policy analysts, with the general public, or with members of the business community—and vice versa. Each needs the perspective of the others.

We do not pretend to offer solutions to the vexing problems of health services today. There are no simple solutions; that is, perhaps, the central historical conclusion to draw from these essays. Nor, as will become clear on reading through the essays, do they convey a single political or strategic message. American health care is segmented, and health policy serves multiple purposes. As the product of independent, strong-minded thinkers, the book is also varied in approach and rich in content. Early in our discussions we tried out possible unifying scenarios for the essayists, such as identifying specific turning points in history or key ideological and organizational themes. The group rejected a single narrative or theme, for none was ultimately satisfying. Health care is so embedded in American culture and politics that to write about it is to write about our country writ large: What we value. How we think. How we govern. How we achieve an ultimately unstable consensus by crafting short-term compromises that paper over structural divisions.

Nevertheless, in reading through all of the chapters, the reader may recognize a cumulative, illuminating similarity in the themes presented and the issues addressed. Notably, rather than one health policy, there is a congeries of separate policies, each with its own internal rationale and sponsoring groups, and an array of policy histories rather than one health policy history. Some policies are intentional, such as the growth of federal funding for biomedical research after World War II. Some, such as the growth of Medicaid expenditures for nursing home care, seem unintentional, though as Colleen M. Grogan points out "unintentional" does not necessarily mean inconvenient to powerful actors. In other cases old problems keep recurring. For example, contemporary experts in mental health policy are repeating the concerns of thirty years ago. Through all the interweaving histories, public and private organizations work together, struggle, negotiate, and attempt to reach consensus.

Charles E. Rosenberg dissects the underlying historical messages of the book in his essay: the intersections of public and private action in the United States; the nature and importance of values that go far beyond today's political concentration on health-care economics and costs; the historical rationality of the health-care system we have invented; and the prevalence of fundamental conflicts and ambiguities. Health policy is indeed a mirror of our society, messy and muddled though it may seem. If, as is sometimes said, we have developed the ideal health system for our purposes, it follows that constructive change may rest on reexamination of those purposes.

These themes reinforce the maxims Lawton R. Burns presents to his Wharton MBA students in including (and justifying) history as a management skill: "I frequently fall back on some famous quotations. Quoting Ecclesiastes, I explain to my students there is no new thing under the sun. The history of the health-care system often repeats itself (for example, the recurrent interest in national health insurance every twenty years or so). If that isn't convincing enough, I quote the late President Harry Truman who said, 'The only thing new in the world is the history you don't know.' Finally, to make it really relevant to the younger generation, I quote the pop singer Shirley Bassey, 'Just a little bit of history repeating.'" It was with his own maxims in mind that he agreed to help in the production of this volume.

In reading the essays, you will be confronted with a key paradox in the history of the health-care system: though the problems and debates remain unchanged, their form changes over time. Thus Amy L. Fairchild demonstrates a two-hundred-year concern about not only the notion of patient privacy, but change in its basic meanings; Beatrix Hoffman shows not just a persistence of crisis in the emergency-room system, but a change in the nature of that crisis;

David Mechanic and Gerald N. Grob chronicle the persistent problems in mental-health policy over the past half century but also describe the new forms the debate has assumed; Nancy Tomes charts the rise in prominence of the health-care consumer without any meaningful change in the consumer's personal responsibility.

In reflecting back on these and other chapters, one gets the sense of seemingly opposing forces, or "polarities," at work in our health-care system. These might be described as "dynamics without change" and "transformation in the face of stability"—observations that are important to business students as well as those in history or other policy fields. Business school researchers have recognized over the past decade or so that the essence of management is managing seemingly opposite things—such as incremental and revolutionary change, centralization and decentralization, large scale and small size, and global operations and local market sensitivity. How to manage these polar opposites in the corporate world has become new field of management research. Such research may also prove illuminating for health-care scholars, health-services researchers, and policy makers in creating workable approaches to the problems in each of the health-care sectors analyzed here.

Even though the essays, overlapping as they do in subject matter and message, do not fit neatly into any topic groupings, with some trepidation the editors have imposed a didactic structure on the book to emphasize underlying perspectives. The first three chapters are grouped as Actors and Interpretations, and include the big-picture essays by Charles E. Rosenberg, Lawrence D. Brown, and myself (Rosemary A. Stevens). Taken together, they show the extraordinary interplay of public and private actors and actions in American health policy, and the sometimes concealing role of ideology in policy making (in this case government expansion masked by political rhetoric that urges government's reduction). As I argue in my essay, policy is expressed by what is *not* legislated as much as by what is; notably, medical specialization is a strong, implicit national policy for health care in the United States, embedded in public and private policies, and marked by the absence as well as the presence of congressional decisions.

The second grouping we have called Rhetoric, Rights, Responsibilities. Nancy Tomes addresses the use (and misuse, historically speaking) of language such as "consumer" and "consumerism" to identify and jump-start new policy initiatives. Amy L. Fairchild explores changing concepts of privacy: how privacy, a matter of concern well beyond the health policy arena, has shifted in its historical meanings while there remain critical questions about public-health protection versus the privacy protection of individuals. And

Gerald Markowitz and David Rosner, taking the greatest advocacy position in the essays, criticize pollution as a health hazard that has come to involve major corporations and question corporate responsibility for the public's health, the measurement of toxins, and the nature of proof.

We would point out that there is path-dependency in health care as in other fields, in that what happens at any one time builds on, rejects, or must at least take account of what was there before, but that nevertheless, there may be strong changes of meaning along that path. We want you, the reader, to ask why, for example, consumers have emerged so strongly in the political rhetoric of the present, and why we often assume that privacy has only one set of meanings. Policy assumptions that may seem clear, such as consumerism, market efficiency, or corporate responsibility, may be clouded with hidden, shifting meanings.

The third grouping, Priorities and Politics, emphasizes that there is not one American health policy (or set of policy assumptions) but multiple policies (or sets) located in many different private and public policy worlds, inside and outside the formal health-care sector. Robert A. Aronowitz examines how the concept of a health "risk" has become something to treat medically and pharmaceutically as if it were the equivalent of a full-fledged disease—and thus part of policy making, including what we count in assessing the population's health. Robert Cook-Deegan and Michael McGeary describe the tremendous growth of the National Institutes of Health as a story of political and technological success, but also a story that carries with it, nevertheless, some troubling questions about the focus of health policy as a whole. Colleen M. Grogan shows how Medicaid has, perhaps inadvertently, become a middle-class source of funding for nursing home care, as well as protecting the poorest members of the population.

Taken together, these essays suggest that American health policy may perhaps best be described as opportunistic. Health risks (such as hypertension) become diseases because they can be treated by a pill—suggesting in turn that disease, a central focus of health-care policy, may be defined opportunistically by the availability of treatment, rather than treatment defined by disease. Biomedical research has prospered as government policy in part because it met multiple national goals, was well supported politically, and was far easier to achieve than alternative, conflicted goals for universal health insurance coverage or more effective health-care organization. Medicaid proved a convenient device for providing institutional care in nursing homes that might otherwise be unavailable while avoiding larger policy interventions into chronic and long-term care. Such approaches may be seen as successful examples of American pragmatism in health care as in other fields; as policies that, by sidestepping difficult but central policy questions of coverage, accessibility, quality, and cost, are cumulatively unsuccessful in offering value for money in health care in the United States; or as both.

The final section includes essays on Policy Management and Results. David Mechanic and Gerald N. Grob depict how states have withdrawn from the direct provision of care for mental health, and how the mentally ill have been shunted around in the wake of policies for the deinstitutionalization of mental hospital patients from the early 1970s, leaving worrying gaps in the care provided for the seriously ill. Beatrix Hoffman shows how emergency rooms have become a "reluctant safety net" for all types of ailments, responsive both to consumer demand and federal requirements to treat emergency-room patients.

Policy making in the private sector has also often produced unexpected results. Only yesterday, it seems, hospital mergers were touted as the future of efficient, competitive hospital systems. In the event, illustrated in the spectacular Allegheny bankruptcy case discussed by Lawton R. Burns and Alexandra P. Burns, policy factors unrelated to hospital change defeated this mission. The authors make the more general point that health-care innovation based on a reigning ideology, such as "mergers are the name of the game," that does not take account of the full range of relevant factors (including the unexpected) can produce costly turmoil for everyone involved. In the final essay Bradford H. Gray reviews the history of another supposedly transforming policy, the birth and transmutation of health maintenance organizations (HMOs). HMOs were heralded as transforming health policy in the 1970s, market provision in the 1980s, and managed care in the 1990s. And indeed managed care did transform the provision of health care, though not in the way originally envisaged for HMOs. Gray concludes that today's organizational structures for providing health care are little more effective than those of 1970.

It would be easy to become despondent in reading some of these histories of narrowly opportunistic or overly enthusiastic choices, derailed (or rerouted) strategies, and dislocated dreams. But these essays also depict extraordinary instances of energy, experiment, and willingness to take risks on behalf of a multitude of participants. Collectively they demonstrate that health care is not on an inevitable trajectory, that choices have been made in the past, and new choices can be made in the future. That future is more malleable than many of us might think.

The last introductory word goes to the great, late policy scholar Aaron Wildavsky—a consummate realist about the limitations as well as the value of policy studies, and about the value of history in defining new policy problems and redefining old ones: "If history is abolished, nothing is settled. Old quarrels become new conflicts . . . . Doing without history is a little like abolishing memory—momentarily convenient, perhaps—but ultimately embarrassing" (Wildavsky 1987, 38). We hope you will be provoked to think more largely and in new ways about health care and policy as you read this book and that you will reassess your views of particular policies, assumptions, and institutions. Imagining possible alternatives for the future is a first step in attaining them.

## Notes

1. See Neustadt and May 1986; Stone 1997.
2. See, for example, Huisman and Warner 2004, especially the essays by the editors and by Allan M. Brandt.

## References

Huisman, Frank, and John Harley Warner, eds. 2004. *Locating Medical History: The Stories and Their Meaning.* Baltimore: Johns Hopkins University Press.

Neustadt, Richard E., and Ernest R. May. 1986. *Thinking in Time: The Uses of History for Decision Makers.* New York: Free Press.

Stone, Deborah. 1997. *Policy Paradox: The Art of Political Decision Making.* New York: W. W. Norton.

Wildavsky, Aaron. 1987. *Speaking Truth to Power: The Art and Craft of Policy Analysis.* New Brunswick, NJ: Transaction Books.

# Part I

# Actors and Interpretations

# Anticipated Consequences

## Historians, History, and Health Policy

Policy is a familiar term. But like many indispensable words, it is not easily defined. In one sense it is descriptive: policy refers to current practice in the public sector. It also has a variety of other meanings: policy may imply an "ought" of planning and strategic coherence—or a real world "is" of conflict, negotiation, and compromise.[1]

As the history of United States health policy makes clear, moreover, the real world is not a very orderly place. Policies on the ground seem less a coherent package of ideas and logically related practices than a layered conglomerate of stalemated battles, ad hoc alliances, and ideological gradients, more a cumulative sediment of negotiated cease-fires among powerful stakeholders than a self-conscious commitment to data-sanctioned goals. But policy outcomes are hardly random; they embody the divergent rationalities and strategies of contending interests. Public-sector outcomes are determined by structured contention and contingency—not the prospective models and metrics of social scientists.[2]

Thus, the familiar dismissal of the historical community's potential contribution to policy seems, at least to this historian, paradoxical. Structured contention and contingency *are* history and so is contemporary policy—even if historians and historical data seem tangential to the demanding (and demanded) task of anticipating the consequences of particular present actions.[3] From the historian's perspective, it is equally clear that recent policy—including ideological invocations of the past—constitutes a comparatively neglected area for research. Health policy tells us a great deal about the relationships among interest and ideology, formal structures and human need, professionalization and social welfare, and technology and its applications. The debates, rationale, and actions of successive generations of American legislators, executives, credentialed experts, and administrators have constituted a sequence of what might be described as recurring social experiments— and thus rich data for the historian and policy-maker.[4]

Some of the key themes in this particular story have become abundantly clear. One is the foundational relationship between public and private functions, peculiarly significant in medicine but far from irrelevant in other areas of American life. Second is the way in which values and ideas shape perceptions of the possible and the desirable and express themselves in the social strategies of institutions, of disciplines, and of interest groups. Third is the way that the policy-making process constantly creates new realities and new choices yet is itself structured by preexisting interests, perceptions, and cumulative decisions. Finally, I would emphasize the persistence of structured—and thus to a degree predictable—conflicts shaping American health care, conflicts that have grown, and will continue to grow, out of interactions and inconsistencies among these three underlying factors.

All of these themes are fundamental not only to health policy, but to American history more generally. Medicine is an indicator as well as a substantive component of any society. It is a cliché to emphasize that all medicine is social medicine and that the provision of health care links individual lives to larger social and cultural realities—but this cliché has not always dictated academic research priorities. The seemingly meandering history of American health policy underlines this instructive if banal truth.

## Public and Private

There is nothing more fundamental in the history of American health care than the mixture of public and private. In this regard, American distinctiveness lies not in some unique devotion to the market and individualism, but in a widespread inattention to a more complex reality. From the canal and railroad land grants in antebellum America to support for the aircraft industry in the twentieth century, from tariff policy to the creation of the corporation in the nineteenth century to today's outsourcing of military functions, the interactive and mutually constitutive mixture of public and private has been so ubiquitous in American history as to be almost invisible; it is as true for medicine as it is and has been for transportation or the military-industrial complex. All have been clothed with a sense of collective responsibility that implies—if not demands—the active role of government. Since the Second World War, the public sector (and especially the federal government) has supported medicine in all of its aspects—basic research and the training of biomedical scientists and clinicians, the provision of care, and the management of medically defined dependency.

It is a tradition with roots older than the nation itself. The Pennsylvania Hospital, for example, was founded in the early 1750s through a mixture of legislative subvention and private philanthropic money and leadership. Similarly, in colonial Virginia, the House of Burgesses created the colonies' first mental hospital to deal with a community responsibility, the dependent insane. Dependency and sickness have always enjoyed a complex and symbiotic relationship in America. Almshouses, for example, always had a medical-care component, even if one not easily distinguishable from their general welfare function.[5] Nineteenth-century localities found numerous ways to support health care—from lotteries to tax policy to cash grants—while states created institutions to care for the insane, the tubercular, and in some states later in the century even the epileptic and the inebriate.

It seemed only natural. Health and medicine have always been seen as clothed with the public interest, as somehow different from—if dependent upon—economic relationships; medicine was in but not entirely of the market. And if pain, need, and sickness have made medicine historically sacred, the relationship between sickness and dependency in another of medicine's aspects has linked the provision of treatment and care to the state's welfare responsibilities as well as to traditional notions of religious benevolence and more contemporary assumptions concerning access to health care as an aspect of citizenship in a democratic society. This unselfconscious yet intricately interdependent relationship between the public and the private, the community and the individual, the spiritual and the material has always characterized health care in America. Public and private are ultimately no more distinguishable in medicine than are art and science or care and cure. In the area of health, government and the market, public and private are hard to imagine as distinct and exclusive domains, except as ideological—if analytically useful—abstractions; in the real world they cannot be understood in isolation one from the other.

It is an historian's task is to understand the structure of such interrelationships. How, for example, are we to think about the creation, the regulation, and the clinical use of pharmaceuticals? Despite an intense contemporary focus on the decisions of corporate actors, the reality is far more complex. Government pays for much of the basic research and the training of laboratory investigators at every level and has for a century played a regulatory role, as well as acting in the market as purchaser (directly or indirectly) through Medicare, Medicaid, and the veterans administration. Patent law and the courts constitute another significant aspect of government involvement in the world of medical therapeutics. The medical profession also plays a fundamental role, serving as a source of intellectual and moral authority in the acceptance and clinical administration of drugs—thus occupying a position at once private yet clothed with public interest and authority.[6] It is within this context that we must view the vexed contemporary question of payment for prescription drugs, an increasingly visible, intractable, political—and politicized—issue that links the private and the public, the corporation and the community.

This pattern of what might be called mixed enterprise in medicine is hardly limited to the world of drugs and their clinical use. The institutional history of American medicine reflects the same pattern; hospitals and outpatient services have always been clothed with the public interest, for example, yet have remained largely in the hands of nongovernmental—not-for-profit—entities. It is assumed that hospitals perform basic social functions in restoring the sick to productive social roles—as well as serving a higher, less instrumental and more spiritual good. As I have just suggested, even the regulation of the medical profession reflects the same pattern. Specialty boards are private entities, yet they assume de facto public responsibilities, and their policies and credentialing activities create social, legal, educational, and even economic realities.

I have argued that for a mixture of instrumental and moral reasons it has long been assumed that the state has some role—and an interest—in protecting the health of its citizens generally and in providing at least minimal care for the helpless and indigent. This generalization is hardly controversial but it is insufficiently precise. Cultural assumptions, institutional forms, and technical capacity are historically specific—as is medicine itself. Until the mid-twentieth century few in the Anglo-American world thought it the responsibility of the public sector to support medical research; and not until the end of the nineteenth century did most laypeople think it important to control access to the medical market by carefully designating legitimate practitioners.[7] But even in America's earliest years as a nation, it was assumed that communities might and should enforce quarantines and a minimum level of urban sanitation as well as provide some care for the chronically ill and incapacitated. (As early as the end of the eighteenth century, for example, the federal government initiated a health insurance scheme to protect merchant seamen, workers regarded as strategically important and peculiarly at risk.) Obviously our social assumptions have changed drastically since the Federalist era—and the role of the state in medicine has been revolutionized, particularly in the last three-quarters of a century.[8] But this theme of a role for the public sector in protecting community and individual health has remained a reality, even if continually redefined, renegotiated, and continuously—if erratically—expanded. And this despite a quarter-century of rhetorical demands for smaller government; the rhetoric has remained just that—words, even if politically resonant words—as the public sector's role in health care has hardly diminished.

A parallel and reinforcing ambiguity surrounds the medical profession and its relationship to the market. Medicine has always been a business, and American physicians have until comparatively recently had to earn their living in a brutally competitive and unforgiving search for paying patients. Yet the professional identity and market plausibility of medicine has rested historically on a special moral and intellectual style, formally transcending the material reality and reflecting the sacredness of human life and the emotional centrality and specialness of the doctor-patient relationship. In the past century, the medical profession's claims to self-regulation and autonomy of action have been justified by mastering an increasingly efficacious body of clinical knowledge. Doctors are no longer priests, as they sometimes were in the premodern world, and many other contemporary professions claim a legitimacy based on esoteric knowledge. Nevertheless, there remains something special about the physician's vocation, about the profession's peculiar configuration of ethical and knowledge-based claims. Even in those centuries when, as gentlemen, physicians could not charge fees but expected honoraria, predecessor versions of this inconsistent but seemingly functional set of values defined the special place of medicine and helped legitimize its guild demands for status and autonomy. One consulted an elite physician in part because of the practitioner's moral stature and gentlemanly bearing, but one assumed that learning and skill were the natural accompaniments of such attributes.

This mixed tradition of moral standing and technical expertise has over time worked to facilitate the mutually reinforcing interconnection of public and private in medicine, even as the scale and scope of such relationships have changed drastically in the past two-thirds of a century. Medicine's traditional identification with the sacred, the selfless, and the public interest has over time blurred and hybridized with the intellectual, the technical, and the instrumental. The merging of these diverse sources of authority has obscured areas of potential inconsistency and conflict. Some of these conflicts are obvious. Are physicians necessarily and appropriately profit maximizers or committed to a selfless devotion to their fellow citizens? Are they healers or scientists?

And how can these inconsistent visions of the profession's social role and responsibilities be made coherent in the categories of public discourse and as components in the setting of health policy? Such questions underline a few of the ways in which public and private values and policy ceaselessly and inevitably interact—and are in a variety of ways mutually constitutive.

## Values and Structures

I have always been dissatisfied with our conventional usage in which the term *health-care system* refers only to economic and administrative components.[9] *System* implies interaction and inclusion—and in the case of health care a myriad of cultural expectations and norms, of institutional, political, and technical as well as economic factors. This portion of my argument might be called the cultural politics of health policy—a necessary parallel to the political economy of health policy. The connections and constraints are ubiquitous. One need hardly elaborate when we have in recent years lived through debates on abortion, on cloning and stem cells, on managing the end of life, on the provision of care and drugs to the aged, and on the expectations surrounding basic and applied science. The list could easily be extended.

It is easy enough to specify cultural values particularly relevant to medicine: attitudes toward life and incapacity, toward the old and young, toward technology and death, toward the bodies of men and women. But health policy has, of course, also been shaped by values and rhetorical strategies reflecting general—that is, not specifically medical—attitudes toward individual responsibility (distinctions among work, poverty, and dependence, between the worthy and unworthy poor), toward government, toward the market as mechanism and optimum allocator of social goods. Similar to these assumptions are the cluster of cultural values and practical expectations placed on technical solutions (or temporary fixes as critics might sometimes call them) to intractable social and policy questions. Such attitudes have unavoidable political implications; technological innovation, for example, can be presented and often understood as politically neutral—and thus more easily funded and adopted. The costs and benefits become apparent only in retrospect.

Most of us harbor a pervasive faith in the world of scientific medicine, a visceral and inarticulate hope of a temporal salvation: modern medicine will extend life, avoid pain, provide a gentle death. Even if we regard it as romantic or delusive, the idealization of research and its presumably inevitable practical applications has always been a part of the emotional and institutional reward system of science—and thus of medicine. Such hopes are widely internalized in lay minds as well. One thinks of Sinclair Lewis's *Arrowsmith* (1925) or Paul de Kruif's *Microbe Hunters* (1926), which glorified bacteriologists and public health workers as selfless warriors opposing infectious disease. One thinks also of a newer generation of hopes surrounding the promise of gene therapy and stem cell research.[10] Recent controversy over the commercial exploitation of academic science has in part mirrored this lingering sense of value placed on what used to be called freedom of research—and to the intuitive notion that knowledge of the natural world is the property of all men and women (and certainly the American taxpayer who has paid for a good portion of that biomedical knowledge). Neither assumption fits easily with market-oriented practices that emphasize private-sector actors, material incentives, and the blurring of lines between academic and corporate identities.[11]

Another value now widely disseminated is what might be called reductionism in medicine. Most patients as well as physicians expect disease to be a consequence of biopathological mechanisms, and thus ultimately understandable and treatable. These views are historically—if perhaps not logically—in conflict with other widely disseminated anti-reductionist ideas such as the interactive relationship between mind and body, the body's natural healing power, the social roots and multicausal nature of disease, the caring as well as curing mission of medicine. Though hardly monolithic in espousing reductionist views, organized medicine generally accepts and rewards the laboratory's achievements, and benefits from the status and—often unrealistic—public expectations that accompany technical innovation. There are a good many social consequences of our tendency to see disease as discrete and mechanism-based. Thus, for example, ailments with behavioral manifestations and no agreed-upon mechanism inevitably occupy a kind of informal second-class status in terms of everything from insurance reimbursement to social legitimacy, while—at the other end of the value spectrum—there are unrealistic or at least premature expectations surrounding the seductive certainties of genetic medicine.

At the same time, however, Americans have not abandoned a pervasive desire to maximize the role of individual responsibility in the etiology and management of illness. Cultural needs to find a logic of moral accountability in health outcomes inform discussions of any ailment that might be associated even remotely with potentially culpable personal choice. I refer here, for example, to such familiar battlegrounds as the appropriate public health response to AIDS or to smoking or to fetal alcohol syndrome or to substance abuse. It is easy enough to fault the alcoholic, the lung cancer patient, or the depressive for their respective failures of will and thus complicity in their own complaint. Society still needs victims to blame.

As all these examples indicate, historically situated cultural assumptions (or values) both legitimate and structure public policy—not because they float in some unanchored cultural space, but because they are reified and acted out in the policies, interests, self-perceptions and moral hierarchies of particular men and women and thus in their choices among policy options. Embedded in particular senses of individual self and institutional notions of corporate selves (medicine and nursing, for example), such values shape assumptions and constitute political constraints and motivations.

### Process, System, Structure

One of the characteristics of policy is what might be called its cumulative, developmental, or process aspect: each decision and its consequences interact over time to define a new yet historically structured reality, often one not anticipated by most contemporary actors. The system moves through visible decision points, elaborated by subsequent administrative practice—with that specific experience along with other relevant variables shaping the next visible shift in public policy. All are linked in a context of periodic confrontation, negotiation, and renegotiation—a setting in which the historian's contextual point-of-view can be particularly helpful. Policy formulation and subsequent implementation provide us with opportunities to see the relevant costs and benefits as perceived by particular men and women as they choose among a variety of available options at particular moments in time.

But, of course, the health-care system is, from one necessary perspective, a dependent variable; it is part of a political system. In the years since Franklin Roosevelt, health has become a substantive and increasingly visible issue in national, state, and even local politics. And I refer not only to the delivery of clinical services, but to policies on the environment, income distribution, and lifestyle: all can have effects on health. Increasingly the world of medicine has reflected, embodied, and been subject to the realm of electoral politics and to changes in party structure, in ideology, and in its relationship to other policy issues and the setting of budgetary priorities. Lobbying, local politics, and legislative committee considerations have all played a role in defining the specific contours of health-care legislation—while creating an ever-expanding bureaucracy with inevitable feedback into the relevant service communities and institutions.[12] Every public program creates or reconfigures an interested constituency: hospitals, pharmaceutical and device manufacturers, nurses, and physicians are all potentially benefited or hurt by changes in government policy; every proposal implies winners and losers. In the largest historical sense, bureaucracy and technology have created a new medicine. And the political system, like the health-care system itself, necessarily incorporates values, perceived equities, available technologies and institutional forms, which collectively define and constitute the possible and map the desirable.

Though much change is gradual, incremental, and elusive, the nature of policy implies periodic public discussion and decision making. How is health care to be financed? hospitals to be reimbursed? dependent children to be cared for? sexually transmitted diseases to be prevented? How are drugs to be certified as safe and efficacious? The discussions and conflicts surrounding such issues and their resolutions (however provisional) tell us a great deal about political goals and tactics. Sequences of events create a constantly revised sequence of structured choices. By following those events the historian can focus on the relevant loci of interest, power, and authority as they configure themselves in the consideration, passage, and consequent administration of particular policies. If the health-care system includes values, individual and group interests, and history, the political process allows us to look at that system and, in a sense, weigh those variables. One thinks, for example, of the roles played by medicine and medical specialties, pharmaceutical companies, patient advocacy groups, insurance companies, and party strategists in the recent discussion of prescription drugs. Such analysis demonstrates that the medical profession is not always monolithic, that specialties may have different interests, that academic and community physicians may similarly have different interests in specific contexts, even if all share certain guild interests and attitudes. Nurses, as we are well aware, have interests that differ dramatically from those of physicians or hospitals. We are equally well aware that for-profit and not-for-profit hospitals may have different interests, as might community and university teaching hospitals—yet all appeal to widespread ideas about technology and clinical efficacy. All also interact with local, state, and national government. The health-care system includes lobbyists and party strategists just as it incorporates cultural norms, hopes rationalized in terms of technology, and the disciplinary identities of physicians and nurses. Nothing ordinarily happens without alliances, and the nature of those alliances may tell us a good deal about underlying structures—as well as the political process. Studying the process of health-care legislation and implementation is a bit like stepping behind the scenes at the proverbial sausage factory; it allows us to study the perhaps less-than-elevating realities of what we delicately call "policy formation." Serious students of health policy are as much obligate political scientists as historians and ethnographers.

Tracking that political process leads us to structure, and analysis of structure permits a finer understanding of sequence, which allows us to configure cultural values and economic and guild interests, and even weigh the input of credentialed experts and the data they collect and deploy. One of the policy questions most needing attention is—in fact—the role of would-be rationalizers and problem solvers. How do we understand the impact of those individuals who work in policy-oriented think tanks, then move laterally into the academy, into consulting, or into government? Do they initiate change or simply provide an ensemble of rationales and models—tools in a toolbox—that can be utilized for particular purposes by strategically situated players?

And perhaps I should have listed demographers among those experts contributing to policy discussions. For, as I have assumed but not stated explicitly, population is itself a key health-policy variable—framing questions, making issues socially visible, and demanding a response. One thinks of the shift from rural to urban, and, especially in the industrial West, the demographic and epidemiological transitions, which—whatever their causes—have produced an older population demanding public-sector responses to ever-increasing levels of chronic and incapacitating disease. (In a similar way, it has been argued, the focus on children in a low-childhood-mortality environment has shaped public-health policies at the local and national levels.) The distribution of potential patients provides not only challenges to the delivery of health care but has, in our advocacy-oriented society, created a powerful pressure group— older citizens who vote.

A parallel argument might be made about globalization, which, as has become clear, threatens to create a social and biological as well as an intellectual, economic, and geopolitical community. AIDS and multi-drug-resistant tuberculosis—and emerging diseases in general—imply and foreshadow a world of risk and interconnection. And that threatening world implies a linked moral and policy dilemma; for mirroring domestic concerns, academic and government researchers and pharmaceutical companies have devoted comparatively little effort to a variety of infectious and parasitic ailments that still kill and disable in the developing world. But as we are well aware, the comparatively recent visibility of the problem has already constituted a novel policy variable.[13]

## Structured Conflict

An overarching theme in my argument is the persistence of structured conflicts in American health care, in some ways a consequence of the very complexity and scale of the system and of the cumulative ad hoc decisions that have helped constitute it. These conflicts are at once products, constituents, and predictors of history.[14] I would like to suggest seven such conflicts:

1. The place of the market as resource allocator in a system legitimated historically in rather different terms. Most of us find it difficult to accept instrumental notions of efficiency and market rationality as the ultimate determinant of available health-care options.
2. The problem of valuing outcomes. How does one measure an effective health-care system, when there is no easy metric for either clinical efficacy or humane outcome—or ultimately for disaggregating the two?
3. The inherent conflict at several levels between global standards of medicine and local contexts of use.
4. The question of boundaries. Where does medicine stop and something else begin?
5. The immanence and omnipresence of technological and institutional change in a system ill-organized to anticipate and contend with the consequences of such often unpredictable yet culturally valued innovations.
6. The problems associated with decentered and fragmented loci of power, and not only in the obvious realm of government(s).
7. The way in which medicine as a fundamental social function reflects, incorporates, and acts out more general aspects of social hierarchy, status, and power.

Such issues will continue to shape the medical care available to ordinary Americans in the foreseeable future. Let me say a bit more about each of these continuing conflicts.

## The Market: Problem and/or Solution

Medicine has always foraged aggressively in the world even as it has consistently invoked and often acted out a heritage of the sacred and the selfless. But in today's highly bureaucratic society, the sometimes uneasy relationship between soul and body, between the selfless and the material has been particularly strained by increases in scale and by relatively novel and in some ways inconsistent claims for the market itself as a rationalizing mechanism. The efficacy claimed for the market's discipline fits uneasily with more traditional ideas about healing the sick and defining humane ends.

This is a conflict that has long been implicit but has become increasingly explicit. As the recent history of managed care or of the pharmaceutical industry have made abundantly clear, it is difficult to implement—and effectively sell to the American public—the notion that private-sector competition provides the best available mechanism for achieving a stable and responsive medical environment. Most Americans feel that health care, especially *their* health care, is a right and not a commodity. Indignant reaction to cuts in traditional employer-based health insurance schemes reflect such assumptions— as well a growing disquietude at the increasing number of uninsured generally. But while this sense of moral entitlement constitutes a political reality, it conflicts with another ideological reality: a powerful suspicion of government and an equally widespread assumption that the market is itself a technology that can solve problems. Free-market advocates assume, if not always explicitly, that value conflicts are illusory because ultimately the market constitutes the best available mechanism for providing the greatest good to the greatest number.

But this argument, I would suggest, constitutes another example of an endemic ill in our society: a reductionist solution to a holistic problem. The market and its decision-making rationality may be a necessary technology in a complex world, but it is clearly not in itself a sufficient or autonomous one. Market incentives may be powerful, but they are not the only incentives; political power as well as institutional interest can distort and in part constitute the market. Hope constitutes another powerful externality. Humanitarian traditions allied with utopian techno-fantasies of life extended and pain forestalled have helped enable an atmosphere of ever-increasing costs and posed the insistent question of how those costs—material and existential—are ultimately to be repaid. The benefits of America's highly technical health-care system are in some dimensions elusive and not easily reduced to consistent, measurable terms.

### Measuring Efficacy

We have neither an easily agreed-upon metric for clinical excellence, nor a metric for misery. The extension of the average life-span and the lowering of infant and maternal mortality are clearly useful and appealingly concrete measures, and they constitute a powerful rhetorical as well as political argument. But in an aging society, beset by anxieties concerning health and seduced by technologies promising cures, such aggregate numbers are clearly insufficient. Thus the creation of concepts such as quality of life or quality-adjusted life years. But such formal constructs inevitably fail to capture and balance the costs and benefits involved in the health-care enterprise—both in terms of individuals and the collective. How does one define "progress" or "efficacy" and how do these relate to actual or projected policies? There is something both dissatisfying yet inevitable about such attempts to provide measurable yardsticks for immeasurable goods.

This is only one part of a much larger difficulty in arriving at consensus in health-care policies. And that is the question of defining success. What is efficacy in health care? And how does it relate to physiological or social function—themselves far from transparent terms? What are the criteria for the physiologically normal? What is to be measured? And against what standard? How does one frame moral and political judgments about the appropriate distribution of resources? How does one implement decisions concerning trade-offs between quality and cost? But one need hardly go on; these are the familiar complaints of health reformers, and a staple of bioethical as well as political angst. No end is in sight.

## Global versus Local

At some level medicine is objective and universal. Most of us think of it that way—as a continually evolving body of accessible knowledge, practices, and tools. Yet we are equally aware that clinical practice varies dramatically from place to place, even within the continental United States, and that not all of these differences can be accounted for by inequality of resources. If we add an international dimension, of course, differences are even more dramatic (one thinks of the Johns Hopkins–trained physician practicing in Lagos or Lima—even if in an elite, well-equipped hospital). Available resources and institutional realities determine the continuing negotiations between a hypothetically possible and the practically achievable. But that inconsistency between the hypothetical best—universal—solution and the implacable contingencies of local circumstance creates a permanent and recurring tension. There is no easy strategy for balancing the generalized truth of the laboratory finding or of the randomized trial against the place- and time-specific context in which that knowledge is applied. Such structured conflicts turn on inevitably contested questions of legitimate authority and the balancing of available resources and social priorities—and thus policy.

## Boundary Tensions

This balance is only exacerbated—intensified—by another dimension of this question. And that is the matter of boundaries, of defining where medicine ends and everything else begins. How much does the goal of health promotion, for example, trump other values and interests? Are cigarettes drugs? When does a nutritional supplement become a drug appropriate for FDA oversight? Is obesity an issue for clinical medicine or a social, structural, and cultural—and thus social-policy—problem? Or is obesity an issue of individual responsibility masquerading as health policy? Is violence a problem for the Centers for Disease Control or for the criminal justice system? Similarly, is substance abuse the responsibility of the psychiatrist, the social worker, the minister, or the police? Such boundaries are bitterly contested at many levels and on many battlefields but the burden remains the same: who is responsible and how much does the need to focus on individual agency trump the determinism implicit in the medicalization of problematic behaviors.

There is also a question of policing. What is the practice of medicine? Is it to be internally policed by our contemporary version of guild authorities, the medical societies and specialty boards? Or is medical practice subject in some measure to government and the courts? We have all been made aware of the controversy surrounding what has come to be called complementary or alternative medicine—and the questions it poses in regard to the institutional boundaries that define the physicians' role and the knowledge that legitimates the regular profession's status.

Preventive medicine in general provides another area for debate. Toxic substances, cigarettes, and fetal alcohol syndrome represent occasions for debate and contestation. Is fetal screening for genetic defects a morally neutral technical option—or an occasion for religious introspection, since abortion is so closely linked with screening? How do we balance individual clinical judgments, cost-benefit calculations, and the ever shifting consensus of evidence-based medicine in justifying particular diagnostic or therapeutic procedures? These are questions of jurisdiction and boundaries, but also occasions for the exercise of social authority. They will continue to remain objects of conflict and contestation.

## Technological Change and Its Discontents

The only thing more predictable than continued technological change in medicine is the debate and conflict surrounding such change. All those social expectations that encourage and support innovation also nurture conflict—over access and specialty control, over economic costs and ethical appropriateness. Humane concerns about the impersonal attributes of high-tech medicine can be traced back to the turn of the twentieth century, when available technologies were, in retrospect, rather crude. Anxieties about cost have an equally long pedigree. More recently, economic and ethical criticisms by most Americans—and not just bioethicists and health economists—have focused on the extraordinary and cost-ineffective technologies involved in preserving life in extremity. The ICU and respirator represent a nemesis that threatens everyone regardless of social class.[15] I could refer as well to the widely discussed dangers of overdiagnosis and the creation of a legion of asymptomatic—yet therapy-implying—ills. And we live with ever-present dystopian fantasies of human cloning and bodies kept alive with an ever-increasing variety of spare parts.

## Loci of Power

The contexts in which medical power is exerted are, as I have implied, fragmented and not always consistent. At one extreme is the bedside—the site of the physician's root legitimacy as healer. Very different sorts of power reside in the intellectual, bureaucratic, and administrative factors that constrain and shape the individual physician in his or her practice. I refer to everything from modes of reimbursement to the practical constraints implicit in disease protocols, evidence-based medicine, and the practice guidelines adopted by large insurers. Physicians have traditionally seen the clinical relationship as theirs to control—citing both ethical and logical reasons to maintain the bedside space as appropriate to the individual physician's control. In today's highly technical and increasingly bureaucratized society, that interpersonal decision-making authority has been increasingly compromised by considerations of efficacy, cost benefit, and all those generalized rationalities that constrain clinical choice. Randomized clinical trials, the conclusions of clinical epidemiology, the algorithms, protocols, and thresholds of managed-care administrators all imply a structured conflict at the level of decision making—a conflict that remains central not only to what might be called the macropolicy of insurance provision or hospital funding, but to the micropolicy of everyday clinical decision making. Yet the patient idiosyncrasy that underlies the intellectual rationale (and, in part, the profession's vision of itself) for the individual physician's clinical authority is now at risk. There is no easy strategy for balancing the generalized truth of the laboratory finding or of the randomized trial against the site- and individual-physician-centered truth legitimated by the patient's particular biological and social circumstances. That conflict between the generalized truth and its specific application will not be solved by some meta-consensus committee or cost-benefit analysis.

The question of appropriate authority in clinical decision making is a question of power and politics—macro and micro—but it is also a question of ethics, political theory, and policy. In America's complex federal system there are some obvious linkage questions. Where is the appropriate balance between state, federal, and local authority? It is a recurrent issue in American history—manifested now in struggles over such visible issues as abortion policy or Oregon's "right to die" legislation or California's medical marijuana statutes. Even more fundamental is the conflict between these traditional definitions of local jurisdiction and the instinctive moral feeling that health care should be universally accessible—and not determined by one's place of residence along with one's income. Who is to set priorities in everything from the distribution of research support to the provision of funds to subvent care for the poor and uninsured? Tax policy as well as randomized clinical trials helps shape the care delivered ultimately to particular patients. The political and administrative realities of health care also demonstrate the complexity of the interactions and interdependencies among local, state, and federal levels of need and responsibility. American federalism implies local differences in social need and available resources—intractable realities that often seem inconsistent with the legitimating vision of medicine as an objective—and thus universal—body of knowledge and practice.[16]

## Medicine as Mirror of Society

Finally, of course, medicine mirrors all the ambiguities and conflicts that characterize and mark our society: welfare policy, specific attitudes toward race as in drug laws and aid to dependent children, attitudes toward sexuality as manifested in AIDS policy and sex education. Changing media and communication realities imply changing social relationships; one need only watch consumer advertising on network television to extrapolate a new world of chronic disease, an aging population, and an ongoing set of political filiations and agendas. The same might be said of the internet with its ability to crystallize and distribute the message of disease advocacy groups, for example, as much as political parties themselves. And with an aging population and the increasing economic prominence of the health-care enterprise, it was inevitable that health issues would be as subject to the same lobbying and tactical political considerations as tax or industrial policy.

## History and Structured Contingency

Policy is always history. Events in the past define the possible and the desirable, set tasks, and define rewards, viable choices, and thus the range of possible outcomes. As we move through time those choices reconfigure themselves and trends may establish themselves—but at any given point the "actionable" options are highly structured. It is the historian's disciplinary task to define those likelihoods. Most important, what history can and should contribute to the world of policy and politics is its fundamental sense of context and complexity, of the determined and the negotiated. The setting of policy is contingent, but it is a structured contingency.[17] There should in this sense be no gap between history and policy—anymore than there is between any of the other social sciences and the making and administration of policy.

But there is. In some ways it is a problem of audience and expectation. Historians make uncomfortable prognosticators. We feel that historians should look backward, while the essence of policy is to look forward—as though the past is not in the present and the present in the future. History cannot predict what will happen; it is a more useful tool for predicting what will not happen. Or to put it another way, defining non-choices is an important way of thinking about choices. But history is not simply a database from which policy makers and policy scientists can mine rhetorically useful bits of admonition or encouragement; history is a complex discipline with its own constraints and necessities—its own notion of contexts and ongoing substantive consensus.

Every participant in the world of policy and practice has his or her own history that creates community and legitimates policy choices. Even the work of academic historians is inevitably a source of decontextualized data for real world actors who deploy it in the context of their particular visions of history. But the historian's primary context is the world of other historians, and it is this very distance from the policy arena that makes the historian's perspective so valuable. It is in this sense that history can best be considered a policy science. To be effective historians must maintain their disciplinary identity, their own criteria of achievement and canons of excellence. We are spectators at the policy dogfight—and may even lay the odd wager—but at least we don't own any of the combatants in the pit.

## Notes

1. In our disciplined and bureaucratic society it also assumes a role for experts (including lobbyists for a variety of interests) interacting with decision makers—both elected and unelected—in what is sometimes called a policy community. Policy may also imply claims to legitimacy based on presumed connections among data, data analysis, and subsequent decisions and practices. And, finally, at the national level, domestic policy presumes a logic of center and periphery, of centralized decision making even if particular decisions mandate the devolution of implementation to the periphery (as in Medicaid, for example, or, in its rather different sphere, specialty credentialing). Even the term *health policy* implies too neatly unified a sphere of action, as though health practices and expenditures could be insulated in a complex and interactive world of political and economic decision-making. On specialism, see Stevens 1998 and Stevens's chapter in the present volume.

2. Which is not to say that such contributions have not and will not continue to have their uses, sometimes central ones, but only in appropriate contexts of power and advocacy.

3. The de facto disdain for history acted out by many policy-makers is itself an historical artifact that demands explanation in historical and cultural, not epistemological, terms. Yet every discipline and every political position has its own proprietary

history: the nurse's history is different from the physician's, the free-market disciple's history different from that understood by advocates of a robust government role in health care. But one thing all such actors share is the willingness to frame and legitimate policy commitments in tactically convenient historical terms.

4. For an example of the use of history to reflect on public policy, see Fox 1986; 1993.

5. On hospitals, see Rosenberg 1987; Stevens 1999.

6. Though the profession is characterized by a historically negotiated self-governing status, that autonomy is itself legitimated in part by medicine's traditional identification with the public interest.

7. There were some other areas in which the federal government did begin to support scientific investigation in the nineteenth century—most prominently agriculture and then engineering (through the Morrill Act colleges and experiment stations), the geological survey, and—indirectly—through the support of higher education.

8. It should be emphasized that American government was at every level erratic and inconsistent in performing these functions.

9. It is not without significance that we conventionally refer to our "health-care" system, not our "medical-care" system, reflecting another usage distinguishing public from private—and thus obscuring the disparate strands that collectively make up these conventional categories; even the "private" practice of medicine has included aspects of what might be called "public" medicine—as in immunizations against infectious disease.

10. There is a countervailing—dystopian or one might call it Frankensteinian—vision of the increasing dangers implicit in technological innovation. But I would argue that such anxieties have always been a minority or oppositional theme.

11. Which is not to say that such relationships are unprecedented, but that they are often *perceived* as somehow radically novel—and morally compromising.

12. I refer to everything from hospitals and outpatient clinics to specialty boards and health maintenance organizations.

13. It should noted that we live to some extent in an increasingly global world of medical personnel and medical education as well as of finance and manufacturing.

14. Most of these conflicts are structured into Western medicine generally and not limited to North America. My argument focuses, however, on the United States.

15. For a defense of the economic and human rationality of continued investment in high-tech medicine, see Cutler 2004.

16. It is striking how studies that demonstrate regional patterns of inconsistency in clinical practice simply presume that the inconsistency speaks for itself—both logically and morally—as indicating irrationality and thus need for change.

17. Paul David's term *path-dependency* has become commonplace in the policy world; to a historian it is in operational terms another word for history—and de facto substitute for it. I have used the term *structured contingency* because I hope to emphasize that key area of contention between the determined and the negotiated—the structured as opposed to the contingent. See David 1985; 1986; Arthur 1994; Goldstone 1998.

## References

Arthur, W. Brian. 1994. *Increasing Returns and Path Dependence in the Economy.* Ann Arbor: University of Michigan Press.

Cutler, David. 2004. *Your Money or Your Life: Strong Medicine for America's Health Care System.* New York: Oxford University Press.

David, Paul. 1985. Clio and the Economics of QWERTY. *American Economic Review* 75: 332–337.

———. 1986. Understanding the Economics of QWERTY: The Necessity of History. In *Economic History and the Modern Economist,* ed. William N. Parker, 30–49. Oxford: Basil Blackwell.

Fox, Daniel M. 1986. *Health Policies, Health Politics: The British and American Experience, 1911-1965.* Princeton: Princeton University Press.

———. 1993. *Power and Illness: The Failure and Future of American Health Policy.* Berkeley: University of California Press.

Goldstone, Jack A. 1998. Initial Conditions, General Laws, Path Dependence, and Explanation in Historical Sociology. *American Journal of Sociology* 194: 829-845.

Rosenberg, Charles E. 1987. *The Care of Strangers: The Rise of America's Hospital System.* New York: Basic Books.

Stevens, Rosemary. 1998. *American Medicine and the Public Interest.* Berkeley: University of California Press. (Orig. pub. 1971.)

———. 1999. *In Sickness and in Wealth: American Hospitals in the Twentieth Century.* Rev. ed. Baltimore: The Johns Hopkins University Press. (Orig. pub. 1989.)

# The More Things Stay the Same the More They Change

## The Odd Interplay between Government and Ideology in the Recent Political History of the U.S. Health-Care System

I see report is fabulous and false.

Shakespeare, *Henry VI, Part I,* Act 2, Scene 3

Disentangling continuity from change in U.S. health-care policy is no task for those who crave instant intellectual gratification. The system is, of course, (in)famously stable: ever inclined to equate specialization and technology with quality, loath to impose planning on the independent institutional fragments of the "supply side state" (Jacobs 1995), unwilling to discard an employer-based approach to medical coverage, unable to acknowledge medical coverage as a right and to make such coverage universal and affordable, and quick to reject every real reform as a formula for "too much government."

The history of this same system, however, also shows much morphing and mutation: a "social transformation" (Starr 1982) brought industrial organization to cottage enterprises; competitive forces wrestled a provider-dominated sector into something more closely resembling a "normal" market; public regulatory innovations proliferated (professional standards review organizations, peer review organizations, health systems agencies, certificate-of-need programs, state rate setting, the prospective payment system and resource-based, relative-value-scale fee schedules in Medicare, the Health Insurance Portability and Accountability Act, and restrictions on managed care); broader coverage for low-income populations advanced (Medicaid expansions); new coverage for lower-income children emerged (the State Children's Health Insurance Program); Medicare finally added limited coverage for prescription drugs; and public dollars now constitute nearly half the funds in the nation's $1.6 trillion annual health-care budget.

Moreover, the confrontation between political ideology and policy history perplexingly parallels that between continuity and change. Three years after Medicare and Medicaid became law and national health insurance basked briefly in unquestioned imminence, Richard Nixon won the presidency and the nation began its rightward political shift. In health policy, as in other arenas, the President and Congress regularly pledged allegiance to deregulation, competition, market forces, correct incentives, and consumer choice, denigrating all the while bureaucracy, regulation, and big government, the era of which, Bill Clinton declared in 1996, was over.

Although this antigovernmental animus has endured, indeed grown, from Nixon to George W. Bush, the recent history of U.S. health policy has seen steady enlargement in the scope and scale of government's programs and presence—not as much as the Left seeks, of course, but much more than the Right can comfortably accommodate in its basket of conservative ideas. In the health realm, political ideology and political practice stand disconnected. This chapter traces the sources of this disconnect and in so doing tries to explain the frustrations that haunt the quest to distinguish continuity from change in the recent history of U.S. health policy.

The basic question is why government's role in health policy grows when "official" ideology says it should not. The following pages explore three of the main reasons for the disconnect: the agenda-shaping powers of technological innovation; the group politics that affirm antistate rhetoric in principle while admitting a long parade of government-expanding "exceptions" in practice; and the ironic invitations extended to public-sector repairs by policies that aim to maintain and enhance the role of market forces in health policy.

**Medical Technology**

The steady growth of innovative medical technology decisively drives health-care policy and—notwithstanding the myth that innovation is a nearly pure product of market-minded entrepreneurs as opposed to fusty public bureaucrats—draws government inexorably into the act. This public role, moreover, spans all stages of the research, development, and deployment of technologies, old and new.

Invention

Technological progress derives from scientific exploration—basic, applied, and mixed in complex and controversial combination (Stokes 1997). Since the mid-twentieth century, Americans have declined simply to leave medical research to the market, preferring instead to encourage and steer it by means of a growing cadre of national institutes of health (NIH) that set research priorities, conduct scientific studies internally, and award grants that shape the character of the nation's academic medical centers. The fundamentals of this tale of government growth are well known (Strickland 1972): before World War II these national institutes were few and small; accelerated medical innovation in service of the war effort dramatized the benefits of research with the muscle of the federal government behind it; the prospect of conquering afflictions such as cancer and heart disease captured the minds of the scientific community, the medical profession, the media, and the public; a network of philanthropists, researchers in NIH and in academic medical centers (AMCs), and enthusiastic congressional leaders enlarged both the number of national institutes and their budgets; and the United States affirmed a commitment to more and better technology, the political economy of which has never wavered. Public investment in the life sciences in the antistatist states far exceeds that of other nations and helps make the financial world safe for the research and development ventures of private firms. Such funding "has created most of the new opportunities for biotechnology and pharmaceutical companies, and it will undoubtedly continue to do so" (Croghan and Pittman 2004, 27). Between 1998 and 2003 the NIH budget more than doubled (Campbell et al. 2004, 69).

## Validation

Once science has spilled its discoveries onto the collective carpet, someone has to decide what drugs, devices, and procedures are fit for human consumption, and under what conditions. That "someone" is often government. At times NIH tackles this validating role by sponsoring and collaborating in clinical studies long after technologies arrive on the scene as "expanding indicators of use" arise (Gelijns 2004). Validation can, moreover, be post-factum as well as prospective. For example, as the panoply of procedures that bear the collective moniker "complementary and alternative medicine" (CAM) gained popularity, purists in NIH grudgingly began supporting research on the scientific merits of acupuncture, meditation, tai-chi, and more. The Office of Alternative Medicine that Congress established in the NIH in 1991 with a budget of $2 million—encouraged by a senator whose allergies responded favorably to bee pollen—is now the National Center for Complementary and Alternative Medicine and was funded at $112.5 million in 2003 (Ruggie 2004).

The major master of ceremonies, however, is the federal Food and Drug Administration (FDA), which oversees the testing of medical innovations and certifies their safety and efficacy. As the scale and pace of medical innovation expands and quickens, the agenda of FDA regulators grows too. That the agency retains a public approval rating of seventy percent while navigating political terrain populated by an estimated 3,100 disease-specific interest groups (Carpenter 2004) suggests a strikingly high acceptance of a big role for big government in mediating the demands of rigorous science, the yearnings of consumers for cures, and the promise of high corporate profit. And illness-based political mobilization is becoming increasingly intense: "to a degree never before witnessed, disease-specific lobbies now press Congress for medical research funding, insurers and state governments for favorable coverage rulings, and the FDA for quick approvals" (Carpenter 2004, 57).

New medical technology need not be particularly "high" in order to launch a steady expansion of the public presence. The arrival of the polio vaccine in the 1950s, for instance, quickly led to federal grants that encouraged states to buy vaccine and give free immunizations to children and pregnant women. In the 1960s vaccines for DPT, measles, and rubella joined the preventive portfolio, followed by a new section of the Public Health Service Act (1970), requirements that the Early and Periodic Screening, Diagnosis, and Treatment program within Medicaid provide immunizations (1979), and federal legislation (1986–1987) to address liability issues surrounding vaccines. A measles epidemic in 1989–1991 triggered a national Vaccine Advisory Committee; a white paper on measles; a federal Interagency Coordinating Committee; a Public Health Service Action Plan with fourteen goals and 120 action steps; an Infant Immunization Initiative; a "national effort"; the preparation of "Immunization Action Plans by states, territories, and large cities"; a Vaccines for Children program (1993); and more, and better, so that the federal government "today plays a central role in the effort to eliminate vaccine-preventable childhood disease" (Johnson et al. 2000, 106, 99).

## Diffusion

Safe and efficacious medical innovations do not automatically find their way to patients. Few view allocating them by ability to pay as equitable, so for most of the population insurance coverage governs access to technological progress. Commercial carriers reach their own conclusions on who should be covered for what, but these are often shaped by government-sponsored studies on cost effectiveness and by lists (often long) of benefits that individual states mandate plans to cover. For nearly half the population (forty-two million in Medicare, forty-three million in Medicaid, forty-five million uninsured), however, what one gets is what government defines as reimbursable. Officials in the Centers for Medicare and Medicaid Services (CMS) and in state Medicaid offices, and innumerable obscure decision makers (and "rationers") in the hospitals, clinics, and health centers of the safety net thus join the NIH and FDA as arbiters between technologies and their beneficiaries.

The relentless march of medical progress expands the scope and complexity of the issues confronting public policy. For example, the feds' resolve to perfect an implantable artificial heart by Valentine's Day 1970 came up short, but an offshoot of that effort, ventricular assist devices, originally viewed as "bridges" to transplantation, have proved to be effective "destination" therapies (Rose et al. 2001). This is good news for heart patients, but a mixed blessing for CMS, which faces potentially vast demand for costly care. Seeking to manage new and complex tasks, CMS has begun defining who will be covered for these devices, how much providers will be paid, and which medical centers may perform the procedure. That agency is also insisting that participating providers contribute data to a national clearing house that will (under joint direction of NIH, FDA, and the Agency for Healthcare Research and Quality) support studies of patient outcomes and the cost effectiveness of the procedure (Bussell 2003; Gelijns 2004).

Sometimes government grows by iterative, interactive steps across "sectors." The exclusion of prescription drug coverage from Medicare in 1965, for example, generated a thriving private MediGap industry, the abuses, limits, and inequities of which encouraged, in turn, both extensive federal regulation and growing pressure for Medicare prescription drug benefits. The recent enactment of these benefits obliges federal officials to promulgate new rules for beneficiaries, the pharmaceutical industry, and government in a game that simultaneously entails a supposed infusion of market forces into Medicare and a sprawling penumbra of new public regulation.

Nor is coverage the sole route that carries government into controlling the diffusion of medical technology. Because such innovations are costly, payers and planners eternally yearn for assurance that their application honors norms of appropriateness and necessity. Since the late 1950s, when Milton Roemer's famous "law" highlighted the induced demand for inpatient care allegedly exerted by the supply of hospital beds, policymakers have thought it not unreasonable to condition the diffusion of costly facilities and equipment on certification by public reviewers that such goodies are indeed "needed." Hence certificate-of-need (CON) programs, which began in New York State in 1964, spread to half the states by 1974, were required by the federal government in all states between 1974 and 1986, and, notwithstanding federal permission to the states to abandon them in a new pro-competitive era of cost containment, endure today (albeit largely unsung and unstudied) in two-thirds of the states.

## Application

In principal, medical technologies that emerge under the close scrutiny of the NIH, FDA, CMS, and other public guardians are applied to patients according to the definitive canons of medical science. In practice, considerable uncertainty haunts medical practice (Gelijns et al. 1998, 2003) and shows up in wide and inexplicable variations in practice patterns across regions and clinical conditions. John Wennberg's small-area analyses are to medical-practice guidelines what Roemer's law was to CON—a research-based alarum to payers that invites policymakers to ponder whether the health system is unnecessarily expensive and what government might possibly do about it. In 1989 the federal government began funding the Agency for Health Care Policy and Research (AHCPR; now called the Agency for Healthcare Research and Quality, AHRQ) in hopes of narrowing the range of medical uncertainty by learning what practices are "best" and then embodying them in "guidelines" to which physicians should be exhorted to adhere. (The Professional Standard Review Organizations, or PSROs, which emerged contemporaneously with Wennberg's first findings, were an early variation on this theme.) This quest, its supporters contended, would not only slow the growth of costs but also improve the quality of care.

Although AHCPR/AHRQ's short life has been full of woe—three federal agencies cast aspersions on its work, surgeons mounted a virulent attack on its guidelines, and its appropriations nearly expired in the mid 1990s—the organization has survived and even enjoyed modest growth (Gray et al. 2003). Attacks from the Right were countered not merely by legislators who viewed research as a tool for more assertive federal shaping of the system, but also by conservatives who recalled the agency's origins in the George H. W. Bush administration and contended that "Republicans created this. It is allowing us to figure out what we are spending money on" (Gray et al. 2003, note 32). Meanwhile, as guidelines and Patient Outcomes Research Teams (PORTs) waned on AHRQ's agenda, inquiries into medical errors and patient safety have waxed, and the demand for "high-quality evidence" as a guide to decisions about clinical care and coverage grows steadily. Pragmatic (or practical) clinical trials, for example, proceed within NIH, AHRQ, the Center for Education and Research in Therapeutics (jointly run by AHRQ and the FDA), and the Cooperative Studies Program of the Veterans Administration—efforts that are said collectively to constitute a mere portion of the potential benefits of high-quality evidence

(Tunis et al. 2003). Guidelines for treatment of ills such as hypertension, arthritis, obesity, and high cholesterol (most of which, if followed, would substantially increase the use of drugs and services) advance under NIH auspices (Kleinke 2004). A prominent health-policy analyst urges that the feds create, fund, and perhaps run a pharmaceutical-research institute to "study and disseminate results on pharmaceutical cost-effectiveness" (Reinhardt 2004, 107). Apparently the quest for evidence, like that for medical innovation itself, is an endless frontier (Bush 1945) the state has a manifest destiny to conquer.

## Withholding

On a growing number of occasions government is obliged to adjudicate claims that particular medical innovations are not truly beneficial and should therefore be withheld or, conversely, that benefits being withheld ought to be made mandatory. Such issues trigger intense moral conflicts that prompt partisans across the political spectrum—most certainly including those persuaded that less government is better government—to drag the state onto the battlefield. As pediatric surgeons multiplied and perfected interventions that might keep handicapped newborns alive, for instance, right-to-life advocates pressured the federal government to forbid parents of these children to decline treatment on the grounds that preserving so damaged a life was not in their child's best interest (Fox 1986). As medical technology enables seriously ill patients to extend their lives, government is urged to help providers, patients, and kin untangle the formal–legal complexities that accompany living wills, do-not-resuscitate orders, and physician-assisted suicide. During the 1980s and 1990s right-to-life organizations fought to keep the FDA from allowing the RU-486 abortion pill to enter the U.S. market.

Few Americans care to watch rapid and dramatic late-twentieth-century advances in cloning, stem cell research, and genetic mapping unfold in a climate of professional and economic laissez faire. Reflecting the widespread view that these breakthroughs "touch the essence of human existence" (Wade 2004) and that the federal government is obliged to set conditions on their diffusion and application, President George W. Bush appointed an expert Council on Bioethics to advise him, studied the issues, and went on television in 2001 to unveil his conclusions about the permissible limits of research with human embryonic stem cells. Each such technical advance invites government to define its scope and limits, and each such definition invites quarrels (including among otherwise placid ideological soulmates) about whether government should be doing more in the face of grave human needs. For example, though Ronald Reagan parlayed pitiless attacks on big government into a fabulous political career, his widow and son now belabor President George W. Bush to soften the above-noted limits on the use of federal funds for stem cell research, which might help scientists to map and combat diseases such as Alzheimer's, from which former President Reagan suffered in the last decade of his life (Kirkpatrick 2004).

Across these stages of policy's life cycle for medical technology run three patterns. First, the march of medical progress yields a fairly steady correlative increase in the governmental regulatory presence—to wit, NIH, FDA, CMS, CON, AHRQ, and more—most of them getting bigger and doing more over time. Second, all these stages are, and have long been, arenas of intense political conflict on big social issues—conflicts, for example, over the merits of basic versus applied research, which groups and conditions deserve research priority, the proper balance between speed and caution in bringing innovative products to market, the definition of cost-effective medical services, the legitimate scope of physician autonomy, rights-to-life versus rights-to-choose, and the sanctity versus the perfectibility of human life. Yet, third, notwithstanding the breadth, depth, and intensity of this catalogue of social conflicts, even conservative circles of increasingly strident antistatist sensibilities have been little inclined to deny the necessity and legitimacy of interventions by "big" (mainly national) government in steering medical progress along the paths of public policy. Public support for, and regulation of, medical technology seems to constitute a sort of water's edge at which ideology (in its more virulent forms at least) recedes.

### Group Particularism

The prominence of the state in the health system grows steadily because government is indispensable to the provision of a range of political and economic benefits that far transcend "mere" technology. That many parties to this provisioning prefer ideologically to keep government's helping hand invisible by no means diminishes either their participation in the political game or the power that the public hand acquires from repeated exercise.

The trans-ideological appeal of public growth in the health sphere spans all three of Theodore J. Lowi's arenas of power (1964). First, government controls roughly half of the nation's $1.6 trillion annual health budget and confers cherished distributive benefits among areas and organizations. As Bruce Vladeck explains, Medicare "spends money in just about every city and town, and in every congressional district, in the United States" (27). Beneficiaries include not only the elderly but also hospitals, physicians, home health-care agencies, clinical laboratories, durable medical equipment suppliers, physical and occupational therapists, health maintenance organizations (HMOs), AMCs, and the private insurers that help administer the program. These providers (broadly defined) are "major sources of employment, political activity, and campaign contributions" across the nation (30–31). Medicaid, though famously a "poor people's program" of supposedly limited political appeal, engages most of the groups that defend higher spending on Medicare and adds nursing homes; coalitions that advocate for children, families, and human services; and local safety-net institutions, which often also enjoy strong political roots and formidable political reach (Brown and Sparer 2003). Conservatives, no less than liberals, like bigger, better AMCs in their states and districts and (as noted in the previous section) extend an equally warm welcome to the technological marvels these entities import and export. Tax expenditure policies for health insurance cost the United States Treasury almost $200 billion annually but sustain enthusiasm among policymakers, notes Daniel Fox, because these sums "subsidize coverage while insulating general government from advocates on all sides of controversies of health policy" (Fox, this volume; see also Howard 1997).

All is not invariably additive, to be sure: for example, Hill-Burton, as frankly distributive a bricks-and-mortar program as ever graced the federal statute book, was phased out in 1974. Its demise owed much to a growing conviction that building more hospitals was inflationary and unnecessary, but it derived also from conflicts within the program's coalition between urban and rural districts and between proponents of inpatient versus free-standing ambulatory facilities. In any case, after 1965 Medicare's generous fiscal handling of hospitals extended a flexible replacement for Hill-Burton's more targeted largesse. Health spending, in short, has much the same ageless political appeal for greedy legislators as that devoted to highways, river and harbor projects, and defense bases.

The regulatory arena grows alongside the distributive because bigger doings in the public, private, and nonprofit sectors trigger new demands by one or another stakeholder for government intervention on its behalf. For politicians who want to claim uncontroversial credit for containing health costs, voluminous rules that purport to deter fraud and abuse in Medicare and Medicaid are highly serviceable. Businesses that prefer not to cope with some government rules—for instance, those the fifty states may impose on corporate health-benefit packages—are happy to defend national Employee Retirement Income Security Act (ERISA) rules that tie the states' hands, but in so doing trigger both extensive litigation over what ERISA means and myriad state regulatory adaptations that aim to skirt its preemptions. Physicians want government to leave health care to medical professionals—after, of course, the state has reduced their exposure to malpractice suits and the fiscal and administrative discipline by which managed care organizations (MCOs) seek to control providers. The public may not endorse a national plan that covers the uninsured but it wants state and federal regulators of health insurance to limit the discretion of insurers to drop enrollees and raise premiums for groups and individuals who hold coverage. Some of the push for regulation comes from organizations that applaud more government steering of the system as a matter of political principle, but no small amount derives from groups that opportunistically insist that government make regulations on behalf of their worthy ends and then go away.

Redistribution, said to be the site of epic ideological and partisan clashes that pit class against class and haves against have-nots, also often blurs and blunts a priori positions on the proper role of the state. As noted above, Medicare and Medicaid cannot very well move money from the haves to buy care for the have-nots without, in the process, lining the pockets of physicians, hospitals, Community Health Centers (CHCs), medical suppliers, drug companies, nursing homes, MCOs, home health agencies, and other interested entities. CHCs appeal as much to conservatives who fancy them an "alternative to government" as to liberals who work to ease access to care for the disadvantaged. Although allegedly inclined to "starve the [governmental] beast," the George W. Bush administration, impeccably conservative and Republican, has expanded funding for CHCs and—much more expensively and dramatically—presided over the enactment of long-deferred legislation introducing a prescription drug benefit in Medicare.

The point here is not that the distributive, regulatory, and redistributive arenas are open roads along which interests advance effortlessly, albeit incrementally, toward bigger government. Were that so, the government's role in U.S. health policy would be much more prominent than it is and more closely akin to that found in other Western nations. The point rather is that although U.S. culture and political structures combine to make the road to public programs rough indeed, groups regularly construct detours around these blocked avenues, that these detours have come increasingly to dot (and blur) political and programmatic landscapes, and that their accumulating presence extends opportunities both for incremental expansion of programs nestled comfortably in the status quo and for innovations by policy entrepreneurs of the Left and the Right. One ends up with a lot of policy—more of it all the time—though little of it exhibits the coherence that presumably would result from a straight march to systemic reform.

## Market Malfunctions

A third reason why the role of government expands in health affairs is simply that various malfunctions ("failures") in the market trigger demands for public repair. One example, ironic on its face, is the call for government to fix unintended and undesired consequences of attempts to make the system behave more like a normal market by means of managed care. A second, ironic in its depths, is government's quiet but steady accumulation of broken pieces picked up from a health system whose market forms no longer honor the functions that workable arrangements for coverage and care presuppose.

Beginning in the late 1960s the wisdom and capacity of government came under mounting attack, and electoral quests to capitalize on these assaults have enjoyed remarkable, indeed barely broken, success to the present day. Atop these ideological and political waves rode an analytic push for the "public use of private interest" (Schultze 1977), meaning strategies to implant consumer choice, competition, and "correct" incentives into public programs that would otherwise suffer under some combination of "professional dominance" and the misfortunes of "command and control" tactics deployed by inefficient, unresponsive, and "captured" government agencies. From the start (that is, from the Nixon administration's embrace of HMOs in 1970), health care has been prime terrain for these experiments. The health system, said the policy analysts, costs too much because it rests on a basic conceptual error, to wit, the combination of fee-for-service medicine and third-party payment, which of course embodied "wrong" incentives that encouraged consumers and providers to run up tabs that insurers cheerfully passed on to purchasers. (How most comparable nations retained this combination and managed to cover all their citizens at lower cost than did the United States was an intriguing question the market reformers apparently did not ask, much less press.) HMOs, later known as MCOs, would reverse these bad incentives by conjoining the financing and delivery of care within their own organizational contours and by imposing economic and managerial controls on the providers in their selectively chosen panels and networks. Managed competition among these MCOs would kick these efficiencies up several notches by obliging provider-controlling MCOs to contest in a disciplined fashion for the business of sharp-eyed purchasers (Brown 1983).

First proposed as a new Part C for Medicare, MCOs became a major, oftentimes dominant, force in private insurance and Medicaid in the 1990s. (Their presence in Medicare remains weak despite repeated federal attempts to expand it.) In some quarters competition, "managed" or not, came to be viewed as a necessary and sufficient replacement, not only for the unhappy conjunction of fee-for-service and third-party payment, but also for such governmental interventions as PSROs, health planning, CON, state setting of hospital rates, and indeed all publicly regulated pricing or premium caps. (A provision for such caps as a "backstop" in the Clinton plan, should managed competition somehow fail to contain costs, quickly drove angry incentive-changers from the template.)

As managed care played on, however, providers and consumers, whose giving and getting of care were newly constrained, took offense, began decrying the allegedly damaging effects of such management on access and quality of care, caught the ears of reporters and politicians, and took to crafting interventions that purported to protect against the public misuse of private interests. The laws enacted and rules adopted by the federal and state governments soon made a long list. Any-willing-provider laws limited the power of MCOs to contract selectively with physicians in their communities. Direct-access laws prohibited plans from requiring that members visit a primary-care gatekeeper before seeing certain specialists. Mandated-benefit laws obliged plans to cover specified services (for example, screening for breast cancer and diabetes, chiropractic care, CAM). Prompt-payment laws penalized plans that failed to pay providers' bills within a set number of days. Requirements for external review of disputes between members and plan managers gave the former more leverage and the latter less incentive to manage care firmly. Provisions setting forth detailed criteria that defined a "solvent" plan aimed to forestall an inconvenient concomitant of market competition, namely, failed competitors that close their doors and leave thousands of consumers to find new coverage and new caregivers. Most of these rules applied to commercial and nonprofit MCOs in Medicaid as well as in the commercial sector. Nor were these measures mere political nibbling around the edges of a "transformed" system. By 2000 or so, some analysts had concluded that these and other curbs on the autonomy of managed care had cumulatively neutralized its economic and administrative discipline, a development that, in turn, is said largely to explain why health-care costs shot up again in the late 1990s and have stayed up (Brown and Eagan 2004).

Meanwhile these regulatory responses to those market responses to the supposedly inherent flaws of bureaucracy have enlarged the agendas of public agencies compelled to grapple with new tasks and roles. Departments of insurance (and sometimes departments of social services and of health), for instance, must figure out how to gauge the implications of plan-provider relations for the fiscal solvency of MCOs and must define administratively when providers' bills are "clean" enough (properly documented) to trigger prompt-payment rules. Each governmental interposition that aims to avert what constitutes market failure in the eyes of some influential organization or coalition increases the play of public power in the system.

Although Republicans have, on the whole, evinced more enthusiasm for managed care as an answer to the system's ills than have Democrats, alleged abuses by MCOs have elicited a fairly bipartisan reaction. Republican conservatives, no less than liberal Democrats, proclaim themselves deeply moved by indignant calls and letters from constituents in their districts; by media exposés of care delayed, denied, or deformed; by the lobbying of supposedly disinterested consumer organizations and by overtly interested but professionally respected groups of medical providers. The countervailing powers of business firms and MCOs themselves, though strong enough to head off more draconian rules at the pass, have failed to block interventions that are, in aggregate, far- and deep-reaching.

Sophisticated architects of market forces in health care (most notably Alain Enthoven) never doubted that responsible and public-interested competition must be managed within extensive and detailed public rules about enrollment practices, setting of premiums, monitoring of quality, and more. As the failure of the Clinton plan proved, the United States is unwilling to admit "too much government" in this guise. Facing the worrisome consequences of unmanaged competition among MCOs, however, policymakers have responded with bits and pieces of regulation that conform to no economic theory or other master plan for a coherent system but rather cater to the multiple complaints and demands of myriad constituencies whose voice and loyalty resound across partisan and ideological divides. While rejecting the doctrine of managed competition, policy has moved toward the political management of competition in (largely incremental and decentralized) practice.

The farthest-reaching embodiment of government repairs to market forces, however, appears not in correctives for market failures in managed care but rather in "developments" that seek to make ex post facto sense of the essential properties of the larger system itself. Rejecting a universal, compulsory, and nationally defined system of coverage like those most other Western nations began implementing in the early twentieth century, the United States entrusted health coverage to arrangements in which insurance entities (mainly Blue Cross and Blue Shield), built by and for providers (hospitals and physicians), sold coverage in local markets to employers, who might choose to buy it if and as they pleased. This approach brought health insurance to millions of workers and dependents from the 1930s on—so much so that when Harry Truman tried to make national health insurance a top issue on the domestic agenda in

the late 1940s, he was easily checkmated by a phalanx of providers and insurers who persuaded the public that the progress of private, local, and voluntary
plans made such recent miscarriages as the British National Health Service
superfluous as well as dangerous for the United States. That a work-based system of coverage did not work for retired and unemployed Americans was duly
acknowledged and in due course addressed by the enactment of Medicare and
Medicaid (1965). Thus was the cultural die cast: government's role in health
coverage was "officially" confined to filling in the gaps of an otherwise robust
private system.

Today the gaps government fills extend to nearly half the population, and
government's role in caregiving reaches not only the uninsured and Medicaid
beneficiaries who have trouble finding providers willing to treat them at prof-
fered public rates, but also a substantial number of privately underinsured
Americans. These groups are often obliged to seek care in the safety net, locally
variable line-ups of public and voluntary hospitals, CHCs, county clinics, free
clinics, and private physicians willing to treat some patients for low or no fees.
As private coverage erodes (that is, fails to keep pace with the number of
Americans who need health insurance) and the public sector struggles to pick
up some, but not all, of the slack, more citizens (not to mention documented
and undocumented immigrants) seek care from the safety net, itself a third sector of mixed public-private pedigree. This trend steadily increases government's prominence in ways not adequately captured by head counts of the
uninsured. Although safety-net providers may gain revenue from commercial
customers and contributions from foundations, the bulk of the money that
keeps them going comes from a motley amalgam of Medicaid payments, Disproportionate Share Hospital Program funds, earmarked county taxes, state
appropriations, federal grants earmarked for Federally Qualified Health Centers, and Medicare subsidies that help teaching hospitals cover the costs of
uncompensated care.

Because their costs run high and their incomes are precarious, safety-net
institutions are perennially in perilous straits; hospitals and centers regularly
edge toward collapse and closure. Yet apocalyptic predictions usually prove
to be wrong as the safety net somehow stays afloat (and in the case of CHCs,
may even expand) because local, state, and federal policymakers contrive to
adjust and augment the cash infusions that keep these providers in business.
While the Left predictably worries about the medical fate of the disadvantaged
should the safety net disintegrate, few to the right of center want to see emergency rooms in their middle-class communities flooded with low-income
patients and trauma and burn centers closed. Many conservatives presumably

understand too that these providers serve as a safety net, not only for poor patients, but also, by validating the contention that people without coverage can nonetheless get care, for the system as a whole. Bigger government, in short, may be all that stands between a functionally challenged employer-based system and really big government. As government's role as the primary source of coverage and care approaches an indeterminate but probably imminent tipping point, the historic division of labor between market and state may be reversed in practice and perhaps eventually revised in theory as employers come to fill "gaps" in mainstream public coverage.

## Conclusion

Historical continuities in the United States health-care system are usually framed and highlighted by comparative reference to glaring spatial discontinuities: to wit, the refusal of U.S. health policy to display the structural features of other Western democracies, which embraced affordable universal coverage long ago and have successfully marshaled the political will to make it work. American exceptionalism is real enough, but the full story also chronicles changes that endow the U.S. system with crude homegrown functional counterparts (though rarely true equivalents) of the state policies that assure coverage and contain costs elsewhere.

The central continuity, of course, is the wide scope the United States extends to nongovernmental (private and nonprofit) forces to supply coverage and curb costs. No other nation expects a private sector, little constrained by public rules on the size and terms of employer contributions, to carry so heavy a burden of coverage, and none asks private insurers to hold the line with providers (including specialists, uncommonly abundant in the United States) on prices outside a framework of public policies that guide the bargaining game (Glaser 1991). The first of these two grand exceptions largely accounts for the nation's high rates of un- and underinsurance; the latter mainly explains why American health spending is so high by cross-national standards.

Change entails public challenges to and inroads against these vast inherited preserves of private power. To grasp the rigors of the challenge, to plumb the cultural and structural depths from which such privatism draws strength, is to understand why the changes charted here usually advance incrementally and take forms exasperatingly distinct from what comparable nations think rational and workable.

The general pattern entails first, an intensifying (since 1968) "official" insistence that a private-centered system for buying and selling coverage and care and addressing costs in local markets is preferable to one in which govern-

ment plays a larger role; second, growing awareness across party and ideological lines of the myriad malfunctions and incapacities of that private-centered
system and an accumulating cadre of ad hoc exceptions to the antigovernment
"rule"; and third, steadily spreading political willingness to act on these perceptions by creating and extending at all levels of government programs that
enlarge the state's role as supplier of care and coverage and, in that capacity,
as container of costs. The fourth act, presumably, will be a "revisioning" that
laggardly admits "official" uncertainty over what is rule and what exception,
over what is the heart of the U.S. system and what are the gaps around it, and
that admits, in turn, more forthright democratic discussion about the is's and
ought's of government's role in health care. Act V, perhaps, will stage a recon-
figuration of the system's sectors, a rearrangement of policy furniture that better fits institutional forms to the essential functions of a modern health-care
system—that is, affordable universal coverage and all it implies. American
health politics being what they are, some will denounce such a denouement
as tragedy, some will dismiss it as comedy, but others may discern in it a more
or less natural progression of the U.S. health-care system's peculiar political
history.

### References

Brown, Lawrence D. 1983. *Politics and Health Care Organization: HMOs as Federal Pol-
icy.* Washington, DC: Brookings Institution.
Brown, Lawrence D., and Elizabeth Eagan. 2004. The Paradoxical Politics of Provider
Reempowerment. *Journal of Health Politics, Policy and Law* 29: 1045–1071.
Brown, Lawrence D., and Michael S. Sparer. 2003. Poor Program's Progress: The Un-
anticipated Politics of Medicaid Policy. *Health Affairs* 22: 31–44.
Bush, Vannevar. 1945. *Science, the Endless Frontier.* Washington, DC: National Science
Foundation.
Bussell, Mary, 2003. Innovation Management: The Politics of Technological Develop-
ment. Ph.D. dissertation, Columbia University.
Campbell, Eric G., Joshua B. Bowers, David Blumanthal, and Brian Biles. 2004. Inside the
Triple Helix: Technology Transfer and Commercialization in the Life Sciences. *Health
Affairs* 23: 64–76.
Carpenter, Daniel P. 2004. The Political Economy of FDA Drug Review: Processing, Pol-
itics, and Lessons for Policy. *Health Affairs* 23: 52–63.
Croghan, Thomas, and Patricia M. Pittman. 2004. The Medicine Cabinet: What's in It,
Why, and Can We Change the Contents? *Health Affairs* 23: 23–33.
Fox, Daniel M., ed. 1986. Special Section on the Treatment of Handicapped Newborns.
*Journal of Health Politics, Policy and Law* 11: 195–303.
Gelijns, Annetine C. 2004. Personal communication.
Gelijns, Annetine C., N. Rotenberg, and A.J. Moskowitz. 1998. Capturing the Unexpected
Benefits of Medical Research. *New England Journal of Medicine* 339: 693–698.
———. 2003. Uncertainty and Technological Change in Medicine. In *Uncertain Times:
Kenneth Arrow and the Changing Economics of Health Care,* eds. P. H. Hammer,

Deborah Haas-Wilson, Mark A. Peterton, and William Sage, 60–70. Durham, NC: Duke University Press.

Glaser, William A. 1991. *Health Insurance in Practice: International Variations in Financing Benefits, and Problems.* San Francisco: Jossey-Bass.

Gray, Bradford H., Michael R. Gusmano, and Fara R. Collins. 2003. AHCPR and the Changing Politics of Health Services Research. *Health Affairs*, web exclusive, 25 June.

Howard, Christopher. 1997. *The Hidden Welfare State: Tax Expenditures and Social Policy in the United States.* Princeton: Princeton University Press.

Jacobs, Lawrence R. 1995. The Politics of America's Supply State. *Health Affairs* 14: 143–157.

Johnson, Kay A., Alice Fardell, and Barbara Richards. 2000. Federal Immunization Policy and Funding: A History of Responding to Crises. *American Journal of Preventive Medicine* 19:3:1: 99–112.

Kleinke, J. D. 2004. Access versus Excess: Value-Based Cost Sharing for Prescription Drugs. *Health Affairs* 23: 34–47.

Lowi, Theodore J. 1964. American Business, Public Policy, Case Studies, and Political Theory. *World Politics* 16: 677–715.

Kirkpatrick, David D. 2004. Bush Defends Stem-Cell Limit, Despite Pressure Since Reagan Death. *New York Times*, 16 June.

Reinhardt, Uwe E. 2004. Perspective: An Information Infrastructure for the Pharmaceutical Market. *Health Affairs* 23: 107–112.

Rose, Eric, Annetine C. Gelijns, Alan J. Moskowitz, Daniel F. Heitjan, Lynne W. Stevenson, Walter Dembitsky, James W. Long, et al. 2001. Long-Term Use of a Left Ventricular Assist Device. *New England Journal of Medicine* 345: 1435–1453.

Ruggie, Mary. 2004. *Marginal to Mainstream: Alternative Medicine in America.* New York: Cambridge University Press.

Schultze, Charles L. 1977. *The Public Use of Private Interest.* Washington, DC: Brookings Institution.

Starr, Paul. 1982. *The Social Transformation of American Medicine.* New York: Basic Books.

Stokes, Donald. 1997. *Pasteur's Quadrant: Basic Science and Technological Innovation.* Washington, DC: Brookings Institution.

Strickland, Stephen P. 1972. *Politics, Science, and Dread Disease.* Cambridge, MA: Harvard University Press.

Tunis, Sean R., Daniel B. Stryer, and Carolyn M. Clancy. 2003. Practical Clinical Trials: Increasing the Value of Clinical Research for Decision Making and Health Policy. *Journal of the American Medical Association* 290: 1624–1632.

Vladeck, Bruce C. 1999. The Political Economy of Medicare. *Health Affairs* 18: 22–36.

Wade, Nicholas. 2004. Human Cloning Marches On, Without U.S. Help. *New York Times*, 15 February.

# Medical Specialization as American Health Policy

## Interweaving Public and Private Roles

> Life usually doesn't just dump truth on your plate, neat and simple. It usually comes with a side of nuance, garnished with paradox.
>
> Chris Satullo, *Avoid the Dreaded Either/Or—Seek the Sweet Bird of Paradox*

What is health policy? On the face of it, there seems a simple answer. Health policy is what governments do, or try to do, to further health care, typically at the national level. As other essays in this volume resoundingly attest, however, seeing health policy only as what government does or fails to do gives a blinkered, partial—and much too tidy—view of the rich, complex, and constantly shifting landscape of health policy in the United States. I want to suggest some of this complexity, nuance, and paradox by examining specialization in American medicine as a vital, yet often neglected, policy issue.

Public and private policy making have long been entwined in American politics. Specialization weaves together several histories: the history of government, to be sure, but also the histories of science and technology, the medical profession, health care, business, consumerism, and other more generic historical fields. I concentrate here on the history of the U.S. medical profession, which is now formally structured—through education, examination, and certification—into thirty-seven primary specialties and ninety-two subspecialties (with more under way). New historical interpretations of the profession are overdue. This is also a particularly important time to reconceptualize the policy role of the medical profession in setting standards in the information-oriented health-care system of the twenty-first century.

In the last quarter of the twentieth century, ruling narratives within the scholarly and medical communities included the rise and current decline of the medical profession, and thus gave negative interpretations of the social role of medicine as a profession. In turn, such perceptions obscured the very real challenges faced by professional organizations, particularly their roles as public agents (Stevens 2001a). Yet, as this chapter shows, during this same period professional organizations in and across the medical specialties struggled successfully to create and legitimate new fields of medicine through a process of private negotiation and organizational consensus—influenced by related government policy but outside the realm of government. Today, twenty-four medical specialty boards, each sponsored by national specialty associations in the field of interest, certify almost ninety percent of all practicing physicians in the United States. For a list of the boards, see Table 3-1 at the end of this chapter.

Through their umbrella organization, the American Board of Medical Specialties (ABMS), these boards embarked in 2000 on a new policy to require board diplomates to not only demonstrate current knowledge in their chosen field but also fulfill specified curricula for life-long learning, periodic self-assessment, and peer and patient assessment as a condition of maintaining board-certified status. (I have served as a public member on the ABMS since 1999.) The formative history behind this movement is part of the larger evolution of medical specialization as a central—if hidden or implicit—theme in American health policy from past to present, coloring options for the future.

These specialty certifying boards, and medical professional organizations in general, have been surprisingly silent in public debates. It is useful to consider why this is. How might professional groups participate more fully in health policy in the future? Should they?

## Twentieth-Century American Medicine:
## Two Overlapping Reform Movements

Specialization as a movement was evident well before the famous Flexner report (1910) became the symbol of reform in American medicine in the early twentieth century.[1] Historians have paid considerable attention over the years to the success of the "Flexner reform movement" as the exercise of professional power: in defining the American Medical Association (AMA) as the central professional institution for organized medicine, a position it held up to the

1960s (Burrow 1963; Fishbein 1947); for demonstrating, in a nation unwilling or unable to enact governmental health policies, the political role of private institutions in effecting social change—not only the AMA, voice of an autonomous profession, but also the charitable foundations that supported professional reform with money drawn from profits in commerce and industry (Brown 1979; Starr 1982; Berliner 1985); and for forming long-lasting, cherished characteristics of America's medical schools as "academic medical centers"— elite, scientific, post-baccalaureate institutions, symbols of a technologically advanced nation (Ludmerer 1985; 1999; Stevens 1971).

But while the Flexner report publicized the enormous variations (and often horrifying deficiencies) in the scientific and clinical quality of America's medical schools in the first decade of the twentieth century, the reform movement paid little attention to what was happening at the same time in medical practice. Professional reform in the early twentieth century was based on the goal of achieving professional *unification* through specifying and enforcing standards for medical education and licensure. Medical licensure, both then and now a function of the states, designated basic standards to be met by all practitioners—no matter whether their field of interest was the eye, the ovary, the psyche, or the skin. It was essentially designed for general practitioners. Difficult, fractious questions of specialism, in contrast, promised a new *fragmentation* within the profession—which would, in the longer run, generate a second movement for professional reform. The two movements coexisted between 1900 and 1920, one coming to fulfillment, the other just beginning. Leading medical professors, who were specialists, led both movements.

In the early twentieth century, a slick city specialist with minimal if any specialty credentials could hold himself (for they were almost entirely male) out as a gynecologist, dermatologist, neurologist, ophthalmologist, otolaryngologist, orthopedic surgeon, or urologist, or, for that matter, as a specialist in rheumatism, fever and catarrh, or hair and complexion (Zeisler 1901)—free to cure or inflict damage on his patients. One Illinois physician declared that the motto of the successful surgeon was: "Practice strictly limited to profitable cases" (Reid 1908).

Besides an initial lack of standards for specialty training and credentials in the United States, there was no enforceable, formal relationship between general practitioners and specialists such as was developing, for example, at the same time in Britain, where national health insurance legislation (1911) shored up the position of the general practitioner as the patient's designated primary doctor (Stevens 1966; Honigsbaum 1979; Weisz 2005). Some American general practitioners limited their practice on scientific grounds, choosing to refer patients to specialists in well-developed fields such as ophthalmology or abdominal and gynecological surgery. There was no defined role for general practice; no effective mechanism to dissuade patients from seeking specialists unnecessarily (from the medical point of view); no standards by which patients could choose well-trained or even minimally competent experts; and, with some notable organizational exceptions such as the Mayo Clinic, practically no coordination among the parties involved.

Did the lack of standards for specialized skills matter? This is a fair question from today's pro-market perspective but irrelevant in the context of the early twentieth century. If one saw medicine, as did thoughtful physicians, journalists, and others of the time, as a science or form of engineering, and thus as naturally associated with standardization and precision as the Rockefeller Institute's pristine research laboratories or Ford's mass production of automobiles, then the question never arose. It was assumed that standards mattered. The motto of the private, nonprofit, professionally engendered National Board of Medical Examiners (established in 1915 to provide a voluntary, national examination for new doctors that states could endorse for licensure) was both progressive and noncontroversial: "Ever More Exactly," signifying a precise, standardized direction for medicine. Illustrating public and private cooperation in pursuit of common policy goals, six senior federal officials were founding members of the fifteen-person National Board, including the surgeons general of the Army, Navy, and U.S. Public Health Service. Meanwhile the state licensing boards were pressing for uniform standards for all medical licenses across the country (Stevens 1971). General medical education and licensing were on an apparently irrevocable march toward bureaucracy and control.

Medical practice, in contrast, was messy and market-driven. By the late 1920s, tonsillectomies and adenoidectomies (necessary treatments in those pre-antibiotic days), hospital-based childbirth, and other surgeries were part of the middle-class American experience. With its well-educated medical profession (at least among the younger generation of doctors), successful surgeries, and gleaming hospitals, American medicine had become a valued social and consumer good, at least for those who could afford its rising costs. Some hospitals offered lines of credit so that the purchase of a surgical operation would be as convenient a transaction as buying a refrigerator (Stevens 1989). As the American public, its entrepreneurial hospitals, and its competitive, fee-for-service medical profession joined together with verve to try new methods, drugs, and surgical solutions, the rambunctious character of American medical care was delineated. Specialism meant all-out competition among physicians, and patients became consumers with the right to consult whichever specialist they wished.

Physicians, in turn, expected to admit their patients to the hospital as they saw fit. Hospital trustees and managers had little interest in antagonizing doctors, for doctors were, after all, the source of hospital patients, particularly those patients who paid. By mutual consent there was a "gauze curtain" between managers and physicians (Thompson 1985); that is, they held themselves aloof. Each was mutually suspicious of the motives of the other—a phenomenon that has unfortunately continued to the present.

The American College of Surgeons, created in 1913, three years after the Flexner report, offered surgeons a new national professional institution and new sources for professional reform. It joined a growing body of specialty associations, journals, medical school departments, professorships, and designated hours in the medical curriculum. Among the college's other activities, it embarked on reforming the technical, qualitative standards of hospitals, which like the medical schools before them were uneven, to say the least—often operating without patient records or with totally inadequate pathological diagnosis (Rosenberg 1987; Howell 1995). The college's hospital standardization program was conveniently analogous to the Good Housekeeping Seal of Approval, another voluntary program for consumers and producers that flowered in the 1920s. Both illustrated the role of noncoercive, private regulation. Today's version of hospital standardization (now known as institutional accreditation) is a direct descendant, the Joint Commission on Healthcare Organizations (for hospitals awaiting inspection, the often feared JCAHO).

What *was* medicine? On the one hand it was a science—an "attempt to fight the battle against disease most advantageously to the patient," as Abraham Flexner put it (Flexner 1910, 23), or "an art which utilizes the sciences," in the words of a later blue-ribbon commission. But it was also, remarked that commission, "an economic activity with definite relations to the cost of living, the distribution of wealth, and the purchasing habits of the people" (Committee on the Costs of Medical Care 1932, 2). Medicine was also a growing network of institutions, including huge city teaching hospitals with medical schools architecturally embedded in them, smaller hospitals that were major employers in their communities, and an increasing complex of professional organizations. Each institution brought its own agenda to the table. Well before World War II, "medicine" had multiple meanings and a variety of constituents.

The medical profession continued its own educational reforms while claiming freedom from external control for fee-for-service private practitioners, whether they practiced as generalists, specialists, or with a generalist-specialist mix (as many did). The organizational and political consequences of specialized medicine were largely ignored. In theory ethical doctors would make sure each individual patient received the right care from the right array of practitioners, and where this turned out to be too expensive for the patient, those physicians would reduce their fees. The AMA Code of Ethics was an important symbol and vehicle of this philosophy (Baker et al. 1998). To protect ethical behavior, the American College of Surgeons made its fellows agree not to engage in "fee-splitting," that is, paying kickbacks to other practitioners for patient referrals. Some specialists were more amenable to changes that favored their own fields and patients. For example, pediatricians were crucial participants in the child-health movement of the early twentieth century, and surgeons saw the benefits of private hospital insurance in the 1930s (Halpern 1988; Stevens 1989). Nonetheless, the AMA forcefully represented the profession to the outside world. As demonstrated in the now-rich historical literature, the AMA objected strongly (and successfully up to the 1960s) to proposals for larger social and organizational change—via health-care organization and health insurance—that came from outside sources (Somers and Somers 1961; Poen 1979; Starr 1982; Engel 2002; Oberlander 2003; Gordon 2003).

The principles guiding post-degree, specialty education from the 1920s through World War II were an extension of those of the Flexner reforms: scientific subdivision of medicine into standardized, discrete fields and formal recognition and training of specialists. By 1942, twelve of the fifteen specialty certifying boards required at least three years of hospital residency training, and the movement to standardize specialty education through hospital residency programs was well under way. It was to be through efforts to identify and certify specialists (and therefore their organized specialties) that the second professional reform movement was to mature in the late twentieth century. By that time, the power of the AMA was on the wane.

### Specialty Certification the American Way

Open competition between professions in the medical market prompted the formation in 1917 of the first of today's twenty-four specialty certifying boards: the American Board for Ophthalmic Examinations (today's American Board of Ophthalmology). The precipitating factor was that non-physician optometrists had organized to push for state licensing in optometry, thus claiming the eye as a legally defined field of work for themselves. Optometry was licensed in all jurisdictions by the end of 1924. Without their own qualification, medical ophthalmologists would have had no means of distinguishing themselves as specialists. Indeed, it is worth remarking in passing that fierce jurisdictional rivalries between different health professions continue to the present, not just over the eye, but also in many other fields. In August 2004, for example, a governmental directive from the Veterans Health Administration (VHA Directive 2004–045) sparked acute concern among ophthalmologists by providing guidelines for the clinical privilege of optometrists to perform therapeutic laser eye procedures at VA medical facilities.

From the beginning, a specialty certifying board was different from a state licensing board. The former was privately organized, the latter governmental. Specialty certifying boards were national rather than state-based, voluntary rather than a compulsory requirement for practice, and designed for specialized groups of doctors rather than for all practicing physicians. For the doctors, formation of a medical specialty board proved a useful vehicle for establishing medical jurisdiction. In patterns that were to recur in other specialty fields through the years, the American Board for Ophthalmic Examinations described its chief functions as establishing standards of "fitness" to practice the specialty, providing examinations to test qualifications, and conferring certificates through a purely voluntary process. The specialty diploma was not to be regarded as a license nor to control practice in the field, and ophthalmologists without the certificate were not to be regarded as "unfit."

In 1924, a second specialty board was founded along the same voluntary, noncoercive, professionally controlled lines: the American Board of Otolaryngology. This coincided with the huge volume of operations on tonsils and adenoids, often done by ill-trained practitioners. The third specialty board was the American Board of Obstetrics and Gynecology in 1930, bringing these two fields together and emphasizing the surgical aspects of obstetrics. The fourth was the American Board of Dermatology.

The flowering of the specialty boards as a new professional movement happened at the same time as the economic pressures of the Great Depression, and was in essence part of it. The economics of the 1930s encouraged medical students to take hospital internships and residencies in a specialty, hospitals to offer these residencies (doctors were typically provided room and board but not paid), and doctors to claim market advantage, including designated specialty skills. Twelve of today's twenty-four specialty boards were established by the end of the 1930s.

Each board was a critical ingredient in defining the specialty in competition with other medical specialties, and each staked authoritative territorial claims. As with the earlier education reforms—and arguably *any* reform—the process was highly political. Groups of doctors claiming they were specialists could only succeed in establishing a successful, institutionalized "specialty" if they had the strength of numbers, could make a reasonable living in the field, had a reason to get together to form a strong organization (for example around the science and technology of the field or to combat common threats), had effective leadership (typically out of the medical schools), and were able to push their claims for legitimacy in the medical schools and through the AMA.

Sometimes the character of the board resulted from strategic compromise. The American Board of Psychiatry and Neurology, for example, joined two distinct fields together, not just because a number of physicians practiced in both fields, but also as a matter of convenience. A speaker at the American Psychiatric Association in 1933 worried that if psychiatrists "sit idly by and do nothing," other groups would intervene (White 1933). Psychiatrists and neurologists recognized a common organizational interest, though they looked at each other with suspicion and wrangled over which specialty should come first in the new board's title. In the end they agreed to combine on the basis of largely separate arrangements for the two fields within the umbrella of a parent board. (The Board effectively runs as two separate boards today.)

The proliferation of specialty credentials in the 1930s raised broad policy questions of whether this fledgling movement toward specialization should be coordinated and who would be responsible for the overall organization—questions we are still grappling with today. There was no organized health-care system to provide functional (on-the-job) definitions of specialty status and standards or to prescribe the specialty distribution of doctors, either through government or private-sector initiatives. Instead the existing boards came together with other medical professional groups in 1933 to form the present ABMS (then called the Advisory Board for Medical Specialties), a kind of club of clubs. The early ABMS provided for communication among the various specialty boards. Its power rested, however, on its assumption of authority over the legitimacy of new claims. The ABMS published its first rules or "Essentials" for the establishment of new specialty boards in 1934, laying out patterns that have come down through the years. Each new board was to represent a "well-recognized and distinct specialty of medicine," to include more than one hundred specialists, and to have the support of the major specialty societies in that field and the related AMA specialty section. Obviously none of these conditions was clear-cut. What is a well-recognized field of medicine? Recognized by whom? These and other questions have generated controversy and fueled negotiations, case by case, over the years. Nevertheless, there was now a forum for wrestling with such questions—housed in the machinery of professional self-regulation.

Three lasting characteristics of the ABMS and its member boards were established by World War II:

1. In the absence of other forms of control the profession had the responsibility to approve new specialties through evaluating applications from specialist groups.
2. New claimants were to be judged by those who were already in the network—thus laying the process open to charges of cronyism and unfair competition.
3. This was a voluntary process for aspiring specialties and individual specialists. There was no compulsion for any specialty group to seek ABMS approval or for any doctor to be "board certified." Any group might call itself a specialty certifying board subject only to common legal strictures, such as fraudulent representation or trademark infringement.

Nevertheless, ABMS approval carried (and still carries) prestige for a specialty, ratified and opened doors to designated hospital residency education and funding programs, and was a valued credential when used by health insurers, hospitals, and now by medical licensing boards. Once inside the charmed circle of approval as a member board of the ABMS, there was little motivation to standardize specialty certification (until recently) or to consider its overall effects.

### Specialization as National Health Policy

By the mid-1940s, when historian George Rosen published a classic study of medical specialization, the topic was ripe for investigation. Specialization was an "essential feature of modern medical practice"; there were more self-styled (full-time and part-time) specialists than full-time general practitioners in the United States, though only a minority practiced their specialty full-time (Rosen 1944; Stevens 1971). Status as a specialist carried social prestige and was advantageous in the medical marketplace. Rosen observed features of specialization that later experience was to make only too familiar. Social and economic factors were at least as important as scientific and technological factors in the successful establishment of specialty fields. Medical specialization thrived because of the confidence of the American public in the authority of experts and the cachet of seeing a specialist who charged high fees or offered esoteric treatments. In these and other ways, Rosen wrote, specialization intensified the social trend to see medicine as an economic transaction, at least in the United States (Rosen 1944, 77).

Specialization was changing the structure of American medicine, shifting its internal balance away from being a profession of general practitioners. Organizationally, a unified profession was giving way to one based on power blocs of specialists.

Government policy during and immediately after World War II stimulated the growth of specialty practice. Such policy was haphazard and inadvertent to be sure, but the message came through loud and clear. Doctors' massive participation in the armed forces during the war convinced them of the functional advantage of concentrated practice in fields such as neurological surgery, urology, dermatology, plastic surgery, and otolaryngology, as well as the practical advantage of credentials, which were (in the military) linked to role, rank, and pay. Leaders of the specialty certifying boards worked with the surgeons general of the Army and Navy to make sure their diplomates were appropriately assigned, and the boards expected a great expansion of residencies in the postwar years. Between 1940 and 1950, the total number of residency training positions more than tripled.

When Congress decided not to pass the Wagner-Murray-Dingle bills to establish compulsory health insurance in the 1940s, it lost an opportunity to create patterns of medical care based on general practice, a beleaguered field which might (or might not) have received powerful support from these bills. There was insufficient congressional support for the health-insurance proposals, as well as rank opposition to them by the AMA among others (Poen 1979; Gordon 2003). Nevertheless, the "what if?" prospect is intriguing. Maybe, if general practitioners had been better organized, able to see further ahead, and truly committed to their own interests, they would have supported national health insurance in the interest of shoring up their status. As it was, the medical market was left wide open to specialty practice, for there were literally no constraints to dissuade any licensed doctor from declaring a specialty in any field.

Other government actions during and after the war stimulated specialization. The federal decision to provide tax benefits for employers who established private health insurance for workers—a form of government-funded "welfare capitalism"—galvanized the growth of private health insurance organized through the workplace (Klein 2003; Starr 1982). As with other (non-health) forms of private insurance, the new plans focused on the largest risks to consumers' pocketbooks: specialized and hospital-based services, not a cozy check-up with a GP. Insurance thus stimulated specialists to woo patients and patients to seek their services. Medicare was to do the same when implemented in 1966.

Three other large-scale federal programs encouraged specialization after World War II, with lasting effects through the twentieth century. The Veterans Administration encouraged returning servicemen to enter specialized residency programs through benefits under the GI Bill. The Hill-Burton Act (1946) provided federal subsidies to build or expand community hospitals, chiefly in rural areas, creating new centers for specialized practice across the United States. And the rapid growth of the National Institutes of Health (NIH) as the national bastion of biomedical research affirmed a compelling cultural message (and the money to support it) about the value of specialized science and techniques in medical education (see Cook-Deegan and McGeary, this volume). Different institutes within the NIH also funded superspecialized research and clinical fellowships—thus adding to the growing cadres of subspecialists.

As with other aspects of national health policy in the United States, these various actions and non-actions were largely unconnected. Anyone who has been involved in the public-policy arena (now or then) will recognize the political process that led to the passage of each piece of legislation: shifting congeries of private-interest groups and legislators come together to support or oppose a cause (such as the AMA in opposing compulsory health insurance or the American Cancer Society in pushing for funds for the National Cancer Institute). Legislative agendas in health may also encompass wider, nonhealth interests, so that very different coalitions may push, for example, for veterans' benefits, rural hospitals, or biomedical research.

For scholars, the political process involved in health legislation has been tailor-made for discussions of power, ideology, and compromise, not to mention legislative failures. Less studied have been the cumulative messages embedded in the grab-bag of legislative initiatives in different periods. The forces of both federal action and inaction represent national policy writ large: to encourage trends toward specialization.

## Specialty Boards as Private Policy Makers

Given this national-policy context, the role of the specialty certifying boards in the second half of the twentieth century can be interpreted from at least three perspectives:

1. National health policy delegated specialty definition to reputable private organizations that represented the exercise of responsible professional self-regulation, most boards being led by medical school professors who had served the nation well in World War II.

2. In the absence of other policy-making directives, specialty organizations seized power in order to advance their own interests, carving up medicine into fiefdoms.

3. The freewheeling medical market for specialty services from the 1950s through the present created its own specialty preferences out of a combination of consumer and provider choices, and the boards responded to the market.

All of these statements ring true. The boards also responded to strong public or private reform proposals from outside of the profession, for example in advancing the cause of family practice and emergency medicine in the 1960s and 1970s, and later in embracing the quality movement (see below).

By 1969, thirty percent of American doctors practiced full-time as surgical specialists, forty-seven percent practiced full-time in nonsurgical fields, and twenty-three percent were general practitioners and/or part-time specialists (Stevens 1971, 181) This was not necessarily an "ideal" distribution from the health-planning point of view, at a time when planning was both in vogue and supported by government funds. "Are enough physicians of the right types trained in the United States?" an official report asked in the late 1970s, suggesting more direct national influence on the distribution of medical residencies. The Department of Health, Education, and Welfare projected an oversupply of doctors in fields such as pediatrics and neurological surgery, and an undersupply in family practice and plastic surgery, among other fields, though opinions differed "as to what constitutes a sufficient supply of specialists and whether too many of certain specialists are being trained" (Comptroller General 1978). But, after all, the United States did not claim to have a planned, or even "ideal," health care system.

The incorporation and renaming of the American Board of Medical Specialties in 1970 suggested it might acquire a stronger, more unified role in the context of federal support for health manpower education and health planning in the 1970s. The new, full-time director wrote enthusiastically about a more active role in raising standards and conducting studies of the "proportionate production of medical specialists, including their relationships with members of the allied health professions" (ABMS 1974, 4). Any such effort assumed a much stronger, centralized ABMS than before. Interest in certification, expressed by government agencies and public consumer groups in the late 1970s, also prompted the ABMS to extend its public gaze, including the addition of three public members in 1978. However, thoughts of activism faded as federal planning gave way to the market orientation of national health policy in the 1980s. Without a strong external stimulus or threat, the boards perceived no need to join forces around a common agenda if this meant giving up any of their own autonomy. Until the late 1990s, there was largely fruitless debate within the ABMS and the member boards as to what the boards represented as a collective. Was the ABMS a "federation," which implied greater power over independent boards, or was it a "confederation," a convenient meeting place for twenty-four independent units?

It was left to the specialty certifying boards, individually and collectively, to signify what a "specialist" was in terms of education and certification. Patients could look up their doctor in the ABMS *Directory of Medical Specialists* (and more recently online, www.abms.org), assuming they had heard of it. Alternatively, or in addition, a doctor could announce a specialist field of practice by choosing among a longer list of fields that appeared (and appears) under the term "self-designated specialty" in the AMA's national medical directory. His or her name was then displayed as such a specialist in the directory.

Other organizations were also in play. The distribution of training programs in different specialties and geographical regions represented (and represents) the combined actions of teaching hospitals across the United States. Teaching hospitals employ residents and pay their salaries in return for work and for the value (in imputed quality and prestige) in serving as a teaching institution. Common sense suggests that the one who pays the piper calls the tune. There has been a long, unresolved debate about how far demands for residents to staff the hospital in different fields or serve the demands of powerful medical constituencies have skewed the production of specialists toward hospital rather than practice needs.

Meanwhile, national accreditation of residency education within each specialty tightened. In 1972 a new Liaison Committee on Graduate Medical Education, sponsored by various professional medical organizations, strengthened private national oversight over the length, content, and standards of residency education in each field. This body was replaced by the Accreditation Council for Graduate Medical Education (the present ACGME) in 1981, and grew even stronger when this became an independent corporation in 2000. The ACGME, acting through residency review committees in each specialty, is organizationally separate from the specialty certification boards, and hence the ABMS, but they work in tandem and have some overlapping membership.

The organizational array may seem confusing. The net result is simple: an interlocking system of professional regulation. Every doctor in the United States went to a medical school accredited by a professional group, moved to a professionally accredited residency in an approved specialty, either did or did not add subspecialty training in an approved field, and sat the appropriate specialty (and subspecialty) board examinations. All of these processes were linked, with overlapping membership and communication, across the various organizations.

By the end of the 1970s, the second professional reform movement (standardizing specialist medical education) appeared to be moving toward completion. The public could rest assured that a board-certified specialist had received professionally designated training and a diploma certifying standards of 'fitness" or "competence" for the field. However, at least until the 1980s, this process applied to only a minority of doctors. Specialties as a group could not claim success as reforming organizations within the house of medicine until they actually represented the "profession."

The boards were also psychologically, if not organizationally, ill equipped to reinvent themselves as consumer-oriented institutions between the 1940s and the 1990s. Moving along the path of professional reform, their vision looked inward to professional organization and improvements in specialty education. Improved quality of care for the patient was assumed, not unreasonably, to be the outcome of this process, as it had been in the first professional reform movement. Americans were not clamoring for further change in the 1980s. Indeed the general public was almost entirely unaware that board certification existed, let alone what "certification" might mean, other than a reassuring official-looking framed document among others on the doctor's wall.

The American Board of Urology provides a good example of the self-defined organizational rationale for the boards, as it appeared in 1946:

> REASON FOR APPLYING FOR A CERTIFICATE; ITS VALUE. The American Urological Association, the American Association of Genito-Urinary Surgeons, and the Section on Urology of the American Medical Association are interested in furthering the cause of Urology and have participated in the formation of this Board. They are sponsoring its activities. The various national medical societies, the public, hospital directors and others, will utilize the certification from this Board as a means of discriminating between those well grounded as specialists in Urology, and those who are not.                    (ABMS 1946, 889)

When (in an influential exercise of public policy) the Federal Trade Commission and the courts began to apply antitrust provisions more generally to professional institutions in the 1970s, legal caution persuaded all of the boards to limit claims for "discriminating" in the marketplace because of actual and potential lawsuits—for example, from aggrieved doctors without a specialty diploma who claimed that the boards represented unfair restrictions on market competition.[2]

The specialty boards were private policy makers that influenced the structure, prestige, and success of American medicine between the 1940s and the 1990s. There was little recognition or call for them to play a broader role in public policy, either inside or outside of the boards.

### Professionalization of the Specialty Boards

To become effective public organizations, the specialty boards had to overcome their history as elitist clubs, or at least balance elitism with highly professional methods (psychometrics) for measuring the knowledge and skills of practitioners. Over the years the boards have become sophisticated agencies for professional evaluation using the most advanced testing methods.

Balancing qualitative (objective) and professional (subjective) goals was, initially at least, tricky. One of the founders of the American Board of Neurological Surgery expressed his strong dismay at their lax, cozy examining procedures in the late 1940s, compared with the much tighter methods used by Orthopedic Surgery. "Board members are ridiculed and are accused of operating secret clubs which permit membership only to those who are 'pets' of the examiners. . . . Have we provided adequate training and conducted an unbiased examination?" (Adson 1948). The implication was that they had not.

Between the 1940s and the 1990s each board worked, with greater or lesser success, to professionalize its administrative operations and to adopt and develop the latest techniques for objective examinations in its field. Professor Howard P. Lewis, chair of the American Board of Internal Medicine from 1959 to 1961, described the early success of board certification in that specialty. When he took the board examinations in 1937, he said, his colleagues in internal medicine "just laughed at me" for wasting time. By 1952, however, certification "had become a very well appreciated indication of competency." Valued by hospitals, medical schools, and insurers, the certificate had acquired material worth, for institutions as well as diplomates (Benson 1994, 22).

But what actually *was* a board, in terms of organizational culture and administration? In the 1960s, the boards were typically low-cost operations run out of the private office of the board's president or secretary (and some still are). These offices were scattered across the United States, moving as the officer changed. The culture was (and is) decided by the unpaid members of the board. The great diagnostician Jack D. Myers, chair of the American Board of Internal Medicine from 1967 through 1970, described that board as a "small club of about a dozen people." Another member of the board remembered it as "the finest dining club in America at the time." Oral examinations offered by the specialty boards in different hospitals across the country brought recognized specialists together for a common, prestigious mission. Examiners bonded together in camaraderie. Quoting Myers again, "The friendships, the mission of the Board, and the learning have made Board service an outstanding part of their careers" (Benson 1994, 54, 68, 56).

The specialties and subspecialties had examining structures that were largely isolated from each other. The specialty boards were autonomous corporations. With time, they became increasingly independent, both from each other and from their sponsoring specialty societies. "We were ferociously independent," recollected a member of the American Board of Internal Medicine. "We felt that independence was the only way we could maintain impartiality and avoid being influenced." Each subspecialty, in turn, developed its own culture and sense of camaraderie within the board system, and where relevant, in relation to its own sponsoring groups. In the 1950s, the subspecialty board chairs in internal medicine did not even meet with the parent board. Each group assumed without question that it was furthering responsible, professional self-regulation (Benson 1994, 23, 37).

How much standardization there should be *across* specialties has remained a problem for decades. It involves issues of professional autonomy, real differences between specialty fields, legal challenges, and the public interest. The AMA gave the first standardization movement strong central direction. Specialty groups, in contrast, relished their independence. Just as individual specialists competed with other specialists for patients, their organizations competed to protect, expand, and modify their fields. The ABMS, representing all the boards, published a directory of certified specialists and held annual meetings for discussions of mutual interest, but remained an organizational convenience for established members rather than a powerful national professional institution. Only now are the member boards seeing collective advantage in making the ABMS a unifying, standardizing force. ABMS archives from the years after World War II show some reluctance by constituent boards to pay the assigned dues of $1 per diplomate to help support the organization. In 1947, the relatively large American Board of Internal Medicine claimed poverty and tried unsuccessfully to cap its annual contribution at $300 instead of paying the actual amount of $482 (Werrill 1947). The ABIM is now a multi-million-dollar-a-year corporate force.

The most critical function of the ABMS has been to review applications for new specialties. This is done by a joint "liaison" committee of ABMS and the AMA Council on Medical Education. In the dance of professional self-regulation, groups of doctors claim they are specialists in a new field and deserve the full professional recognition assured by an "approved" certifying board—approved, that is, by the ABMS, representing the incumbent boards, and the AMA, representing doctors in practice. Approval of a new board rests on the strength of a formal proposal and negotiations with boards already in the system, who have clear perceptions of their own actual and would-be jurisdictions.

There were sixteen approved specialty boards in 1948, with many more contenders—in addition, of course, to general practice, which was by then a declining field. How many formal specialties should there be? In a market system we might perhaps say as many as the market would bear. Restrictive professional actions against new specialties could be labeled monopolistic and unfair. At the same time, never-ending splintering of medicine into specialties could pose serious economic and organizational problems for hospitals, where specialists are trained as residents and specialty practitioners seek staff appointments, as well as for the medical schools, which tend to recognize new fields with new departments or divisions. Splintering medicine further by adding new certifying boards *ad infinitum* would probably destabilize the existing specialty-board system, plunging it into constant turf wars, self-righteous rhetoric, and never-ending bickering. More importantly, from the public perspective, national professional regulation of specialists (the second medical reform movement) might well fail—and there is no plausible alternative in the wings.

In a remarkable show of unity the ABMS imposed a moratorium on the approval of new boards in 1949, which held firm for the next twenty years. Two more were approved before the moratorium took effect, bringing the total to eighteen (see Table 3-1). The general posture has remained conservative, reflected by the existence of only twenty-four boards today, despite years of change in the science and practice of medicine and in the organization and financing of medical care. New fields have been incorporated as subspecialties within the established boards (Stevens 2004).

### Everyone a Specialist

Specialty education and certification were becoming normal practice in the United States by the early 1960s. In 1961 more than two-thirds of all active, self-reported neurological surgeons, ophthalmologists, otolaryngologists, pathologists, radiologists, and thoracic surgeons were board certified; and the average across all specialties was fifty-three percent (Stevens 1971, 545). Through ABMS approval of two new specialty boards in family practice and emergency medicine—areas publicized by medical, political, community, and other groups as important for the health of the nation—the circle of specialization was completed. Every field of medicine was now a "specialty." Every doctor was a specialist. And the specialty boards, collectively, defined educational, if not practice, standards across the whole of medicine.

The establishment of the American Board of Family Practice in 1969 (at the time of writing being renamed the American Board of Family Medicine) broke the ABMS moratorium on the approval of new boards. It also demonstrated the power of the cultural environment to influence organizational change. The American Board of Emergency Medicine, founded in 1976 and approved in 1979 after a period of substantial hostility from established specialties, also reflected social and political concerns—in this case, about the poor service and lack of standards of emergency services in the United States.

The American health-policy establishment of the 1960s—including federal and state officials, practitioners in the growing fields of health planning and health services research (also in part federally funded), and the staff of charitable foundations and national commissions on primary care—regarded the future role of the generalist as the single most important organizational issue for the health care of the American population. General or family practice had its own professional societies, residencies, and a legitimate, if sometimes contested, place in at least some medical schools (often stimulated through state tax support). Given the evident success of other fields, self-designated family practitioners sought to advance their field through the well-established route of specialty credentials.

Most specialties and subspecialties were built around concepts of disease. In contrast, family practitioners presented their field as a professional response to growing concerns about health care in the 1960s, particularly the lack of access to primary care. Leaders in the new specialty of family practice saw themselves as involved in a more general movement for social reform, stimulated by federal and state tax funds for medical education and perhaps eventually by national health insurance. Gale Stephens used the evocative term "counterculture" to describe family practice as a counterweight to the biomedical culture of leading medical schools (Stephens 1979). Nicholas Pisacano, a major force behind the establishment of the family practice specialty board, reportedly held conversations with the ABIM as a possible home for the new field. However, that board apparently expressed no interest in including family physicians in its ranks (Pisacano 1964).

Reacting to a policy environment that was in favor of primary care, opposition among the incumbent specialty boards weakened. One influential speaker during the approval process, William Willard, urged the gathering of ABMS and AMA representatives to "do the right thing." He also suggested there would be unfortunate repercussions if they failed to do so. If the new board were not approved, Willard said, "then I think they are going to be a rebel group in organized medicine among the general practitioner group," and this would not look good for the profession (Adams 1999, 62). Family practice leaders, in turn, were anxious not to appear as second-class citizens in terms of the scientific message they sent out. They wanted to both set rigorous standards for certification and avoid identification with old-style general practice, which was looked down upon as relatively "unscientific" in the leading medical schools. The establishment of the American Board of Emergency Medicine followed a similar course. In the early 1970s a number of doctors involved in emergency care coalesced into what one critic called a "large emergency-medicine politicoeconomic establishment." (Leitzell 1981) Despite the doubts expressed among other specialists within ABMS as to whether emergency medicine was scientifically justified or even a discrete field of practice, broader policy agendas prevailed. Board certification ratified, advanced, unified specialists, and arguably invented the specialty of emergency medicine. Emergency physicians stressed their critical role in health-service delivery by choosing an hourglass as the board's symbol, to represent the importance of time in the management of care in the emergency room. While family medicine is a specialty defined by access to and continuity of care, emergency medicine is one of time and place.

With the establishment of these boards, the array of specialties offered to medical students covered a full range of medical careers. Entering a specialty had become a routine choice. If all doctors were to be recognized as specialists, it could only be a matter of time before the profession was distributed across the very fields that were marked out as specialties by the certifying boards. This has, indeed, been the case.

The American Board of Family Practice also heralded an important professional policy shift for the role of specialty boards in the future. Family Practice was the first specialty board to impose time limits on its certificates, requiring reexamination of every candidate every ten years, instead of giving a lifetime certificate. Two other boards established such certificates in the 1970s, six in the 1980s, and one in the 1990s. While the total, ten out of twenty-four boards, was a monument to slowness, *voluntary* periodic certification was endorsed as an alternative by all the boards in 1982. A major problem of compulsory recertification for the older boards was a feeling of unfairness to younger doctors. New diplomates would be caught by time-limited requirements, but the mass of older specialists in the same field had lifetime certificates to which they felt entitled. "Lifers" accounted for about half of all diplomates as late as 2004, varying in proportion from board to board. Nevertheless, with these moves the second medical reform movement of the twentieth century had gone well beyond the Flexner reforms into measuring the knowledge of doctors out in practice.

Family practice was largely an invention of the 1960s, as emergency medicine was of the 1970s. As a result, more so than in other fields, the fortunes of its members rose and fell with the successes and failures of the specialty in the sociopolitical milieu and what we might call the "expert" context of health care—that is, the prevailing views of the health policy establishment. Emergency physicians gained monopoly positions in hospital emergency rooms. Family practitioners were more vulnerable, for their success depended on restructuring consumer behavior that had long been encouraged in the medical market, away from disease-centered or organ-specific specialties toward comprehensive advice and primary (even managed) care.

The mood of euphoric idealism that distinguished the establishment of Family Practice turned to gloom as the 1960s "counterculture" and the resources of government were overtaken by political conservatism and market-oriented messages in the late 1970s (Stevens 2001b). The managed care movement of the 1990s attempted to reinvent primary care through rules incorporated into private insurance—notably, recognition of physician "gate-keepers" and rules for specialist referrals—but this effort largely failed (see Gray, this volume). Emergency physicians have been critical participants in the development of first-rate trauma services and are necessary to fulfill expressed public desire for on-call medical care twenty-four hours a day, seven days a week, in hospital emergency rooms. Today the specialties of both primary and emergency care are once again in "crisis" (see Hoffman, this volume). Outside the hospital, consumers still flock to specialists.

### The Growth of Subspecialties

As the number of specialties remained relatively constant, the number of subspecialties grew. Subspecialty education, via a hospital residency or university fellowship, follows a period of education in a primary specialty (such as internal medicine). The method for approval of a subspecialty mirrors that of new primary boards; each requires a formal, written presentation, debate, and ABMS imprimatur. In recent years much of the work of ABMS as designer of American specialty divisions has thus shifted to considerations of claims for approval of subspecialty certificates.

The subspecialties themselves are not new. Three of today's ninety-two subspecialties were formally approved in the late 1930s, and all fell within the American Board of Internal Medicine: gastroenterology, pulmonary disease, and cardiovascular disease. Pathology sprouted subspecialties in the 1940s and 1950s: neuropathology, medical microbiology, chemical pathology, hematology, and forensic pathology. Psychiatry first issued certificates in child and adolescent psychiatry in 1959; Pediatrics, for pediatric cardiology, in 1961. Ten subspecialties went into business before 1972, eighteen in the 1970s, seventeen in the 1980s, twenty-eight in the 1990s, and so far nineteen in the 2000s. Since medicine is constantly changing, many more claims are to be expected in the future.

To some extent one can trace new developments in medical science and practice over the years (and sometimes cultural and market interest in newly defined medical problems) by charting the course of the approved subspecialties. Among the fields that appeared in the 1970s were endocrinology, oncology, and pediatric surgery; in the 1980s, critical care, geriatric medicine, and clinical immunology; in the 1990s, sports medicine, interventional cardiology, vascular and interventional radiology, and medical toxicology; and in the early 2000s, pain management, developmental/behavioral pediatrics, and plastic surgery within the head and neck.

The rapid growth of overlapping subspecialties from the 1970s challenged boards with interests in competing areas. The American Board of Internal Medicine offered six additional subspecialty certificates in 1972–1973, and reorganized its field conceptually and organizationally into general internal medicine and subspecialties. General internists competed head-to-head with family practitioners in primary care. Increasingly, too, a proposal for a new subspecialty by one board might engage the territory claimed by others. Fundamental questions had become conceptually problematic. For example, if each doctor was a specialist, was that individual also necessarily a generalist? How were generalism and specialism to be negotiated within the overall board structure? Was medicine a set of scientific divisions or of practice roles or of neither of these? And what did any of these terms mean?

Pediatricians, like internists, wrestled for years with the future of their field as a general specialty or as a collection of experts in different fields whose primary connection was the care of children. Pediatrics sheltered three subspecialties in 1973, but these seemed limited in function to highly trained pediatric consultants, rather than career choices for the average practitioner. In fields like pediatric nephrology, pediatric hematology-oncology, and pediatric cardiology, certification could be seen as the badge of an esoteric specialist, someone who had completed a subspecialty fellowship and was working at a major children's hospital. The role of subspecialties became more problematic as they blossomed within different certifying boards. As with the earlier development of the primary boards, the subspecialties had a domino effect. Contextual changes and public visibility of a particular field might lead that specialty's board to recognize a subspecialty, making it difficult for a second board to resist making a similar move, whatever its philosophy of nonproliferation. Oncology was a good case in point. The ABMS approved oncology as a subspecialty of internal medicine in 1972, of pediatrics in 1973, and of gynecology in 1974. The movement for subspecialties was thus pushed in two ways: by groups within a wider field (such as geriatricians in internal medicine or pediatricians specializing in adolescent medicine) and as part of a reaction to an emerging field by multiple boards.

The latter is well illustrated by the increased importance of intensive and critical care in the 1970s. Advocates of critical-care medicine as a defined field achieved recognition of the subspecialty under the auspices of several different boards, including anesthesiology, pediatrics, internal medicine, OB/GYN, and surgery. Newly visible fields like geriatrics, sports medicine, toxicology, pain management, and adolescent medicine sparked the natural interests of more than one board. Five boards came to offer immunology as a subspecialty, four boards sports medicine, and so on. With the expansion of knowledge across traditional specialty boundaries, the definition of a "specialty" was not as clear-cut as it once seemed to be.

### Professional Responsibility and Public Policy

Left open was a raft of new questions. In the context of an increasing critique of the authority of the medical profession in the 1970s and 1980s (Freidson 1970; Starr 1982), and increasing oversight of clinical work through the managed-care movement of the late 1980s and 1990s, the specialty boards could no longer expect to be left alone indefinitely to wrestle with their own problems. There were, indeed, problems enough: how to deal with the proliferation of subspecialties as professional societies pressed for new certificates; how to design better, secure examinations (to avoid allegations of cheating); how to give oral examinations in hospitals when major hospitals were becoming reluctant to donate their resources; how to design testing techniques to effectively measure clinical skills without the need for face-to-face examinations; and how to continue to attract the best examiners to donate their time without pay. In the 1980s, with medicine overtly regarded as "big business" in the United States, and with recertification challenged by specialty societies on behalf of their members, legal (antitrust) challenges loomed as a threat. Through the 1970s, 1980s, and 1990s each board remained fiercely independent.

The boards' administrative offices are still scattered across the country, depending on the convenience of past or present specialty leaders. Today's twenty-four boards are located in twelve different states. In the information age, this may not matter for formal communication, though in the past it undoubtedly encouraged the continuance of organizational isolationism and distrust of joint efforts, discouraged informal communication across boards, and made ABMS meetings more contentious than they might otherwise have been. Some of the boards have invested in beautiful multi-million-dollar buildings befitting their status as august, establishment institutions with a steady stream of income; others are relatively poor.

Organizational inertia among the established member boards and lack of power or resources at the center distinguished the ABMS into the 1990s. However organizations, like individuals, tend to band together in the face of common threats. In the late 1990s groups outside of organized medicine expressed concerns about the competence of physicians. These included groups interested in quality measurement, the overall quality of care, medical licensing for practicing doctors, and accreditation of organizations in health care. Responding to these pressures and recognizing an apparent shift of public interest to the question of "competence," the ABMS established an ambitious Task Force on Competence in 1998. Error in medicine became enormously visible in 1999 with the publication of an influential report from the Institute of Medicine, *To Err Is Human* (Kohn, Corrigan, and Donaldson 2000). Concurrently some states (notably Florida and Texas) have shown interest in specialist credentialing. Whether they liked it or not, the boards were thrust into the center of debates about medical quality and what it now means to be a profession. This history is still being written.

Specialty board leaders are currently moving toward common goals through the establishment of "maintenance of certification" (MOC) programs for physicians; that is the replacement (or extension) of existing certification procedures by a more continuous process of learning, evaluation, and self-evaluation over an individual's whole career. All the boards are now committed to the principle of examining doctors based on six general competencies designed to encompass quality care: patient care, medical knowledge, practice-based learning and improvement, interpersonal and communications skills, professionalism, and systems-based practice. These areas have been identified jointly by the ABMS (for continuous certification through an active career) and

ACGME, so that graduate education in medicine, via a specialty, is standardized from an individual's graduation from medical school through retirement. The movement toward MOC is supported by numerous other organizations, including the AMA, the Federation of State Medical Boards (state licensing boards), the American Hospital Association, and JCAHO.

Many hurdles remain. While all twenty-four boards are developing their programs for implementing MOC, and while those in the lead have developed elegant and sophisticated proposals designed to place specialty certification firmly within the current health-care quality movement (see, for example, Brennan et al. 2004), MOC will be implemented in a health-care market in which many practicing physicians feel overwhelmed, overworked, underpaid, and over-regulated. Marketing MOC requires a major effort to publicize it as a successful move toward enhanced quality for patients, without imposing unfair burdens on practitioners. Currently, such marketing is falling mainly on the unpaid board members of the specialty certifying boards and ABMS, whose own hard-pressed medical schools are reluctant to recognize voluntary national professional service as beneficial. The MOC program remains divisive for certain specialties, because no effort is being made, at least initially, to require diplomates with lifetime certificates to enter MOC. Nevertheless, despite such problems, the opportunity is there for creative, responsible, and publicly useful professional change.

Yet, even in 2006, as this book goes to press, this message is rarely remarked on (or perhaps even known about) in policy debates outside of the profession. It is still possible that specialty testing and credentialing may devolve in the future to licensing boards, insurers, and employers of physicians, and that the specialty boards will cease to have a central role in quality evaluation. If so, should one care? The answer is unequivocally yes. Let us leave aside the costs for both doctors and taxpayers (and ultimately patients) if the current activities and accumulated experience of the boards had to be reproduced by organizations outside of the profession, including paying for the boards' armies of highly skilled volunteers, who create and manage policy and examinations and negotiate specialty and subspecialty fields. There will be potential benefits to patients if their doctors are seriously engaged in specified programs of lifelong learning and assessment of their skills; thus MOC offers a consumer-oriented opportunity for better care. MOC should make medicine more interesting for practicing doctors by putting them on the frontline of knowledge in their fields. Doctors could, however, subvert these opportunities by defining MOC in hostile terms, as just one more unwanted and unnecessary intrusion into their practice. Quality advocates outside the profession may also passively subvert MOC by not recognizing or supporting it. The second "professional reform" movement is now at a crucial stage.

## Conclusion

Medical specialization is, and has long been, American health policy. The boards (with their sponsoring specialty associations) have become de facto public agents, with authority effectively delegated (or ceded) by government. A weaker, but related interpretation is that they are filling a policy vacuum caused by lack of government health-care policy making. This chapter shows, however, that a simple story line is insufficient to explain the centrality of specialization in American health care.

The cultural, political, and policy roles of the specialty credentialing organizations (the specialty certifying boards) changed with the growth in the proportion of doctors who became specialists; indeed individual boards have been exquisitely attuned to messages in the larger policy environment. The idea of a specialty also changed over the half-century following World War II. In the 1940s it was still possible to see a specialty as an avocation. In the 1990s the specialty was more like a brand name and the credential a property acquisition. When only a minority of doctors were full-time specialists (up though the 1950s), specialty certification could be seen as the mark of an elite group or even a clique. By the end of the century, with virtually all practicing physicians certified by an ABMS-approved specialty board, the organized specialties had come to define American medicine and to evaluate the standards of individual doctors.

In the 1940s the specialties were at the periphery of power in organized medicine; by the 1990s they were central. Exercising the privilege of professional self-regulation without government involvement, American specialty groups created and sustained a complex and evolving array of examinations based on approved residency education and began to grapple with the challenge of extending this system into one of life-long education and evaluation, from first-year residency to the end of a career.

Unlike the earlier educational reforms, the specialty movement was not centrally directed. In some ways this makes its history more remarkable than the history of the Flexner reforms. The history of specialty certification in the late twentieth century demonstrates the motivating strength of two cultural beliefs: that a standardized, educated profession serves the public and that the provision of national standards is a hallmark of an organized profession. Whether these beliefs and assumptions continue to be held by the public or indeed by the profession and how far they are accepted, rejected, or ignored by the larger health establishment, consumers, and/or the general public are policy questions for today.

Is this history a story of success, demonstrating responsible self-regulation, and thus offering a good, as well as a strong example of public-private regulation? Perhaps. Much depends on what happens next. Some scholars have recently stressed the rising social importance, even the ascendancy, of the professions as a whole (Perkin 1996; Freidson 2001). In the world of health care, in contrast, the rising authority of managers and other health-care experts has challenged that of doctors, and the sources of the profession's "reduced legitimacy" have been documented (Schlesinger 2002). The history of specialties is one of power plays: the exercise of professional dominance over segments of the medical machine and a means for specialties and specialists to attain market power (Starr 1982; Light 1988; Light and Levine 1988; Halpern 1988; Larson 1977). Specialty boards are at the same time competitors, monopolists, and public heroes.

My interpretation of the history of specialty certification as the second professional reform movement of the past hundred years or so—the first being the Flexner reforms—recognizes the importance of specialization in the history of the American medical profession. The specialty-board movement could be described in other ways. Turf-war stories, riven with internecine conflict, would make a dramatic central narrative. Specialty formation could (and should) be put more firmly into the context of patient care, of changes in scientific practice and technology, and developments elsewhere in American culture, politics, and economy. Government "manpower" and funding policies deserve close attention in relation to professional development. Even the "rise and fall" story could be brought usefully to bear on the decline of the AMA (in membership at least) and the rise of specialty organizations. Viewing the history of specialties as part of the longer history of professional policy making, education, and standardization has, however, both strategic and scholarly resonance in our present.

The Flexner reforms succeeded because various interests aligned, including members of leading medical school faculties, state licensing boards, the AMA, federal bureaucrats, and experts on quality methods (standardization) in disparate cultural and commercial fields. Today's specialty certifying boards have achieved a remarkable unanimity of purpose. Yet the standardization movement for specialty education represented in MOC is fragile. The volunteers who make certification work have taken on the huge additional assignment of MOC at a time when demands on faculty and practitioner time are heavy. Lost reimbursable time because of extensive voluntary work, such as

Table 3-1  **Medical Specialty Boards Approved by the American Board of Medical Specialties by Date of Approval**

|  | Incorporated | Approved |
|---|---|---|
| American Board of Ophthalmology | 1917 | |
| American Board of Otolaryngology | 1924 | |
| American Board of Obstetrics and Gynecology | 1930 | |
| American Board of Dermatology | 1932 | |
| American Board of Pediatrics | 1933 | 1935 |
| American Board of Radiology | 1934 | 1935 |
| American Board of Psychiatry and Neurology | 1934 | 1935 |
| American Board of Orthopedic Surgery | 1934 | 1935 |
| American Board of Urology | 1935 | 1935 |
| American Board of Pathology | 1936 | 1936 |
| American Board of Internal Medicine | 1936 | 1936 |
| American Board of Surgery | 1937 | 1937 |
| American Board of Neurological Surgery | 1940 | 1940 |
| American Board of Anesthesiology | 1938 | 1941 |
| American Board of Plastic Surgery | 1937 | 1941 |
| American Board of Physical Medicine and Rehabilitation | 1947 | 1947 |
| American Board of Preventive Medicine | 1948 | 1949 |
| American Board of Colon and Rectal Surgery | 1935 | 1949 |
| American Board of Family Medicine | 1969 | 1969 |
| American Board of Thoracic Surgery | 1950 | 1970 |
| American Board of Allergy and Immunology | 1971 | 1971 |
| American Board of Nuclear Medicine | 1971 | 1971 |
| American Board of Emergency Medicine | 1976 | 1979 |
| American Board of Medical Genetics | 1980 | 1991 |

Source: American Board of Medical Specialties

Notes

The American Board of Medical Specialties (ABMS) was established in 1933. Boards established before then were founding members.

Present titles of boards are given. Each board also formally includes Inc. after its title.

Five boards offer more than one primary certificate; for example, Psychiatry and Neurology offers three certificates: in psychiatry, neurology, and neurology with special qualifications in child neurology.

Eighteen of the boards offer subspecialty certificates following general certification in the specialty and approved additional training. The boards not currently offering subspecialties are Colon and Rectal Surgery, Neurological Surgery, Nuclear Medicine, Ophthalmology, Thoracic Surgery, and Urology. Half of the 92 subspecialties reside in three boards: Pediatrics, Internal Medicine, and Pathology.

board service, is more difficult to justify to partners, hospital or university employers, and other interested parties than it was in earlier years, when medical fees were more flexible and professional service carried more prestige. Perhaps of more importance, other obvious interests are not (yet) fully lined up—notably the growing ranks of managers and policy and quality experts. The success of MOC may well depend upon their understanding of its goals, their enthusiasm, and their support as part of the present quality movement.

For each group, interpretations of history affect action in the present. The health-services management and research communities have long seen the physician community as the "other" and the relationship between them as one of public-private confrontation (the AMA's opposition to government health insurance, for example) rather than mutual cooperation to improve health care for the future. Meanwhile the medical profession has long assumed that professional responsibilities, including medical education and certification, are no one else's business. Indeed, the reason that MOC is as yet so little known or, alternatively, discounted as a public-policy initiative may simply be the continuation of these two mind-sets, drawing on different historical conceptions of the present. Both are overdue for change.

Yet, if this second professional revolution fails—and it might without strong external support—who in the specialty-driven medical marketplace of the United States will step up to examine, educate, encourage, improve, and maintain certification of the three-quarters of a million doctors in training or in practice in 130 or so specialties and subspecialties?

## Notes

Research for this paper was funded in part by a Robert Wood Johnson Foundation Investigator Award in Health Policy Research. I would like to thank Renée C. Fox, Stephen H. Miller, and Charles E. Rosenberg for very helpful comments.

1. Abraham Flexner was commissioned by the Carnegie Foundation for the Advancement of Teaching to investigate the profession of medicine as part of the foundation's wider inquiries into problems of higher education. Educational leaders in medicine, organized through the newly reformed American Medical Association, welcomed this spur to their own efforts to upgrade educational standards in medical schools at a time of rapid expansion in medical science, technology, and surgical skills. Early twentieth-century schools ranged from scientific institutions such as at the Johns Hopkins University to night schools and small, rudimentary, sometimes dirty schools that were run for profit by practitioners.

   Working in tandem with increased requirements for medical licensure in the states, the AMA Council on Medical Education cooperated with Flexner and concurrently rated (accredited) all the schools,. The result of these interlocking efforts transformed American medical education through the closure of schools that could not compete with new accreditation or licensing requirements, removed the earlier variety of pathways into medicine, homogenized medical education, and increasingly defined medical education as a profession to be entered with at least some undergraduate education as a prerequisite. By 1920, the United States could claim world leadership in scientific medicine. Not least, on the home front the reform movement signaled the AMA's growing authority as the voice of a unified profession.

2. Hospitals, medical schools, and insurers, however, do, of course, use board certification as a criterion for decision.

## References

Adams, David P. 1999. *American Board of Family Practice: A History*. Lexington, KY: American Board of Family Practice.

Adson, A. W. 1948. Open Letter to Members of the American Board of Neurological Surgery (no specific date). Evanston, IL: American Board of Medical Specialties, Archives. History IV.

Advisory Board of Medical Specialties (ABMS). 1946. *Directory of Medical Specialists Holding Certificates by American Boards*. Chicago: A. N. Marquis.

———. 1974. *Annual Report, 1973*. Evanston, IL: ABMS.

Baker, Robert, Arthur L. Caplan, Linda L. Emanuel, and Stephen R. Lathan, eds. 1998. *The American Medical Ethics Revolution*. Baltimore: Johns Hopkins University Press.

Benson, John A. 1994. *Oral Histories: American Board of Internal Medicine Chairmen 1947–1985*. Philadelphia: American Board of Internal Medicine.

Berliner, Howard S. 1985. *A System of Scientific Medicine: Philanthropic Foundations in the Flexner Era*. New York: Tavistock.

Brennan, Troyen A., Ralph I. Horwitz, F. Daniel Duffy, Christine K. Cassel, Leslie D. Goode, and Rebecca S. Lipner. 2004. The Role of Physician Specialty Certification Status in the Quality Movement. *Journal of the American Medical Association* 292:1038–1043.

Brown, E. Richard. 1979. *Rockefeller Medicine Men: Medicine and Capitalism in America*. Berkeley: University of California Press.

Burrow, James G. 1963. *AMA: Voice of American Medicine*. Baltimore: Johns Hopkins University Press.

Committee on the Costs of Medical Care. 1932. *Medical Care for the American People. Final Report of the Committee on the Costs of Medical Care*. Chicago: University of Chicago Press.

Comptroller General of the United States. 1978. *Are Enough Physicians of the Right Types Trained in the United States?* Report to the Congress of the United States. HRD-77–92. Washington, DC: United States General Accounting Office.

Engel, Jonathan. 2002. *Doctors and Reformers: Discussion and Debates over Health Policy, 1925–1950*. Columbia: University of South Carolina Press.

Fishbein, Morris. 1947. *A History of the American Medical Association, 1847 to 1947*. Philadelphia: W. B. Saunders.

Flexner, Abraham. 1910. *Medical Education in the United States and Canada*. Bulletin Number 4. New York: Carnegie Foundation for the Advancement of Teaching.

Freidson, Eliot. 1970. *Profession of Medicine: A Study of the Sociology of Applied Knowledge*. New York: Dodd Mead.

———. 2001. *Professionalism, the Third Logic: On the Practice of Knowledge*. Chicago: University of Chicago Press.

Gordon, Colin. 2003. *Dead on Arrival: The Politics of Health Care in Twentieth-Century America*. Princeton: Princeton University Press.

Halpern, Sydney A. 1988. *American Pediatrics: The Social Dynamics of Professionalism 1880–1980*. Berkeley: University of California Press.

Honigsbaum, Frank. 1979. *The Division in British Medicine: A History of the Separation of General Practice from Hospital Care 1911–1968*. New York: St. Martin's Press.

Howell, Joel D. 1995. *Technology in the Hospital: Transforming Patient Care in the Early Twentieth Century*. Baltimore: Johns Hopkins University Press.

Klein, Jennifer. 2003. *For All These Rights: Business, Labor, and the Shaping of America's Public–Private Welfare State*. Princeton: Princeton University Press.

Kohn, Linda T., Janet M. Corrigan, and Molla S. Donaldson, eds. 2000. *To Err Is Human: Building a Safer Health System*. Institute of Medicine. Washington DC: National Academy Press.

Larson, M. S. *The Rise of Professionalism: A Sociological Analysis*. Berkeley: University of California Press.

Leitzell, James D. 1981. An Uncertain Future. *New England Journal of Medicine* 304: 477–480.

Light, D. W. 1988. Turf Battles and the Theory of Medical Dominance. *Research in the Sociology of Health Care* 7: 203–205.

Light, D., and S. Levine. 1988. The Changing Character of the Medical Profession. *Milbank Quarterly* 66: 10–32.

Ludmerer, Kenneth M. 1985. *Learning to Heal: The Development of American Education*. New York: Basic Books.

———. 1999. *Time to Heal: American Medical Education from the Turn of the Century to the Era of Managed Care*. Oxford: Oxford University Press.

Miller, Stephen H. 2003. Personal communication.

Oberlander, Jonathan. 2003. *The Political Life of Medicare*. Chicago: University of Chicago Press.

Perkin, Harold. 1996. *The Third Revolution: Professional Elites in the Modern World*. New York: Routledge.

Pisacano, N. J. 1964. General Practice: A Eulogy. *GP* 19: 173–181.

Poen, Monte M. 1979. *Harry Truman versus the Medical Lobby: The Genesis of Medicare*. Columbia: University of Missouri Press.

Reid, David W. 1908. Influence of Specialism on the General Practitioner. *Illinois Medical Journal* 14: 580–586.

Rosen, George. 1944. *The Specialization of Medicine with Particular Reference to Ophthalmology*. New York: Froben Press.

Rosenberg, Charles E. 1987. *The Care of Strangers: The Rise of America's Hospital System*. New York: Basic Books.

Satullo, Chris. 2004. Avoid the Dreaded Either/or—Seek the Sweet Bird of Paradox. *Philadelphia Inquirer*, 27 June.

Schlesinger, Mark. 2002. A Loss of Faith: The Sources of Reduced Political Legitimacy for the American Medical Profession. *Milbank Quarterly* 80: 185–235.

Somers, Herman Miles, and Anne Ramsey Somers. 1961. *Doctors, Patients and Health Insurance: The Organization and Financing of Medical Care*. Washington, DC: Brookings Institution.

Starr, Paul. 1982. *The Social Transformation of American Medicine: The Rise of a Sovereign Profession and the Making of a Vast Industry*. New York: Basic Books.

Stephens, G. G. 1979. Family Medicine as Counter-Culture. *Family Medicine Teacher* 11: 14–18.

Stevens, Rosemary. 1966. *Medical Practice in Modern England. The Impact of Specialization and State Medicine.* New Haven: Yale University Press. Reissued 2003 with new introduction, New Brunswick, NJ: Transaction Publishers.

————. 1971. *American Medicine and the Public Interest.* New Haven: Yale University Press. Reissued 1998 with new introduction, Berkeley: University of California Press.

————. 1989. *In Sickness and in Wealth: American Hospitals in the Twentieth Century.* New York: Basic Books. Reissued 1999 with new introduction, Baltimore: Johns Hopkins University Press.

————. 2001a. Public Roles for the Medical Profession in the United States: Beyond Theories of Decline and Fall. *Milbank Quarterly* 79: 327–353.

————. 2001b. The Americanization of Family Medicine: Contradictions, Challenges, and Change, 1969–2000. *Family Medicine* 33: 232–243.

————. 2004. Specialization, Specialty Organizations and the Quality of Care. In *Policy Challenges in Modern Health Care,* eds. David Mechanic and David C. Colby, 206–220. New Brunswick, NJ: Rutgers University Press.

Stone, Deborah. 1997. *Policy Paradox: The Art of Political Decision Making.* New York: W. W. Norton.

Thompson, John D. 1985. The Uneasy Alliance. In *Physicians and Hospitals: The Great Partnership at the Crossroads,* eds. Duncan Yaggy and Patricia Hodgson. Durham, NC: Duke University Press.

Weisz, George. 2005. *Divide and Conquer. A Comparative History of Medical Specialization.* Oxford: Oxford University Press.

Werrill, W. A., to B. R. Kirklin. 1947. Letter, dated 6 December. Evanston, IL: American Board of Medical Specialties, Archives. History IV.

White, William A. 1933. Statement. Proceedings 89th Annual Meeting, the American Psychiatric Association. *American Journal of Psychiatry* 13: 387.

Zeisler, Joseph. 1901. Specialties and Specialists. *Journal of the American Medical Association* 36: 1–6.

# Part II

# Rhetoric,
# Rights,
# Responsibilities

# Patients or Health-Care Consumers?

## Why the History of Contested Terms Matters

Since the 1980s, the use of the term *health-care consumer* as a synonym for patient (along with its doctor analogue, *health-care provider*) has become commonplace in the United States. For many observers today, especially physicians, this linguistic transformation has come to represent the worst consequences of American medicine's growing market orientation. As one doctor quoted by the columnist Ellen Goodman quipped, "Every time a patient is referred to as a health-care consumer, another angel dies," while another cited by William Safire observed, "The managed-care organizations call people *consumers* so they don't have to think of them as *patients*" (Goodman 1999; Safire 2000; emphasis in original). Such visceral dislike of the term *health-care consumer* reflects not only the loss of physician autonomy that has accompanied the coming of managed care, but also a deeper sense of violation: a conviction that applying the base language of the marketplace to the sacred realm of the doctor-patient relationship is fundamentally wrong.

In the introduction to his 1998 book *Some Choice,* George Annas makes a strong case against referring to patients as consumers on just such grounds. Market models of competition do not work when applied to health-care choices, he argues, "because patients are not consumers who pick and choose among physicians and treatments on the basis of price and quality." The legal principles derived from the United States Constitution and the Bill of Rights are a surer foundation for protecting patient interests than any economic theory, Annas suggests; it has been in the courtroom and the legislature, not the marketplace, that entitlements to informed consent, privacy, emergency care, and the like have been most effectively secured. In contrast, consumer rights have focused "not on the context of diagnosing and treating patients, but on the purchase and sale of a health-care policy," with far narrower and less beneficial results. Annas concludes, "Market language, with its emphasis on choice, tends to marginalize the sick and treat the practice of medicine as just another occupation, and medical care itself as just another commodity, like breakfast cereal" (xii).

Such criticisms of consumer rhetoric are common among thoughtful health-care analysts today. While I share their concerns, I aim in this chapter both to dispute the widely held belief that managed-care advocates began the practice of referring to patients as consumers and to provide a broad historical perspective on this linguistic shift. In fact, it was patient activists, not market enthusiasts, who initially embraced the phrase *health-care consumer* in the 1960s and 1970s. They chose that language as a liberating alternative to a traditional doctor-patient relationship they believed to be hopelessly mired in paternalism. The 1970s concept of the empowered patient-consumer was part of a wide-ranging critique of both medical paternalism and the "new medical-industrial complex" so famously described by Arnold Relman in 1980. Activists embraced a consumer-oriented rhetoric in order to redress the growing imbalance of power between patients and caregivers and to ensure that "people come before profits," a favorite slogan of that era (Ehrenreich and Ehrenreich 1970).

Thirty years later, it is tempting to dismiss the 1970s embrace of consumer rights as naive and misguided. But before throwing the consumer baby out with the managed-care bath water, we need better to understand why patient advocates adopted this rhetoric as well as why their grand visions of reform eventually failed. As policymakers continue to ponder how to cross the "quality chasm" toward a more patient-centered model of health care (Institute of Medicine 1999; 2001), the history of what might be termed the first consumer health revolution deserves a closer look. Such reflections are particularly timely, given the current enthusiasm in some policy circles for "consumer-oriented" or "consumer-driven" policy mechanisms such as defined-contribution health insurance plans and medical savings accounts (Herzlinger 1997; Gabel, LoSasso, and Rice 2002).

While the historical analysis presented here helps explain the political appeal of such measures, it also provides little reason to hope that these consumer-driven mechanisms will succeed any better than their managed-care predecessors in transforming the troubled U.S. health-care system. My skepticism about the latest generation of so-called consumer-controlled policies reflects two conclusions based on my historical research. First, that modern conceptions of patients'—and consumers'—rights are best understood as responses to long-term *contractions,* not *expansions,* of patients' powers of therapeutic and economic self-determination. Second, that models of consumer "sovereignty" based on patients' ability to discipline the health-care marketplace through individual choices have historic limitations that will likely never be overcome.

By putting contemporary conceptions of patients' and consumers' rights in historical perspective, this chapter seeks to analyze some of those limitations. Although our modern understanding of those rights dates from the turbulent 1960s, patient-consumers have a much longer history of trying to shape medical institutions to their liking. Tracing the historical antecedents of contemporary notions of patient/consumer entitlements helps to identify long-term shifts in how patients thought of themselves as exercising influence over the cost and course of their treatment. It also reveals changing patient expectations about the rights they should enjoy in their dealings with doctors.

To date, historians have written most extensively about the right to health care itself and the long-running debate Americans have had over the proper form of health insurance in a modern society (Hoffman 2004; Gordon 2003; Klein 2003). I focus instead on the historical antecedents of a different set of rights that came to the fore in the 1960s and 1970s: "the right to safety, the right to be informed, the right to choose, and the right to be heard," as they were enumerated in John F. Kennedy's famous 1962 consumer bill of rights (Preston and Bloom 1986, 38). In other words, I examine rights having more to do with the quality and experience of health care than with its availability.[1]

In this historical mapping exercise, I am not primarily concerned with those rights of safety, information, choice, and self-determination as abstractions in the way that philosophers and bioethicists formulate them, nor in formal definitions that an individual plaintiff might assert in a court of law, although I try to take those into account. I am more interested in the messier uses of "rights talk" in personal and political domains, as in an angry patient's claim that "you have no right to treat me this way" flung at a doctor, or the more measured claim that "people have a right to affordable medical care." These popular uses of rights talk certainly reflect changing philosophical and legal principles, but they also have roots in traditional notions of moral economy and fair play (Thompson 1971; Okun 1986).

With these caveats in mind, let me expand on my working conceptions of the distinctions between patient and consumer roles and identities. Eleanor D. Kinney offers a useful place to begin: "Consumer rights, it has been said, 'focus on purchasing decisions before a provider relationship is formed,' while patient rights 'focus on the relationship between patients and physicians (and other providers) and the type and quality of care provided'" (9) But while Kinney's emphasis on timing is crucial, this formulation assumes too clean a separation of patient-consumer interests. Obviously, the kind of thinking one does on the way to the emergency room is fundamentally different from the sort of deliberation done while pondering different health-insurance plans. Patients, however, do not stop thinking about the therapeutic and economic consequences of their treatment choices after they choose a doctor. Prevailing models of professionalism have encouraged the assumption that patients and physicians check their economic interests at the examining room door, but in reality, the roles of doctor/provider and patient/consumer are hard to disentangle (Rodwin 1993; Tomes 2003). So while it is important to differentiate between therapeutic and economic concerns, I prefer to think of them as distinct but overlapping orientations, as summarized in Tables 4-1 and 4-2.

**Table 4-1   Patient versus Consumer: Roles and Identities**

| Patient role/identity | Consumer role/identity |
|---|---|
| Main concern: relief from illness | Main concern: effective use of resources to maximize personal goals |
| Assumption: MD and patient share same goals | Assumption: buyer and seller have some inherently different interests esp. in regard to price |
| Therapeutic, professional values dominate decision making | Economic values (cost, profit) influence choice of treatment |
| Economic concerns muted (little concern for price, competitive "shopping") | Economic concerns paramount |
| Main protections: professional ethics, law, regulatory policy | Main protections: "rational" shopping, regulation of marketplace (voluntary and involuntary) |

**Table 4-2   Patient versus Consumer: Comparative Conceptions of Rights**

| Patient | Consumer |
|---|---|
| Traditional fomulations in physicians' ethical codes | Regulation of marketplace to ensure competitiveness and product safety |
| Tort law: medical malpractice | Antitrust and product-liability law |
| Extension of Constitutional rights, such as privacy, self-determination, into medical decision making | Consumer law: protection versus misleading product claims  Access to accurate information about goods and services |
| "Right" to choose doctor | "Right" to choose provider |

The comparison of legal versus economic rights inevitably raises the question of which provides the stronger platform for political advocacy. Health-care issues are particularly revealing of the gap between formal definitions of legal and constitutional rights and the broader definition of social rights or entitlements. Since neither the U.S. Constitution nor the Bill of Rights explicitly mention a right to health care, patient/consumer advocates have been forced to improvise arguments about why and how such care should be provided. As Annas (1998) argues, one such strategy rests on extending the reach of basic citizenship rights—for example, the right to self-determination or to privacy—into the doctor-patient relationship. Another strategy has been to cast patient entitlements in the language of the market and to argue that patients' rights to certain economic choices must be protected. While originating in different spheres—citizenship rights tied to Enlightenment political and legal notions, consumer rights to modern economic theories—these arguments have often overlapped. Popular uses of "rights talk" regarding health care reflect this messy intertangling of political and economic issues.

While legal protections can be very powerful, Annas underestimates the appeal that the weaker, more diffuse conception of consumer rights has long had in American political discourse. As historians such as Cohen (2003), Donahue (2003), and Glickman (2001) have shown, the ideal of the "consumer citizen" has figured importantly in twentieth-century politics because it links the goals of political and economic democracy. The superiority of the American way of life has often been equated with the power of "consumer sovereignty," that is, the belief that consumers' choices in a free-market economy serve to direct that economy to provide more of the goods and services that people truly need and/or want. In order for this sovereignty to be exercised, consumers must be able to choose freely among a range of competitive providers who contend for their business in terms of price, quality, and service (Slater 1997). The centrality of this belief is apparent in the faith, frequently voiced in discussions about health-care policy today, that simply providing patients more choice will bring about structural changes favorable to their economic and therapeutic interests.

As any health-care policymaker well knows, however, there are enormous difficulties inherent in applying traditional economic models to the doctor-patient relationship (Sloan 2001). These problems were identified by economists as early as the 1930s (Tomes 2003), three decades before Kenneth Arrow's famous paper (1963) on the subject. The connection between supply and demand in the health-care field remains one of the most notoriously complicated of all modern economic problems precisely because the market conditions under which doctors, hospitals, pharmaceutical companies, and medical technology firms offer their services do not conform to the classic requirements of open competition over price and quality. So even though the consumer health revolution of the 1960s and 1970s has expanded important facets of patient choice, their decision making continues to operate within a uniquely constructed, highly specialized marketplace over which they have comparatively little control.

## Historical Perspectives on the Problem of Patient Choice

A long-term historical perspective on patients' roles as decision makers helps to make this fundamental point clear. The only time conditions even remotely resembling the classic concept of "consumer sovereignty" existed in the United States was in the first half of the nineteenth century, when in a fit of democratic fervor, local and state governments set aside medical licensing laws and allowed a competitive free-for-all among health-care providers (Shryock 1967; Starr 1982). It might fairly be said that these patients exercised choice among treatments, none of which "worked" by contemporary standards of efficacy. But the fact remains that this system provided citizens with a much greater degree of economic and therapeutic self-determination than they would ever possess again. In this sense, the mid-nineteenth century represents the one and only point in the nation's history when a comparatively free market for medical services really existed.[2]

Ironically, the elaboration of patients' rights and responsibilities grew out of physicians' growing determination to close down that free market. As the business of healing grew increasingly competitive in the early 1800s, orthodox medical societies began to develop stricter codes of professional ethics designed to distinguish their members from sectarian rivals (Warner 1999). To this end, the AMA's first code of ethics, written in 1847, spelled out the basic duties and obligations physicians and patients owed one another. Doctors were to be prompt, skilled, discreet, and benevolent in their provision of services; in return, patients were to be loyal, obedient, and honest in disclosing their symptoms. But as various scholars have noted, in this and subsequent revisions of the AMA code prior to 1980, much more attention was given to how doctors ought to behave toward other doctors than toward their patients. This emphasis did not reflect physicians' lack of concern for their patients' well-being, but rather reveals their automatic assumption that their own and their patients' interests were identical and that physicians could always be counted upon to act wisely on the latter's behalf (Katz 1984; Baker et al. 1999).[3]

Early nineteenth-century patients did not necessarily share these assumptions, yet they had no great need to pen any sort of "patients' bill of rights," in that they had little cause to defend a therapeutic and economic power that they already possessed. In an era marked by the hearty embrace of the "every man his own doctor" philosophy, most laypeople felt themselves quite capable of managing their own health affairs (Risse et al. 1977). In their clinical relations, doctor and patient shared a common set of therapeutic assumptions that helped the latter understand and participate in treatment choices (Rosenberg 1979). In their economic relations, the traditional fee-for-service relationship gave patients, at least those with money, considerable power of the purse. As Rosenberg (1999) notes, "Fee-paying patients did not need to be 'empowered'—to use late twentieth-century jargon; they were empowered by their family's social position, by their often sophisticated knowledge of medical thought and practice, by their ability to judge a physician's character and competence, and—perhaps most importantly—by their ability to pay the fees that constitute the physician's sole source of income" (208).

Of course, the early to mid-nineteenth century represented no patient-run utopia; then (as now), sick people who were poor, foreign born, nonwhite, or otherwise socially disadvantaged had less power in their dealings with medical authority. But in many ways, patients enjoyed an unprecedented degree of parity in their relations with physicians well into the late 1800s, the point at which legislatures started to pass new, more stringent medical licensing laws. When they encountered a doctor whose treatment was unsatisfying, patients had no compunction about "voting with their feet" and doctor shopping until they found one more to their liking (Rothman 1994; Morantz-Sanchez 1999). And while often holding their personal physician in high regard, many Americans regarded doctors as a group with the same suspicion they felt toward all forms of collective authority. Medical societies, particularly the American Medical Association, were often denounced as undemocratic and uncaring (Risse et al. 1977).

The first patient-initiated (as opposed to physician-initiated) efforts to define patients' rights and responsibilities developed in areas of mid-to-late-nineteenth-century medical practice where the traditional balance of power between doctor and patient seemed particularly threatened. A new kind of patient sensibility, characterized by demands for safe, effective, and fair treatment, developed in response to particularly aggressive medical therapies and assertions of institutional power. Three examples suggest this association between advancing medical authority and increasing patient consciousness and resistance: the rise in medical malpractice suits, protests against involuntary confinement in mental hospitals, and protection of alternative practitioners' status in the new wave of medical licensing acts passed by state legislatures in the late 1800s.

Medical malpractice suits, whose numbers rose sharply beginning in the 1840s, were one arena in which patients expressed a growing sense of entitlement to safe and effective treatment. As doctors started to operate more as "individual entrepreneurs in an intensely competitive marketplace," in the words of James Mohr (1993, 112), patients began to sue doctors, particularly surgeons, with increasing frequency. Rooted in the common-law conception of a tort, or civil wrong, medical malpractice suits offered an important forum for articulating patients' entitlements to an "ordinary standard of care, skill, and diligence" from their doctors (De Ville 1990). But while the publicity surrounding such cases may have contributed to laypeople's willingness to think of themselves as having certain kinds of rights in relation to their caregivers, malpractice remained a highly individualized form of quality control that required time and energy that many patients did not have (Mohr 1993; 2000).

The rapid expansion of public and private mental hospitals in the first half of the nineteenth century created another arena for articulating patient rights. As involuntary commitment became increasingly common, so too did political and legal concerns about its legitimacy (Mohr 1993). Because of the often-contested nature of mental alienation, patients frequently protested their admission to mental hospitals (Tomes 1984). While most mental patients lacked the personal and social resources to translate that resistance into political action, two—Elizabeth Packard and Clifford Beers—made asylum medicine a forcing ground for a new kind of patients' rights discourse and would later be hailed as forerunners of the modern patients'-rights movement (Himelhoch and Shafer 1979; Dain 1980; Tomes 1999).

Invoking the natural-rights traditions used by many nineteenth-century reformers, first Packard and later Beers argued that those who suffered from mental disease should not forfeit their rights as citizens and as human beings. In advocating for mental patients' rights, they both focused on easily identified wrongs, such as the denial of a jury trial before commitment and the loss of the right to send and receive mail. In response to Packard's campaigns in the 1870s, over twenty states passed so called Packard laws establishing more formal procedures for involuntary commitment and safeguarding inmates' rights to communicate with the outside world (Grob 1983; Sapinsley 1991). Thirty years later, Beers suggested the need for "a Bill of Rights for the Insane" with a similar set of entitlements (Beers 1953, 198–199), and became a leading figure in the early twentieth-century mental hygiene movement (Dain 1980).

Although these initiatives yielded some impressive results, patients' demands for their rights ultimately weakened in the face of an increasingly robust medical professionalism at the turn of the century. Scientific advances such as the germ theory, x-rays, antiseptic surgery, and the like slowly shifted the balance of power, in legal and institutional terms, in the doctor's favor. Physicians gained greater autonomy over the terms of their own education, licensure, and practice. Confronted by medicine's assertive restatement of the "doctor knows best" philosophy, Progressive era reformers arguing for patient-citizens' parity with the new white-coated "men of science" had far less success than their Jacksonian era predecessors.

As the case of alternative medicine suggests, however, the new medical professionalism did have its limits. As the "regular" practitioners pushed for medical licensing laws unfavorable to their alternative competitors, they met with stiff opposition in many states, first from homeopaths and later from osteopaths and chiropractors.[4] In successfully appealing to state legislators to protect their claims to be legitimate healers, alternative practitioners depended heavily on their patients' support, expressed through petition campaigns and fund raising (Rogers 1998; Whorton 2002). They succeeded by representing the choice of one's personal physician as both a basic citizenship right and also a consumer's right to purchase a desired service.

## The Birth of the "Medical Consumer"

The articulation of the right to choose one's doctor at the turn of the twentieth century clearly reflected a closing down, not an opening up, of the nineteenth-century medical marketplace. As historians and sociologists have amply documented, between 1880 and 1930, the rise of scientific medicine and the growing professional power of organized medicine ushered in a new era of increasingly unequal doctor-patient relations (Starr 1982). While better-trained doctors practiced a more scientifically informed, technologically sophisticated medicine than their nineteenth-century predecessors, the dawning of medicine's "golden age" disadvantaged patients, both therapeutically and economically, in some important ways. In clinical terms, the new scientific medicine widened the gap between physician and patient understandings of disease. Treatment rationales became harder for patients to comprehend at just the point when medical care was growing more specialized and more expensive. The cost of medical care rose sharply between 1900 and 1940, costs that patients had to assume with no assistance from third-party payers such as employers or local governments. Now familiar patterns of under- and over-treatment began to emerge as a result: affluent urban dwellers encountered difficult choices among increasingly expensive forms of treatment, while poor patients in rural areas had little access to the new medicine (Tomes 2003).

Significantly, this same era produced the first explicit discussions of patients' dilemmas as consumers, that is, as purchasers and users of goods and services in a modern consumer-oriented capitalist economy. The growing interest in patients' roles as consumers reflected the profound economic and political disruptions that accompanied the Industrial Revolution. Families and communities were moving from a predominantly agricultural, producer-oriented economy, where most goods were locally made and buyers and sellers knew each other well, to a more impersonal economy based on mass industrialization and mass consumption, where goods came from anywhere and buyers and sellers no longer met face-to-face. By the early twentieth century, the emergence of a national (and in some respects international) economy based on mass production and mass consumption had begun not only to transform workplace relations but also spawned important new cultural phenomena, such as national advertising campaigns and innovative forms of mass media. As mass consumption figured more and more centrally in economic growth, what and how much consumers purchased became matters of great significance. Economists began to think seriously about the consumer's role in fostering growth and innovation, while reformers tried to articulate the political rights of consumers as key issues in a democratic polity (Donahue 2003).

Health issues figured centrally in these new conceptions of consumer interests and rights. More specifically, the use of the term *consumer* for patient became common in two important arenas between World War I and World War II: the subspecialty of economics known as "medical economics" (renamed health economics in the 1960s) and the organized consumer movement. Medical economists were among the first groups to begin thinking systematically about patients as a special kind of consumer (Tomes 2003). But it was primarily consumer advocates, rather than economic theorists, who started to formalize conceptions of consumer "rights," that is, the rules of fair political and economic engagement required to preserve economic democracy in a mass consumer economy. In the discussion that follows, therefore, I will focus primarily on the organized consumer movement.

## The Ideal of Consumer Citizenship

The first wave of consumer-oriented theorizing and activism occurred during the Progressive era, as so-called consumers' leagues were dominated by white middle-class women, who tried to use the power of the purse to offset their lack of the vote. The first consumer movement linked the problems of unsafe workplace conditions with tainted products, such as the canned food described in *The Jungle* or sweatshop-made garments supposedly infected with TB and smallpox (Tomes 1998). Their weapon of choice was the "white label" campaign, in which consumers were urged to patronize only those manufacturers who agreed to the consumer league's fair-workplace standards (Sklar 1995). Among the major achievements of the early consumer movement was passage of the first great piece of national consumer legislation in American history, the Pure Food and Drugs Act of 1906, which created the Food and Drug Administration (Hilts 2003).

In the conservative, comparatively affluent 1920s, this Progressive-style consumer advocacy faltered, as large corporations co-opted consumer group appeals to worker safety and product cleanliness, and reformers found that even mild criticisms of market behavior earned them the label of "Bolshevik." During the Great Depression, however, the ideal of consumer citizenship once again became attractive as political groups sought a regulatory counterweight to the growing power of Big Business and Big Labor. As a higher standard of consumption came to be equated with the democratic way of life, as distinguished both from communism and fascism, protecting consumer rights became an increasingly important aspect of American political discourse (Cohen 2003).

Led now by white professional men, including engineers, economists, and journalists, the interwar consumer movement increasingly focused on consumer protection as an end in itself, not as a vehicle for improving labor relations. Consumer advocates wrote best sellers such as Chase and Schlink's *Your Money's Worth* (1927) and Kallet and Schlink's *100,000,000 Guinea Pigs* (1933), alerting middle-class readers to the dangers of unsafe products and deceptive advertising. In 1930, consumer activists in the New York City area banded together to found Consumers' Research, a nonprofit organization that began to publish *Consumers' Bulletin,* a periodical designed to help readers evaluate different products. After a nasty battle over unionization, a rival group broke off in 1936 to found the Consumers Union, which began to publish its own periodical, *Consumer Reports* (Glickman 2001). Consumers Union became the far more successful of the two organizations, remaining an important source of consumer information and advocacy to this day.

Despite their differences, both Consumers' Research and Consumers Union argued that Americans needed more objective information about the quality of goods they were purchasing, and pressured the federal government to act more aggressively to protect consumers against irresponsible business

interests. Health issues figured importantly in their reform agenda: consumer activists helped to pass the most important of New Deal consumer-
oriented reforms, namely the 1938 bills extending and strengthening the
powers of the Food and Drug Administration and the Federal Trade Commission respectively to regulate drugs and their advertising (Jackson 1970).
Although they were disappointed in the legislation's pro-business slant, consumer advocates at least saw some form of legislation succeed, a success that
eluded contemporary efforts to enact national health insurance (Gordon
2003; Klein 2003).

The expanding vision of interwar consumer advocacy, however, stopped
short at challenging the growing authority of physicians. Until the 1960s, consumer activism remained heavily product oriented, focusing chiefly on the
manufacture, labeling, and advertising of food, drugs, and cosmetics, rather
than the power relationship between doctor and patient. The focus on products
as opposed to services reflected the inherent difficulties that consumer advocates faced in setting themselves up as critics of the doctor-patient relationship. In private, consumer advocates expressed great resentment over what
they perceived to be physicians' professional arrogance (Tomes 2003). Yet they
had no independent, scientific testing process with which to measure and critique the increasingly specialized, technical world of medical practice. While
Consumers' Research and Consumers Union could do "consumer research" on
household products and automobiles, they lacked the means to do comparable
tests on drugs or medical procedures. Instead they had to rely on the testing of
drugs and devices done by other groups, such as the AMA (one reason they
could not afford to antagonize that group) and the FDA.[5]

Still, despite its limited focus, the interwar consumer movement's
approach to product testing and protection laid the foundation for later conceptions of patient safety, information, and choice. The pre-1960 model of
consumer advocacy advanced four important premises of modern consumerism that would subsequently be applied to health care more generally:
that economic democracy requires strong governmental regulation to protect
the consumers' interests; that objective scientific testing is necessary to guarantee the efficacy and safety of consumer goods and services; that consumers
need access to objective test results and other forms of unbiased information
in order to make wise choices about how to spend their money; and that
given corporate domination of the economy and government, consumers
must be ever vigilant in protecting their interests. As shown in the next section, these ideas all became fundamental to the health consumer revolution
of the 1970s.

## The Making of a Consumer Health Revolution

Dramatic changes in the post–World War II health-care system created the conditions for the previously distinct conceptions of "patients' rights" and "consumers' rights" to converge in the 1960s. The expansion of what later commentators would christen the "medical-industrial complex" (Starr 1982) further reduced consumers' control over the terms of their health care.

Underlying the new post–World War II medical economy was a rising level of governmental investment in the health-care system. As Starr (1982) has shown, in the 1950s and 1960s, the federal government began to invest heavily in medical research, hospital building, and, after the 1965 creation of Medicare and Medicaid, direct subsidies for medical care. This public funding came with few strings attached; physicians and hospitals continued to operate largely as independent entrepreneurs, beholden to no one but themselves for how they spent these funds. Not surprisingly, this new medical infrastructure concentrated on highly specialized, technologically sophisticated acute care, that is, the types of medicine most lucrative to practitioners and hospitals alike.

As postwar medicine became increasingly specialized and technology-oriented, the information asymmetry between doctor and patient continued to widen. Armed with powerful new drugs and medical technologies, postwar physicians became even more confident that the less patients knew, the better, while patients found it harder to evaluate their treatment choices. Patient-consumers also faced new economic dilemmas. The growth of private health insurance plans made the new medicine more affordable for the upper ranks of American workers but left uncovered those most in need of medical assistance, namely the poor and the elderly (Gordon 2003). Moreover, while the new insurance plans allowed enrollees to choose their own doctors, they set the terms for reimbursement in ways that greatly favored the doctors' over patients' economic interests (Hoffman 2004). In addition, the postwar pharmaceutical boom made consumers increasingly dependent on expensive medications available "by prescription only," and gave the highly competitive, profit-conscious pharmaceutical industry a growing influence over medical practice (Tomes 2006). All these changes made it more difficult for patients to "shop" effectively for medical care, as Kenneth Arrow pointed out in his classic 1963 article on the welfare economics of health care.

Equally dramatic shifts in the political climate gave these therapeutic and economic problems new ideological significance. Against the backdrop of Cold War ideology, in which every facet of American market economy was to be measured against communist regimes in the Soviet Union and the People's

Republic of China, inefficiencies in how U.S. health-care institutions delivered the sacred goods of doctors' care and miracle drugs took on special political significance. In addition, the horrors of the Holocaust generated a new kind of "rights consciousness," manifest not only in revulsion against Nazi medical experimentation but also in the burgeoning civil rights movement. Slowly the idea that any kind of expertise, including medical knowledge, was sacrosanct began to crumble (Rothman 1991).

In this climate, a new generation of activists far less deferential to medical authority came of age in the 1960s. Drawing upon the increasingly radical energy supplied by the civil rights, antiwar, feminist, and environmental movements, they brought this heightened rights consciousness to debates over health-care policy. The assault on the traditional doctor-patient relationship came from many directions: from physician whistle-blowers (Rothman 1991) and legal activists (Katz 1984) as well as angry groups of former mental patients (Tomes 1999), feminists (Weisman 1998; Morgen 2002), and advocates for the poor (Ehrenreich and Ehrenreich 1970). While pursuing different goals, these groups shared a common conviction that patients needed to reclaim certain essential rights lost to them as a consequence of medicine's professionalization process, including the right to make informed choices about their treatment (Swazey 1979; Annas 1989).

Once again, psychiatry proved to be an early forcing ground for patients' rights advocacy. After decades of studies documenting the failings of the state hospital system, new political and judicial activism combined to bring about a fundamental restructuring of the mental-health-care system (Mechanic and Grob, this volume). Congress passed the Community Mental Health Centers Acts of 1963 and 1965, which allocated federal funds for the construction and staffing of community mental-health centers, designed to provide a less restrictive treatment milieu. As the civil rights movement widened to include disabled Americans, public interest lawyers and patient advocacy groups began to employ the classic natural rights tradition with much greater success than previous generations. For example, in 1966, in a series of influential decisions, District of Columbia Judge Daniel Bazelon articulated the legal doctrine that mental patients had a right to appropriate treatment in the least restrictive environment possible. A wave of lawsuits on behalf of the mentally ill produced a new generation of "Packard laws" that gave the mentally disabled a whole range of new legal protections regarding involuntary commitment and the right to refuse treatment (Grob 1991; Tomes 1999).

It was in the context of these sweeping challenges to medical authority that the term *health consumer* first came into popular usage in the late 1960s and early 1970s.[6] That term was one among several, including *victim* and *survivor*, proposed as alternatives to the word *patient*. The ex-mental patients at the forefront of this linguistic transformation into consumers hardly cut a conservative figure; as one participant in the anti-psychiatry movement recalled, consumer advocates "dressed like hippies and talked like militants" (Clay 2002). Following suit, other groups mounting sweeping critiques of medical paternalism, including the women's health movement and the health-care Left, began to substitute the term *consumer* for *patient* in their calls for radical change in the American health-care system.

That the term *consumer* could take on such a militant edge reflected the birth of a more confrontational consumer movement in the 1960s. Inspired by the same upswellings of protest, a new generation of consumer activists developed a much more aggressive critique of modern capitalism than had their predecessors. The arrival of consumerism as a more potent political force was signaled by President John Kennedy's landmark "Consumer Message" of 1962, which articulated the first consumer bill of rights: the right to safety, information, choice, and governmental recognition of the consumers' voice. The exemplar of the new hard-hitting brand of consumer activism was Ralph Nader, whose celebrated *Unsafe at Any Speed*—an exposé of that sine qua non of the "democracy of goods," the American automobile—appeared in 1965 (Mayer 1989).

Unlike previous consumer activists, Nader and his associates did not hesitate to attack the medical establishment. Drawing on youthful discontent within the medical profession (Rogers 2001) as well as the new legal activism of the era, the Nader-led consumer movement developed a broad-ranging critique of the medical "establishment." The first branch of Nader's organization Public Citizen was the Health Research Group, headed by the physician Sidney Wolfe. (Both Wolfe and the Health Research Group remain important players in current health advocacy efforts.) Among the first publications of Nader's Center for the Study of Responsive Law was a scathing indictment of the nation's mental-health policies (Tomes 1999).

The 1970s consumer critique of health care stressed the negative consequences of the medical profession's uncontested control over physician training and practice. Patient/consumer advocates argued that this medical "monopoly" threatened their health by refusing to share vital information with them, ignoring their rights to therapeutic self-determination and subordinating professional ethics to economic gain. They stressed the tremendous incentives that the "new medical-industrial complex" gave doctors, hospitals, and other health-care industries to emphasize expensive acute care rather than inexpensive preventive measures. They charged that federal regulatory agencies were doing too little to protect citizens against this monopoly power. To correct this dangerous imbalance of power between doctor and patient, consumer activists sought to undermine medical authority by opening up the floodgates of information. If consumers could not trust either the federal government or their health-care providers to watch out for their health, they had to educate themselves in self-defense. This approach gave rise both to a remarkable explosion in self-help literature and growing political pressure on the federal regulatory agencies to rein in medicine's powers of self-governance.

Thus, far from seeming antagonistic, the languages of patients' rights and consumers' rights seemed complementary in the 1970s. Legal and regulatory activism would serve to extend constitutional rights into the doctor's office and the hospital ward; ideals of self-help and personal empowerment would equip patients, as individuals and in advocacy groups, with the tools they needed to negotiate more effectively with health-care providers. Perhaps the greatest strength that the consumer movement brought to its patients' rights counterpart was the model of objective information as a prerequisite to wise choice.

### Assessing the First Consumer Health-Care Revolution

Embedded as it was in a broad critique of the new medical-industrial complex, the initial use of the term *health consumer* differed markedly from the conservative associations the term would later assume in the 1980s and 1990s. While certainly more moderate in tone than the language of "victims" and "survivors" championed by some members of the psychiatric counterculture, the rhetoric of empowered patient/consumers still had plenty of bite in the 1970s. Advocacy groups on the health-care Left, including psychiatric survivor groups and Health PAC, used the term to refer to patients with no apparent sense of selling-out. For example, George Annas himself used the term "medical consumer" in his landmark handbook of hospital patients' rights first published for the American Civil Liberties Union in 1975.

The achievements of the 1960s and 1970s health-consumer revolution were considerable. The fusion of patients' and consumers' rights arguments worked far more effectively than advocacy tradition had on its own prior to 1960. Activists' vision of an empowered patient/consumer brought about fundamental changes in the doctor-patient relationship and the role of patient/consumers in health-care policy making. Starting in the 1970s, the balance of power patients exercised in their encounters with doctors and hospitals clearly shifted in the former's favor.

The list of important changes that date from this era is impressive; it includes improved procedures for involuntary commitment of mental patients; measures for gaining informed consent for medical treatment; stronger oversight of drug safety and efficacy; improved labeling and instructions for both prescription and over-the-counter drugs; increased protection of patient privacy; greater efforts to prevent discrimination against the mentally and physically disabled; and reforms of medical education designed to improve physician communication skills and increase sensitivity to gender, race, ethnic, and class differences.

Viewed in retrospect, there is no question that the 1970s marked a significant turning point in the evolution of more patient-centered treatment. These changes were apparent not only in therapeutic relationships, such as those involved in childbirth (Morgen 2002), cancer treatment (Lerner 2001), and AIDS research protocols (Epstein 1996), but also in the architectural and spatial transformation of hospitals and clinics (Sloane and Sloane 2003).

But while successfully undermining the old "doctor knows best" philosophy of treatment, patient/consumer advocates proved far less effective in their calls for more fundamental economic and institutional changes. In large part, their failures resulted from a monumental instance of bad timing. The patient empowerment movement ran straight into the twin drives for privatization and cost containment that began what McLean and Edwards (2004) have dubbed health care's "Thirty Years' War" over the principles of managed care. The long-term implications and achievements of the managed-care movement are now the subject of lively debate among policy analysts (see for example Havighurst 2002b). Let me suggest briefly how my historical perspective fits with contemporary efforts to understand "how the health revolution fell short" (Havighurst 2002a, 55).

First, the empowered patient/consumer movements coincided with fundamental economic changes in the American health-care system that ultimately worked to limit their power (Relman 1980; Starr 1982). What Ginzburg (1985) termed the "monetarization" of health care created growing numbers of corporations seeking large infusions of capital in exchange for big profits to their share holders. As both the federal government and private employers continued to spend more heavily on health care, the field became increasingly attractive to corporate entrepreneurs. By making medicine more businesslike, these entrepreneurs claimed they could both give investors a higher return on their investment and improve the quality of health-care services. For example, for-profit hospital chains, such as Humana and Hospital Corporation of America, claimed that by eliminating waste and making doctors more businesslike,

they could make hospitals simultaneously more profitable and more responsive to patients' needs. As it turned out, the for-profit hospital chains proved
much less successful than initially hoped, but the idea that more market discipline would improve health care continued to be very popular, and remains so
even now. Likewise, private investors remained convinced that health care was
a good profit sector in a post-industrial "service economy."

In this rapidly changing, extremely competitive economic environment,
both for-profit and nonprofit entities saw the advantages of increasing their
appeal to affluent consumers. To this end, they softened the activists' language
of consumer interests and rights to turn discontent into profitable new "product lines," such as more woman-friendly forms of maternity care and more
prevention-oriented diagnostic services (Imershein and Estes 1996). Not surprisingly, these new consumer-friendly services were designed primarily with
high-end, affluent patients in mind.

At the same time entrepreneurs were discovering the value of the health
consumer "sell," the health-care sector generally faced growing pressures for
cost containment. These pressures came first from the federal government, as
it tried to slow the skyrocketing cost of Medicare and Medicaid in the 1970s,
then by private industry as firms struggled to cover the rising cost of employees' health benefits in the 1980s. Both government and industry began to experiment with payment mechanisms designed to give physicians and hospitals
more incentive to practice cost-effective medicine and to compete openly with
each other, strategies often justified in the language of patient/consumer empowerment made popular by health-care activists (Agrawal and Veit 2002).

Initially, many policy analysts hoped the simultaneous trends toward
decentralization and professionalization would open "new possibilities for
translating diverse consumer desires into provider performance," and thus
lead to a health-care system "more compatible with American pluralism and
democratic ideals," as Havighurst wrote in 1987 (129, 162). Advocates of
market-driven measures portrayed them as part of the historic trend toward
giving Americans more information, choice, and quality-assurance regarding
their health care. But although managed-care measures achieved more in the
way of cost control than some critics acknowledge, more market-oriented medicine most assuredly did not a usher in an era of greater patient satisfaction or
safety (Havighurst 2002b).

While the reasons for that failure are many, the flaws inherent in the concept of patient/consumer empowerment certainly played an important role.
Amidst the crossfire of pressures to make health care both profitable and cost
effective, consumer advocate groups proved much too fragmented to protect

patient interests in any strong or coherent way. First, the rapid multiplication of advocacy groups quickly made it evident that there was no single consumer interest to advance; rather different groups of consumers promoted varied and often conflicting agendas. The mental-health field was a case in point: consumer groups splintered not only along issues of therapeutic faith (for and against a biomedical model of mental illness) but also into patient versus family groups (Tomes 1999). As a series of discrete, sometimes mutually antagonistic camps, consumer advocacy groups proved no match for the better organized and funded lobbies maintained by the medical profession, health insurers, and pharmaceutical companies.

Nowhere were the weaknesses of the consumerist approach better illustrated than its faith in expanded information as a powerful tool for consumer empowerment. On the one hand, consumers gained much easier access to many sorts of health-related information, especially with the coming of the internet. Yet consumers' requests for information also served to increase the volume of health-related advertising. The regulatory equation of information and advertising was reflected in important changes, such as the FTC's successful lawsuit forcing the AMA to lift its ban on physician advertising, and more recently, the FDA's decision in 1997 to loosen its historic strictures on direct-to-consumer advertising of prescription drugs. Measured in terms of volume and accessibility, advertising was far more dominant than the kind of objective information envisioned by consumer advocates. In addition, as pharmaceutical companies began to play a bigger role in funding clinical research, troubling new questions arose about how objective even scientific research could be. Meanwhile, other information that consumer advocates requested, such as a database showing how often and how successfully individual providers had been sued for malpractice, remained unavailable (Tomes forthcoming). As Schuster (1999) noted, "More information is available on the quality of airlines, restaurants, cars, and VCRs than on the quality of health care" (231).

In sum, patient/consumer empowerment movements had difficulty sustaining a focus on the larger macroeconomic dynamics of the medical-industrial complex. Their efforts succeeded far better at securing specific rights and critiquing specific treatments than in fostering systemic change in the health-care system. Activists poured their energies into discrete changes, such as setting up new procedures for involuntary commitment of mental patients, publicizing the benefits of a lumpectomy over a radical mastectomy, or pushing for low-cost generic versions of prescription drugs. While accomplishing a great deal on specific issues, they found it much harder to confront the macro-problems of a highly complex health-care system prone to simultaneously overtreat some and undertreat others based primarily on their economic resources rather than their health status.

Not surprisingly, perhaps the greatest flaw in the health-consumer revolution lay in its inability to address the problems of the "underconsumers," particularly poor and uninsured patients. Historically, the model of the well-informed, politically connected voter-consumer has always worked best for affluent, white, educated Americans (Preston and Bloom 1986; Cohen 2003), and the health-care sector proved no different. Deregulation and privatization only exacerbated differentials in service and access already evident in the patchwork of public and private care created in the 1960s. As the post-1970 American workforce settled into a two-tier system, with highly paid technical, professional, and administrative workers with good coverage at one end and poorly paid, low-skilled workers with little or no coverage at the other end, the ideal of a broad based consumer "sovereignty" in health care proved illusory (Gordon 2003). In its absence, the empowerment of patient/consumers served primarily to privilege the health needs, and increasingly luxuries, of affluent Americans.

**Policy Implications**

The late twentieth century health-consumer revolution did not produce the kind of structural, patient-centered changes envisioned by 1970s activists. While it has succeeded in slowing the growth of some health-care costs, the drive to make medicine more market conscious has not dramatically reduced the overall level of health-care spending. Even more disappointing, the vast changes of the last two decades have not improved the overall quality of patient care (Institute of Medicine 1999; 2001). Many Americans remain uninsured, while those with insurance face higher charges and more restrictions on treatment choices. Although consumer representatives continue to participate in policy councils and legislative hearings, the politics of contemporary policy making are clearly dominated by other, more coherent and more powerful political stakeholders. The problematic choices produced by such a system were well illustrated in the latest, as-yet-unsuccessful congressional efforts to pass a Patients' Bill of Rights establishing a right to emergency care and setting minimum standards for existing health-care plans. Meanwhile, analysts forecast steep rises in the amounts patients pay for their health-care premiums and co-pays within the next five years.[7] Consumers' rights, demands, and needs will undoubtedly continue to hold a central place in the continuing policy debates about how to simultaneously control health costs, improve the quality of care, and extend health insurance to all Americans. Policymakers will continue to argue about which parties are most to blame for the high cost of health care, and whose choices should be limited in order to contain its rise: should it be the doctors who order the treatments, the insurance companies who determine what services are covered, or the pharmaceutical and medical technology industries whose profits are tied to producing new and more expensive product lines?

While seemingly more sinned against than sinning, consumers have not escaped their share of the blame for the current health-care crisis. Consumer irrationality and ignorance have become popular explanations for the health-care system's seeming inefficiency. Indeed, the 1970s patient/consumer empowerment movement now figures centrally in some accounts of this crisis. According to this line of argument, it is the insatiable American demand for more and better health care that makes its costs so difficult to contain. Consumers demand more and better prescription drugs, diagnostic techniques, and surgical procedures, all of which require substantial investments in scientific research and technological innovations to deliver. Patient expectations of quicker, better, safer treatments have spawned a costly infrastructure of protections, from informed consent and privacy protocols to malpractice insurance and drug safety trials. Finally, as government and private industry subsidies to health care have grown, they have created what economists refer to as the "moral hazard problem": simply because health care is available, people will use it even when they don't really need it, an argument beautifully illustrated in a recent *New York Times* piece on healthy retirees in Boca Raton who spend their days visiting expensive specialists at Medicare's expense (Kolata 2003).

At the same time, critics often portray cost-containment measures as heartless efforts to deprive Americans of the sacred goods of lifesaving medicine. Complaints about drive-through mastectomies and gravely ill children denied emergency care helped stall the 1990s move toward managed care; the cost and safety of prescription drugs emerge as major issues in Presidential campaigns. In today's rough-and-tumble world of health-care politics, every major stakeholder, including physicians, insurance companies, and pharmaceutical manufacturers, now jockeys to position itself as the "true" defender of patients' rights. The resulting politics of health consumerism are highly complex, to say the least. For example, pharmaceutical companies have become major patrons of mental-patient advocacy groups. As another recent story in the *New York Times* reported, a patient-consumer protest against the state of Kentucky's decision to leave an expensive antipsychotic drug, one whose therapeutic superiority to older, cheaper drugs has not been definitely established, off their list of preferred medications for Medicaid patients turned out to be financed by the drug's manufacturer, Eli Lilly (Harris 2003).

Perhaps because other stakeholders have more political and economic clout, the idea of disciplining consumers continues to figure as one of the more promising strategies for containing health-care costs. Stories like the ones about the Boca Raton retirees and the Kentucky consumer protestors support the image of Americans as unreasonable in their demands for low-cost, risk-free medicine and as unwilling to pay their fair share of health-care costs. Many policy analysts argue that in order for true reform to occur, consumers must be educated about the "true costs" of their health care and thus become more willing to shoulder their share of the burden. There is certainly considerable validity in those complaints, at least as applied to patients with health insurance. Most Americans do have very fuzzy ideas about how much health care their paycheck deductions, co-pays, and tax dollars can buy; in this, as in many other areas, they indulge in a kind of magic thinking about what their contributions entitle them to consume.

But given the historical analysis presented here, it seems highly misleading to portray patients as the *prime* source of irrationality and inefficiency in the workings of the health-care marketplace. As this history suggests, the conditions necessary to sustain a real sense of patient/consumer sovereignty—that is, the ability of individuals to influence market forces through the mechanism of personal choices—have continually eroded over the last century. The loss of clinical and economic independence has been particularly pronounced since World War II. As a consequence, patients find themselves today interacting with a complex system of health insurance (should they be so lucky as to have it) which determines what goods and services are available to them. Although undoubtedly better informed than their parents' generation, patients still have to rely heavily on physicians in their choice of specific goods and services. It is the doctor, not the patient, who decides whether the latter receives an x-ray or a MRI, a coronary angioplasty or a bypass operation, a new diet or a prescription for a cholesterol-lowering drug. Moreover, the price of the goods and services that patients so "choose" is governed by complex externalities—for example, the cost of research and development for new drugs, the nature of American patent law, the evolution of medical malpractice law—over which they have virtually no control. Finally, many of the most expensive choices about care come at the end of life when patients are often least able, physically and mentally, to perform the work needed to be a wise "shopper" (Stone 2004).

To make real progress toward the goals of a patient-centered system in the twenty-first century, future policy solutions need to be based on a more realistic understanding of what "empowered" patients can and cannot do as agents of therapeutic and fiscal discipline. In the 1960s and 1970s, models of patient-doctor decision making radically changed, raising expectations that these long-standing asymmetries in access to information and autonomy might be reversed. But despite the many positive ways in which patients have become more engaged in their treatment decisions, they remain deeply dependent on other parties when making key health-care decisions. Thus while patients undoubtedly have many more protections and treatment options than four decades ago, the *process* of choosing and paying for them is no less complicated (MacStravic 2000). Moreover, their collective ability as voters to influence the broad mechanisms that shape the process of choosing and paying remains fundamentally limited. Notwithstanding the frequent invocation of their interests, independent groups representing patient/consumers' perspectives are the most fragmented, poorly financed presence among the major stakeholders involved in health-care policy making today.

At the same time, American voters are becoming more, rather than less, aware of the ways that health-care politics work to their therapeutic and economic disadvantages. The rancorous debates of the last decade, starting with the failed Clinton health plan and continuing with recent passage of the Medicare prescription drug benefit bill, have provided a detailed look at the political underpinnings of the so called free-enterprise health-care economy. If asked to accept steep increases in their payroll deduction and co-pays, patients are likely to ask more, rather than fewer, questions, about the government-industry negotiations that determine the price levels and profit margins they are being asked to support. Not all of them will quietly accept further constraints on their health-care choices without asking some hard questions about whose interests are truly being served by the management of the health-care marketplace. As a result, it seems unlikely that policy solutions presented entirely in a "blame the consumer for making foolish choices" register are likely to appeal to them, particularly the aging baby boomers who grew up in the 1960s and 1970s during the heyday of the consumer health revolution. As they enter the Medicare system, they may well take a more skeptical look at the politics of health-care reform than their parents and grandparents.

Moving the national conversation about health care forward is clearly not going to be easy. But within the historical constraints identified here, some strategies for achieving a more patient-centered system seem more promising than others. Reforms that link quality improvement to cost containment are likelier to succeed than those focused solely on cost containment. If patients feel they are getting the best quality of care, not merely the most expensive, they may be more willing to accept a greater economic burden for its purchase, whether in the form of higher payroll taxes, co-pays, or income taxes. Moreover, for all the upheavals in the doctor-patient relationship that have occurred over the last thirty years, patients still trust their doctors much more than their insurance companies to determine the proper balance between cost and effectiveness. Thus the kind of fundamental redesign of the health-care system proposed by the Institute of Medicine (2001), which attempts to link quality assessment and payment mechanisms, seems more likely to achieve meaningful change than proposals designed only to make consumers more cost conscious in their choice of health insurance plans.

Whether we call the beneficiaries of these changes patients or consumers, the scope of change required is daunting. It requires setting up extensive, complex systems to measure treatment effectiveness so that caregivers can quickly evaluate the deluge of new drugs and procedures constantly being offered as better (and usually more expensive) than last year's versions (Millenson 1997). Meaningful reform also necessitates revolutionary changes in how care is delivered: for example, greater continuity and coordination among caregivers and more patient-friendly information about self-care (Institute of Medicine 2001).

Reaching these goals requires more intelligent and critical thinking by policymakers, voters, providers, and patients about protecting and advancing the interests of patient/consumers. Given the many, sometimes misleading, ways that the language of consumerism has come to be used in current health-care debates, it is understandable that its terminology has become suspect in the eyes of many. But let us not jettison the language of the empowered patient/consumer until we have better alternative in place.

## Notes

I would like to thank Walter Lear for sharing material on patients' rights from the Institute of Social Medicine and Community Health Archives; Beatrix Hoffman, George Makari, Christopher Sellers, and Susan Strasser for helpful comments on early versions of this paper. My thanks also to members of the Stony Brook University History Department, the Robert Wood Johnson Foundation history of medicine group, and the Ackerman Symposium on Professional Values in an Age of Consumer Medicine (especially Arnold Relman), for their comments on later drafts. The research and writing of this project have been supported by the National Humanities Center and the Robert Wood Johnson Foundation

1. I by no means intend to imply here that access is not an important issue, only that it is not the only issue that merits historical attention in understanding the evolution of patients' rights movements.

2. Shorter (1985) explores similar issues, but he focuses more on the experience of illness and the doctor-patient dialogue concerning symptom recognition and disease

definition. He is less interested in the economic dimensions of the doctor-patient relationship that concern me here.

3. This emphasis changed in the 1980 revision of the AMA code, the first to reflect the modern patients' rights movement.

4. Note that untrained female healers such as midwives did not survive the regulars' onslaught. See Borst 1995.

5. My observations on the leadership of Consumers' Research and Consumers Union here are based on my research in their respective archives at Rutgers University and at the Consumers Union headquarters in Yonkers, New York.

6. By "popular," I mean to distinguish here between the use of the term *consumer* for patient in grass-roots political efforts, as opposed to the more specialized use of the term *consumer* in medical economics and consumer publications prior to 1960.

7. The U.S. House and Senate passed different versions of the bill, which they have been unable to reconcile. For a summary of the provisions of the two bills, see A Patients Bill of Rights, downloaded from http://democrats.senate.gov.pbr.pbrdoc .html March 8, 2003.

## References

Agrawal, G., and H. Veit. 2002. Back to the Future: The Managed Care Revolution. *Law and Contemporary Politics* 65, no. 4: 11–53.

Annas, G. 1975. *The Rights of Hospital Patients: The Basic ACLU Guide to a Hospital Patient's Rights.* New York: Sunrise Books/E.P. Dutton.

———. 1989. *The Rights of Patients: The Basic ACLU Guide to Patient Rights.* Totowa, NJ: Humana Press.

———. 1998. *Some Choice: Law, Medicine, and the Market.* New York: Oxford University Press.

Arrow, K. 1963. Uncertainty and the Welfare Economics of Medical Care. *American Economic Review* 53: 941–973.

Baker, R., et al. 1999. *The American Medical Ethics Revolution.* Baltimore: Johns Hopkins University Press.

Beers, C. 1953. *A Mind that Found Itself: An Autobiography.* Garden City, NY: Doubleday. Reprint of 1908 edition.

Borst, C. 1995. *Catching Babies: The Professionalization of Childbirth 1870–1920.* Cambridge, MA: Harvard University Press.

Chase, S., and F. Schlink. 1927. *Your Money's Worth.* New York: Macmillan.

Clay, S. 2002. A Personal History of the Consumer Movement. http://home.earthlink.net/ ~sallyclay/Z.text/history/html (accessed 8 March 2003).

Cohen, L. 2003. *A Consumers' Republic: The Politics of Mass Consumption in Postwar America.* New York: Knopf.

Dain, N. 1980. *Clifford W. Beers: Advocate for the Insane.* Pittsburgh: University of Pittsburgh Press.

De Ville, K. 1990. *Medical Malpractice in Nineteenth-Century America: Origins and Legacy.* New York: New York University Press.

Donahue, K. 2003. *Freedom from Want: American Liberalism and the Idea of the Consumer.* Baltimore: Johns Hopkins University Press.

Ehrenreich, B., and J. Ehrenreich. 1970. *The American Health Empire: Power, Profits, and Politics.* New York: Random House.

Epstein, S. 1996. *Impure Science: AIDS, Activism, and the Politics of Knowledge.* Berkeley: University of California Press.

Gabel, J., A. LoSasso, and T. Rice. 2002. Consumer-Driven Health Plans: Are They More Than Talk Now? *Health Affairs* Web Exclusive, 20 November. http://www.healthaffairs.org (accessed 13 January 2004; 10 October 2005).

Ginzburg, E. 1985. *American Medicine: The Power Shift.* Totowa, NJ: Rowman and Allanheld.

Glickman, L. 2001. The Strike in the Temple of Consumption: Consumer Activism and Twentieth-Century American Political Culture. *Journal of American History* 88: 99–128.

Goodman, E. 1999. We've Become Health Care Consumers—And We're Getting Indigestion. *Boston Globe,* 17 June.

Gordon, C. 2003. *Dead on Arrival: The Politics of Health Care in Twentieth-Century America.* Princeton: Princeton University Press.

Grob, G. 1983. *Mental Illness and American Society, 1875–1940.* Princeton: Princeton University Press.

———. 1991. *From Asylum to Community: Mental Health Policy in Modern America.* Princeton: Princeton University Press.

Harris, G. 2003. States Try to Limit Drugs in Medicaid, but Makers Resist. *New York Times,* 18 December.

Havighurst, C. 1987. The Changing Locus of Decision Making in the Health Care Sector. In *Health Policy in Transition,* ed. L. Brown, 129–167. Durham, NC: Duke University Press.

———. 2002a. How the Health Care Revolution Fell Short. *Law and Contemporary Problems* 65, no. 4: 55–101.

———. 2002b. Is the Health Care Revolution Finished? Special issue of *Law and Contemporary Politics* 65: 4.

Herzlinger, R. 1997. *Market-Driven Health Care: Who Wins, Who Loses in the Transformation of America's Largest Service Industry.* Cambridge, MA: Perseus Books.

Himelhoch, M., and A. Shafer. 1979. Elizabeth Packard: Nineteenth-Century Crusader for the Rights of Mental Patients. *Journal of American Studies* 13, no. 3: 343–375.

Hilts, P. 2003. *Protecting America's Health: The FDA, Business, and One Hundred Years of Regulation.* New York: Knopf.

Hoffman, B. 2004. Claims Denied: Consumers and Private Health Insurance. Paper presented at the Annual Meeting of the American Historical Association, Washington, DC.

Imershein, A., and C. Estes. 1996. From Health Services to Medical Markets: The Commodity Transformation of Medical Production and the Nonprofit Sector. *International Journal of Health Services* 26: 221–238.

Institute of Medicine. 1999. *To Err Is Human: Building a Safer Health System.* Washington, DC: National Academy Press.

———. 2001. *Crossing the Quality Chasm: A New Health System for the 21st Century.* Washington, DC: National Academy Press.

Jackson, C. 1970. *Food and Drug Legislation in the New Deal.* Princeton: Princeton University Press.

Kallet, A., and F. Schlink. 1933. *100,000,000 Guinea Pigs.* New York: Grosset and Dunlap.

Katz, J. 1984. *The Silent World of Doctor and Patient.* New York: The Free Press.

Kinney, E. 2002. *Protecting American Health Care Consumers.* Durham, NC: Duke University Press.

Klein, J. 2003. *For All These Rights: Business, Labor, and the Shaping of America's Public-Private Welfare State.* Princeton: Princeton University Press.

Kolata, G. 2003. Patients in Florida Lining Up for All that Medicare Covers. *New York Times,* 13 September.

Lerner, B. 2001. *The Breast Cancer Wars: Hope, Fear, and the Pursuit of a Cure in Twentieth-Century America.* New York: Oxford University Press.

MacStravic, S. 2000. The Downside of Patient Empowerment. *Health Forum Journal* 43: 30–31.

Mayer, R. 1989. *The Consumer Movement: Guardians of the Marketplace.* Boston: Twayne Publishers.

McLean, T., and E. Richards. 2004. Health Care's 'Thirty Years War': The Origins and Dissolution of Managed Care. *New York University Annual Survey of Law* 60: 283–328.

Millenson, M. 1997. *Demanding Medical Excellence: Doctors and Accountability in the Information Age.* Chicago: University of Chicago Press.

Mohr, J. 1993. *Doctors and the Law: Medical Jurisprudence in Nineteenth-Century America.* New York: Oxford University Press.

———. 2000. American Medical Malpractice Litigation in Historical Perspective. *JAMA* 283: 1731–1743.

Morantz-Sanchez, R. 1999. *Conduct Unbecoming a Woman: Medicine on Trial in Turn-of-the-Century Brooklyn.* New York: Oxford University Press.

Morgen, S. 2002. *Into Our Own Hands: The Women's Health Movement in the United States, 1969–1990.* New Brunswick, NJ: Rutgers University Press.

Morone, J. 2000. Citizens or Shoppers? Solidarity under Siege. *Journal of Health Politics, Policy and Law* 25: 959–968.

Okun, M. 1986. *Fair Play in the Marketplace: The First Battle for Pure Food and Drugs.* Dekalb: Northern Illinois University Press.

Packard, E. 1873. *Modern Persecution, or Married Woman's Liabilities.* New York: Pelletreau and Raynor.

Preston, L., and P. Bloom. 1986. Concerns of the Rich/Poor Consumer. In *The Future of Consumerism,* eds. P. Bloom and R. Smith, 37–57. Lexington, MA: Lexington Books.

Relman, A. 1980. The New Medical-Industrial Complex. *New England Journal of Medicine* 303: 963–970.

Risse, G., R. Numbers, and J. Leavitt. 1977. *Medicine without Doctors: Home Health Care in American History.* Madison: University of Wisconsin Press.

Rodwin, M. 1993. *Medicine, Money, and Morals: Physicians' Conflicts of Interest.* New York: Oxford University Press.

Rogers, N. 1998. *An Alternate Path: The Making and Remaking of Hahnemann Medical College and Hospital of Philadelphia.* New Brunswick, NJ: Rutgers University Press.

———. 2001. 'Caution: The AMA May Be Dangerous to Your Health': The Student Health Organizations (SHO) and American Medicine, 1965–1970. *Radical History Review* 80: 5–34.

Rosenberg, C. 1979. The Therapeutic Revolution. In *The Therapeutic Revolution: Essays in the Social History of Medicine,* eds. M. Vogel and C. Rosenberg, 3–25. Philadelphia: University of Pennsylvania Press.

———. 1999. Codes Visible and Invisible: The Twentieth-Century Fate of a Nineteenth-Century Code. In *The American Medical Ethics Revolution,* eds. R. Baker, A. Caplan, L. Emanuel, and S. Latham, 207–217. Baltimore: Johns Hopkins University Press.

Rothman, D. 1991. *Strangers at the Bedside: A History of How Law and Bioethics Transformed Medical Decision Making.* New York: Basic Books.

Rothman, S. 1994. *Living in the Shadow of Death: Tuberculosis and the Social Experience of Illness in American History.* New York: Basic Books.

Safire, W. 2000. On Language: No More Patients. *New York Times Magazine*, 23 January, 14.

Sapinsley, B. 1991. *The Private War of Mrs. Packard*. New York: Paragon House.

Schuster, M. 1999. The Quality of Health Care in the United States: A Review of Articles Since 1987. In *Crossing the Quality Chasm: A New Health System for the 21st Century*, Institute of Medicine, 231–308. Washington, DC: National Academy Press.

Shorter, E. 1985. *Bedside Manners: The Troubled History of Doctors and Patients*. New York: Simon and Schuster.

Shryock, R. 1967. *Medical Licensing in America, 1650–1965*. Baltimore: Johns Hopkins University Press.

Sklar, K. 1995. *Florence Kelley and the Nation's Work*. New Haven: Yale University Press.

Slater, D. 1997. *Consumer Culture and Modernity*. Cambridge: Polity Press.

Sloan, F. 2001. Arrow's Concept of the Health Care Consumer: A Forty-Year Retrospective. *Journal of Health Politics, Policy and Law* 26: 899–911.

Sloane, D., and B. Sloane. 2003. *Medicine Moves to the Mall*. Baltimore: Johns Hopkins University Press.

Starr, P. 1982. *The Social Transformation of American Medicine*. New York: Basic Books.

Stone, D. 1993. When Patients Go to Market: The Workings of Managed Competition. *American Prospect* 13: 109–115.

———. 2004. Shopping for Long-Term Care. *Health Affairs* 23: 191-196.

Swazey, J. 1979. *Health, Professionals, and the Public: Toward a New Social Contract?* Philadelphia: Society for Health and Human Values.

Thompson, E. 1971. The Moral Economy of the English Crowd in the Eighteenth Century. *Past and Present* 50: 76–136.

Tomes, N. 1984. *A Generous Confidence: Thomas Story Kirkbride and the Art of Asylum Keeping*. New York: Cambridge University Press.

———. 1998. *The Gospel of Germs: Men, Women, and the Microbe in American Life*. Cambridge, MA: Harvard University Press.

———. 1999. From Patients' Rights to Consumers' Rights: Historical Reflections on the Evolution of a Concept. In *Making History: Shaping the Future*, 8th Annual Conference of the Mental Health Services of Australia and New Zealand, 39–48. Balmain, Australia: THEMHS (The Mental Health Services).

———. 2001. Merchants of Health: Medicine and Consumer Culture in the United States, 1900–1940. *Journal of American History* 88: 519–547.

———. 2003. An Undesired Necessity: The Commodification of Medical Service in Interwar America. In *Commodifying Everything: Relations of the Market*, ed. S. Strasser, 97–118. New York: Routledge Press.

———. 2006. The 'Great American Medicine Show' Revisited. *Bulletin of the History of Medicine* Winter 2006. Forthcoming.

———. Forthcoming. *Impatient Consumers: American Medicine Meets American Consumer Culture in the Twentieth Century*. Book manuscript in progress.

Warner, J. 1999. The 1880s Rebellion against the AMA Code of Ethics: 'Scientific Democracy' and the Dissolution of Orthodoxy. In *The American Medical Ethics Revolution*, eds. R. Baker et al., 520–569. Baltimore: Johns Hopkins University Press.

Weisman, C. 1998. *Women's Health Care: Activist Traditions and Institutional Change*. Baltimore: Johns Hopkins University Press.

Whorton, J. 2002. *Nature Cures: The History of Alternative Medicine in America*. New York: Oxford University Press.

# The Democratization of Privacy

## Public-Health Surveillance and Changing Conceptions of Privacy in Twentieth-Century America

The right to privacy has never been regarded as absolute. In the late nineteenth century, health officials adopted the practice of name-based reporting for infectious diseases in order to isolate cases, quarantine the exposed, and monitor the health and behavior of the diseased and their contacts as a means of reducing morbidity and mortality. Public-health surveillance has persistently called into question the appropriate limits of privacy ever since. Despite the inherent tension between surveillance and privacy—that is, between a public and a private good—the nature of the conflict has changed, reflecting radical changes in the conception of privacy over the course of the twentieth century.

From the 1890s through the 1960s, privacy concerns were embedded in a medical and public-health culture that was both paternalistic and authoritarian. The prevailing conception of privacy yoked the patient's well-being to the physician's authority: physicians represented the gatekeepers to the patients and protected them from unwarranted interference by public-health authorities. Health officials accommodated physician demands to determine when they might intervene—a concession that privileged "respectable" middle-class or wealthy patients. The 1960s and 1970s were witness to extraordinary challenges to the authority of medicine broadly understood. The paternalistic authority of physicians was brought into question by a new culture and ethics that gave pride of place to the concept of autonomy (Rothman 1991). Privacy ceased to be instrumental to the clinical relationship and became a right that belonged exclusively to the patient. Dovetailing with the "my body, my business" ideal in the clinical setting, some patients ultimately challenged the public-health practice of surveillance as a violation of individual privacy rights.

## Paternalism and Public Health Reporting

The centrality of bacteriology to both medical and public-health practice helps to explain the instrumental nature of public-health privacy as it developed in the late nineteenth century. By the 1870s and 1880s, a scientific revolution began to alter the practice of medicine and place public health on a new footing. Louis Pasteur, Robert Koch, and others laid the foundations for understanding that diseases were caused by germs, microbes too small to see with the human eye but capable of spreading from person to person. In the 1880s and 1890s, medical schools successfully began to incorporate bacteriology and basic science—the hallmarks of a new scientific medicine—into their curricula as a means of transforming medical education and increasing the status of the medical profession (Fee 1987). Scientific medicine promised to shore up the professional authority of the physician, who was almost always male, and fortify him against irregular medical practitioners (Starr 1982; Latour 1988; Ludmerer 1985; Warner 1986). One of the consequences was that a new "scientific reductionism" replaced a more holistic environmental, social, and moral view of the patient (Rosenberg 1979). In the wake of these changes, the physician-patient relationship became highly paternalistic and characterized by deference to scientific authority (Pernick 1982).

Bacteriology also heightened a sense of authority over disease among a new cadre of public-health practitioners, many of whom were physicians educated in northeastern medical schools and further trained in European laboratories (Duffy 1990; Starr 1982). Within the field of public health, bacteriology justified new public-health strategies such as isolation, contact tracing, and house-to-house inspections as measures to control disease in the population on a day-to-day basis. But the bedrock of public-health practice was disease notification: again and again public-health officials argued that without the name and location of diseased individuals they might "as well hunt birds by shooting into every green bush" (Trask 1915, 2).

If reporting was the foundation of public-health practice, it was the responsibility of physicians to report cases of disease. Thus, surveillance created a struggle between public-health and medical practitioners over power and authority—a struggle largely couched in terms of the limits of privacy (Fox 1975). The histories of tuberculosis and venereal disease surveillance—the first instances in which surveillance was mandated and hotly contested—allows us to map the contours of privacy as it was shaped by physicians and public-health officials from the late nineteenth century through the 1960s.

## Tuberculosis

The prospect of TB reporting had been discussed in New York City as early as 1868, but it did not become mandated until the 1890s, at the very moment when Samuel Warren and Louis Brandeis famously framed privacy as the "right to be let alone" (Knopf 1922). Although explicitly concerned with the way in which "instantaneous photographs and newspaper enterprise have invaded the sacred precincts of private and domestic life," Warren and Brandeis noted the traditional sanctity of the medical secret and defined the "difficult task" as being that of determining the "line at which the dignity and convenience of the individual must yield to the demands of the public welfare" (Warren and Brandeis 1890, 214).

In 1893, Hermann M. Biggs—in his capacity as chief inspector of the Division of Pathology, Bacteriology, and Disinfection—recommended that public institutions be *required* to report cases of TB. Private physicians and institutions were *requested* to report the names of the infected (New York City Department of Health 1895). Although it was clear that the city planned to investigate cases and that reporting was intended as a means of allowing direct intervention by the health department, every effort was made to assuage the fear of physicians regarding encroachments upon their professional authority (*New York Medical Journal* 1894). Biggs thus proposed that "This information will be solely for the use of the Department, and in no case will visits be made to such persons by the Inspectors of the Department, nor will the Department assume any sanitary surveillance of such patients, unless the person resides in a tenement-house, boarding-house or hotel, or unless the attending physician requests that an inspection of the premises be made." But even in these situations the health department agreed to take no action if the physician requested that health officials make no visits and agreed to deliver informational circulars regarding the prevention of TB (New York City Department of Health 1895, 322).

The city's inspection plan amounted to a system of active surveillance for TB at the city's various TB clinics, which served the poor and working classes. Although the surveillance regime would expand and contract as funds were available, the city was, in general, divided up into districts, and a nurse (typically female) was assigned to each district. Every day the nurse visited the district TB clinic, collected the names of all newly admitted and discharged cases, and reported these names to the local borough health office by telephone. The local health office, in turn, gave her the names of any new cases that it had received from private physicians or other institutions. The expectation was that the nurses would visit each new case and conduct a monthly follow-up visit unless the report came from a private physician: for private patients she kept a record "for information only," not actually contacting the patients but visiting the locality "to ascertain if there is a house at the address given, and its character—i.e., private one family house, tenement, etc." Whereas in 1909 nurses made some 23,583 visits to patients, in 1911, they made 226,859 (Billings 1912, 90). Thus, while the city certainly monitored trends in the prevalence of tuberculosis from year to year, case reporting was intended primarily as the foundation of an ongoing system of patient supervision on the part of health officials (New York City Department of Health 1919).

The concept of privacy was shaped by the nature of clinical and scientific authority, which demanded medical guardianship of patients. Privacy was not a right of individuals. It existed in the context of the clinical relationship, where paternalistic privacy—in which the physician controlled the terms of privacy in an instrumental way, that is, in a fashion that represented good medicine—prevailed. In making decisions about divulging medical secrets, as in making decisions more generally about the patient's welfare, it was the physician's "own judgment" that was of paramount importance (Faden, Beauchamp, and King 1986; Robertson 1921). The patient, like a child, was in the "caring custody" of the physician, who, like a father, made decisions in the best interests of his family members (Katz 1984).

For the middle and upper classes, physicians were the primary arbiters of medical decision making and hence privacy, which they saw largely in terms of protecting both themselves and their patients from unwarranted and unwanted interference, giving a literal meaning to privacy understood as "the right to be let alone." Accordingly, as the health department extended its reach over TB surveillance and ultimately made case reporting compulsory for private physicians, those medical organizations that endorsed the practice underscored that access to the patient must be mediated by the physician. The Standing Committee on Hygiene of the Medical Society of the County of New York, for example, endorsed the proposal for mandatory reporting with the proviso that "inspectors are forbidden to visit or have any communication with the patient without the consent of the attending physician, believing that the attending physician is capable of giving all the necessary instruction" (Winslow 1929, 145, 46). Likewise, when the Association of State and Territorial Health Officers strongly endorsed name-based TB reporting in 1904, it rejected using surveillance as a trigger for isolation and quarantine—the health department, in other words, might know the identities of patients but should not be the agents of intervention (State and Territorial Health Officers with the United States Public Health and Marine-Hospital Service 1904).

Such an understanding—that privacy represented a protective shield from all manner of interference on the part of health officials in the liberty and lives of the patients of private physicians *rather than* limitations on the disclosure of information to such officials—helped to increase practicing physicians' acceptance of reporting (*New York Medical Journal* 1904). Indeed, disclosures of personal information by private physicians were widespread and unquestioned. Physicians disclosed information at their discretion. Such revelations were defined by their obligations to the family as a unit. The responsible physician felt ethically bound, for example, to report a case of syphilis in a prospective groom to the bride's father or in a domestic servant to the master of the household (Robertson 1921). A 1924 AMA pamphlet on medical ethics meant to be carried in a shirt or jacket pocket described the physicians' responsibilities toward protecting a patient's "delicacy and secrecy" when the health of another was at stake: "a physician should act as he would desire another to act toward one of his own family under like circumstances" (American Medical Association 1924; see also Konold 1962).

Health officials stressed the confidentiality of disease registries, but this did not mean that medical information was sacrosanct, that privacy was absolute. This was, after all, an era in which it was deemed appropriate for the physician to disclose information to the head of the household. Likewise, health officials had long broadcasted the names and addresses of those with contagious diseases in order to fulfill a duty to warn the public. This practice persisted after the advent of notification. In the instances of diseases like diphtheria and polio, health officials placarded the homes of the infected and published in the local newspapers a daily tally of all the afflicted by name and address (Emerson 1917; Cope 1904). Polio primarily struck the children of upper- and middle-class parents. It is remarkable that there is no evidence that members of these classes made any objection to publishing the names of the sick in the papers. While health officials observed greater strictures on medical information in the instance of more highly stigmatized diseases such as tuberculosis—where the registry was explicitly described as "solely for the use of the department" and not to be used for "notification to the community at large"—their mandate to protect the public health continued to warrant disclosure (Biggs 1900, vi). Homes vacated by a resident with tuberculosis, for example, would be placarded by health officers if the homes had not been disinfected. In this instance, placarding was viewed as an essential means of exerting pressure on landlords who failed to comply with regulations. But even though the placard did not state the name of the sick individuals, it necessarily revealed the diagnosis to any friends, acquaintances, or neighbors who viewed the notice (New York City Department of Health 1895; Biggs 1900; Biggs 1894). Such practices did not raise formal objections on the part of private physicians or their patients.

Health officials had considerable leeway regarding disclosure of confidential information, but this is not to say that the health department never kept the secrets of the poor. Health officials felt bound by the same clinical and ethical norms that governed privacy within the physician-patient relationship and defined it as something essential to good medical care. In 1913, for instance, as he countered medical objections to registries of stigmatized diseases, Hermann Biggs explained that health officials were "all medical men and well versed in medical ethics" (Biggs 1913c, 150). Like the private physician, the health department was widely counted on to use its "wise discretion . . . to determine what safeguards and regulations should protect the privacy of its records" (In the Matter of William H. Allen 1912). Thus, as would any physician, health officials emphasized the instrumental importance of privacy when admonishing patients to defer to the judgment of medical authorities regarding medical disclosure: "Do not talk to anyone about your disease, except your physician," the department warned patients in its standard informational circular published in a number of languages and given to all patients registered with TB. It further admonished its team of sanitary inspectors to take steps not to broadcast the patient's diagnosis beyond the proper scope of the household: "In tracing cases on first visit or, if unable to obtain admission, when making a revisit, no messages are left with neighbors. The reason for the nurse's visit (i.e., that there is a consumptive on the premises) is only to be given to the family." Ultimately, the health department framed privacy in terms of the "rights of both physicians and patients" (Billings 1912, 12, 55).

The New York City experience with TB paved the way for the extension of reporting in other major cities. The city had always played a paradigmatic role for the nation. Just as the city's careful documentation of its "technological" conquest of infectious disease shaped social, health, and urban policy in cities and states throughout the U.S., the nation looked to the experience of New York City in extending surveillance to tuberculosis (Illinois Medical Journal 1904; Smith 1913). TB also opened the door to reporting for other diseases, most controversially, venereal disease. As Biggs remarked in 1913, "The ten year long opposition to the reporting of tuberculosis will doubtless appear as a

mild breeze compared with the storm of protest against the sanitary surveillance of venereal disease" (Biggs 1913c, 136).

## Venereal Disease

In 1911, Dr. Prince Morrow, a New York City physician at the forefront of inves-
tigative and educational efforts regarding venereal disease, argued that it was
time to treat venereal diseases like other infectious threats (Brandt 1987).
"Within recent years sanitary science has been markedly aggressive in attack-
ing all other infectious diseases—even tuberculosis," he wrote in 1911, but
"the sanitary forces have paused irresolute, baffled, and driven back" in the
instance of "the great venereal plague." In Morrow's analysis, "secrecy and privacy have been placed above the interests of the public health" and "sanitary
control has been represented as invasion of the private rights of the individual." In contrast to privacy, which implied a freedom from public-health interference, secrecy referred to information that was "personal and concerning
only the individual," meaning, of course, the individual and his or her physician (Morrow 1911, 130). But for Morrow, when secrets were of a venereal
nature, they warranted protection neither from disclosure nor interference
because of the danger they posed to others.

Nonetheless, whereas TB infection was ultimately made reportable by
name for both private and clinic patients—thus, limiting the secrecy of all
patients—public health's accommodationist stance toward physicians'
authority dictated that officials take cognizance of the moral opprobrium
that surrounded sexually transmitted conditions, the "stigma [placed] upon
the moral character of the person involved" (Biggs 1913c, 144). Accordingly,
public-health authorities specified the terms under which physicians could
appropriately keep their patients' secrets. This touched on not only themes of
responsible individual behavior but class expectations.

As in the case of tuberculosis, New York City was the national leader in
instituting VD reporting and, indeed, applied its experience in TB to the task.
In 1911, Biggs, in his last major initiative as city health commissioner, proposed a system of confidential reporting. It reflected the department's orientation toward using surveillance as a wedge for public-health intervention rather
than as a statistical or epidemiological tool undertaken "in order to keep clerks
or adding machines busy" (Biggs 1913c, 150). It was not, however, a wedge that
the department intended to apply universally. Biggs stressed that while "those
in comfortable circumstances who are afflicted with" venereal diseases will
certainly "make every possible effort to be cured," this was not the case with
the "poorer classes, the dispensary and hospital patients" (135). This class of

venereal disease cases would only take treatment until their symptoms were relieved or their treatment was "more or less interrupted by the necessities of their occupation." Therefore, he argued that the city required a hospital to provide for "their free and continuous treatment" (135). And "when a person . . . is being treated in a public institution, or is being cared for at the public expense, there is really no reason whatsoever for not at once reporting the case to the public-health authorities" (145). In contrast to TB, however, where health officials would placard homes, albeit under delimited circumstances, Biggs placed great emphasis on securing VD records, which were to be "regarded as *absolutely* confidential" (Biggs 1913b, 1009). VD was not TB, and public warnings could serve no legitimate purpose.

Reasoning that venereal diseases "should be treated as other infectious and communicable diseases dangerous to the public health are treated," New York City formalized a two-tiered regime of VD reporting: all institutional cases (diagnosed in hospitals, clinics, etc.) were to be reported by name and address; private physicians, however, could withhold the name and address of their patients when reporting new cases (Biggs 1913c, 144). Some classes of patients not only remained free from public-health monitoring and intervention, but also kept their secrets (*Journal of the American Medical Association* 1989). The recommendations were adopted by the Board of Health in 1912 and between May 1 and December 31 of that year, more than 40,000 cases were reported (Biggs 1913b).

Similar formulations of secrecy and privacy characterized the broader national story as both federal funds and patriotic fervor accompanying the outbreak of World War I moved the majority of states to follow New York City's lead and institute reporting (*Public Health Reports* 1916; Dublin and Clark 1921; *Illinois Medical Journal* 1918). In 1916, twenty-two states required venereal disease notification. With war, reporting became part of the nation's defense. The struggle against venereal disease—and the vice that was thought to drive it—became an urgent matter of national security and industrial well-being. The campaign against venereal disease was necessary "for the sake of protecting not only soldiers and sailors, but the industrial army as well—the men behind the men behind the guns" (Seymour 1919, 61).

Anticipating a rush of legislation, the Western Social Hygiene Society in Tacoma passed "resolutions of a very radical nature" calling on state legislatures to adopt venereal disease reporting (*Illinois Medical Journal* 1918, 28). World War I provided the occasion for the passage of a congressional enactment—the Chamberlain-Kahn Act—authorizing the United States Public Health Service (PHS) to provide states with $1,000,000 per year in 1918 and

1919 to fund their anti-venereal-disease control efforts (Moore 1919). To be eligible for such support, state boards had to meet three surveillance-related criteria: venereal diseases had to be made reportable to local health authorities; reported cases had to be investigated in order to determine the source of infection; and penalties had to be imposed on those who failed to meet reporting requirements (American Association for Study and Prevention of Infant Mortality 1919). The PHS followed up on this legislation with a campaign to win the cooperation of physicians, urging them to "pledge" to report venereal diseases according to state law (Cole 1919; *Social Hygiene* 1919).

By 1919, all states required venereal disease notification. Forty-two had adopted variations on the model public-health act that had been proposed by the PHS (Seymour 1919). But strikingly, only six states—Colorado, Indiana, Maryland, New Jersey, Ohio, and Vermont—required reporting by name (*Social Hygiene* 1915). The remainder of states explicitly permitted reporting by "serial number" or patient initials (American Medical Association 1918). In California, for example, private patients were given a pamphlet upon diagnosis informing them that reporting was anonymous unless, of course, they failed to respect the social compact with physicians: "If you want your name kept secret," the booklet instructed, "follow these instructions carefully" (*California State Journal of Medicine* 1918, 375). Coded reporting constituted the "usual method" and names were reported only if "the patient discontinues treatment prior to reaching the noninfectious stage or the patient willfully or carelessly fails to observe the precautions necessary to prevent the spread of infection to other persons" (*Public Health Reports* 1919, 223, 228).

Only rarely was the model challenged. One editorial in the *Illinois Medical Journal* denounced the "loop hole" allowing "escape for the rich and influential, who do not wish their cases and particularly their names, reported" (*Illinois Medical Journal* 1917, 293). But, reflecting the broader, shared understanding of public-health privacy on the part of health officials, medical practitioners, and the lay public, another editorial countered, "Only prostitutes need be reported in full and no sane man"—much less a "patriotic physician"—"will question the wisdom of that" (*Illinois Medical Journal* 1918, 343). With only a few exceptions, reporting by key, serial number, or patient initials continued in most states through the 1930s and into the 1940s (Godfrey 1937; Johnson 1938).

Again, however, advances in medical science served to alter the public-health stance on privacy. With the introduction of penicillin as a highly effective treatment for syphilis and gonorrhea in 1943, "case-holding no longer was the problem. Emphasis was gradually shifted to case finding" (Venereal Disease

Branch, DHEW 1962). On the grounds that "Every existing case of syphilis or gonorrhea was caught from someone who had that disease," the PHS, in conjunction with the American Social Hygiene Association, launched its 1947 campaign: "Find the Missing Million—And Help Stamp out VD." Thus, the new public-health dictum was that "it is essential to *find* these infected people—the 'contacts'—who may have transmitted or acquired the disease" (Clark 1947, 374).

But therapeutic advance alone does not explain the evolution of thinking about privacy. It is noteworthy that the PHS launched its contact-tracing campaign in the broader context of the onset of the Cold War and the domestic crusade against subversion. In 1947 the House Un-American Activities Committee (HUAC) began its intensive investigatory efforts to find Communists within government and private industry. But while the practice of "naming names" was hotly contested in the context of HUAC investigations, seeking out individuals with syphilis drew little criticism. In the case of public health, it was the related issue of search and seizure—not disease surveillance or contact tracing—that drew much critical challenge. In the 1959 case of *Frank v. Maryland,* the United States Supreme Court upheld the right of the health department to arrest and fine a homeowner who refused a search for rat infestation because the health inspector had no warrant. Justice Felix Frankfurter, writing for the majority of the court, recognized the right of privacy, particularly against "arbitrary" search and seizures, as being "fundamental to a free society." But he was impressed by the "safeguards designed to make the least possible demand on the individual occupant," which caused "only the slightest restriction in his claims on privacy," and concluded that the "particular context and . . . social need" legitimated the public-health law.

In his dissent, William O. Douglas, joined by Chief Justice Earl Warren and Justices Hugo Black and William Brennan—the core of what would become the famously liberal Warren Court—remarked that "health inspections are important," but "many today would think that the search for subversives was even more important than the search for unsanitary conditions. It would seem that the public interest in protecting privacy is equally as great in one case as in another." They linked their dissent to the 1957 decision in *Watkins v. United States*—a case revolving around the HUAC attempt to compel the naming of names for the purpose of drafting legislation to combat communism in which the Court sought to protect citizens against "governmental interference," particularly interference that would subject individuals to "public stigma, scorn and obloquy." Douglas and his dissenting brethren thus rejected the "official's measure of his own need" as not "squar[ing] with the Bill of Rights" at a time "when politically controlled officials have grown powerful through an ever increasing series of minor infractions of civil liberties" (Douglas 1958, 104; *Frank v. Maryland* 1959).

The significance of the Douglas dissent was that it began to articulate new procedural protections for the individual and would provide the foundations for a broader social critique of medical paternalism that would come to fruition two decades later (Whyte 1956; Mills 1951). For the time being, however, paternalistic notions of privacy held fast in the context of public health.

### The Precedence of the Public Good

As the death rate from venereal diseases began to drop during the national eradication effort, medical triumph turned to complacency. With the new ease of treatment, therapy was increasingly managed in the offices of private physicians rather than public clinics, and it became more difficult to continue aggressive contact tracing. At the same time, federal funding for VD programs was cut back. While death rates steadily declined, however, in the late 1950s and early 1960s the number of cases began to increase (Brandt 1987; Baumgartner 1962).

In 1961, the United States surgeon general created a Task Force on Syphilis under the leadership of New York City Health Commissioner Leona Baumgartner. Members of the task force were dumbfounded by "the shockingly inadequate reporting of the disease" (Baumgartner 1962, 29–30). Speaking for the task force, Baumgartner argued that "the spread of syphilis can be stopped by vigorous efforts to build a bridge, a highway, a transmission line, between the laboratory, the doctor and the public" (27). Thus, the primary recommendation of the task force was to aggressively enhance reporting and contact investigation: "The individuals who have syphilis have *got* to be found. . . . It is *not* enough for the physicians to treat those who come to them. They must report their cases to the health officials who are in a position to follow up all contacts." Moreover, "since it is clear that in many instances the physician does not report all his cases of syphilis, health authorities must go to him" (30).

In 1962, Congress responded to these recommendations with an appropriation of $6.2 million for the Nationwide Syphilis Eradication Effort (Venereal Disease Branch Chief's Statement 1963). A major thrust of the program was laboratory-based reporting. In other words, rather than relying on physicians to report cases, laboratories sent results indicative of venereal disease to health departments when they sent the results back to a physician. At least half and possibly two-thirds of the states and some eighty localities had adopted mandatory lab-based reporting for venereal diseases by 1966, accounting for sixty-two percent of reporting (American Public Health Association et al. 1966; U.S. Department of Health, Education and Welfare, Public Health Service 1966).

Significantly, the PHS pressed for mandatory lab-based reporting legislation not as a means to gain direct access to patients, but rather to contact physicians in order to solicit reports (Sunkes 1962; Kampmeier 1962). California—one of the first states to adopt mandatory lab-based reporting—forbade health officials "under any circumstances" from contacting either patients or their potential contacts directly "until a diagnosis has been reported to the local health officer by the attending physician" (Venereal Diseases Branch, CDC 1964). Public-health personnel had to make contact with physicians for a very practical reason: though a laboratory test might indicate the *possibility* that a patient had a venereal disease, it was the clinician who had to make the final diagnostic determination. The prohibitions against contacting patients without physician consent even when the patient was positively diagnosed reflected the continuing hegemony of medical paternalism.

Health officials had full access to names, protected only in as much as officials depended on physicians to confirm which patients were true cases. The field manual for contact investigators stressed that they should use information regarding the patient's name, address, marital status, occupation, and medical history "during your conversation with the physician to convey to him that everything you do professionally is done in a personalized confidential manner" (Venereal Disease Branch, DHEW 1962). If the physician failed either to confirm the case or allow health officials to interview the patient, the contact investigator retained the individual's name and other personal information, but simply lacked recourse to *act* on that information until that that person was reported as a contact by another individual (Havlak 2003).

## The Rise of Democratic Privacy

In 1957, Supreme Court Justice William O. Douglas warned against "the searching eyes of government" (Douglas 1958, 108). In 1966, he declared that "We are rapidly entering the age of no privacy, where everyone is open to surveillance at all times; where there are no secrets from government." More ominously, he continued, citizen dossiers are now "being put on computers so that by pressing one button all the miserable, the sick, the suspect, the unpopular, the offbeat people of the nation can be instantly identified" (*Osborne v. U.S.* 1966, 13, 14).[1] In the era of the electronic database, the very existence of centralized lists—both governmental and commercial—and not simply government action based on those lists, created profound cultural anxiety (Packard 1964; Brenton 1964; Westin 1967).

The specter of such abuse fueled congressional debates beginning in 1965 about what personal information to protect and how best to protect it (Regan 1995). Policymakers and lawmakers flirted with the notion of obtaining consent from individuals when it came to obtaining or using personally identifiable records (Regan 1995). More specific to surveillance, President Jimmy Carter's Privacy Commission could not see why public-health officials would need access to names in any kind of surveillance (Assistant Secretary for Planning and Evaluation 1977).

Despite such gestures, privacy as an individual right did not immediately become a stumbling block to public-health surveillance (Regan 1995). In large measure, it was protected by the enduring cultural authority of medicine and popular belief in the sanctity of medical confidence (Packard 1964; Westin 1967). The concept of privacy began, however, to be linked to individual autonomy in a series of landmark U.S. Supreme Court cases involving marital sexual relations and reproduction. As patients' and women's rights advocates began to question the model of medical paternalism as part of a the larger consumer rights movement that Nancy Tomes so trenchantly analyzes in this volume, patients at last raised a constitutional challenge to surveillance.

In 1977, the U.S. Supreme Court heard arguments in *Whalen v. Roe,* in which patients and physicians challenged a New York statute requiring physicians to report the names of patients who obtained prescriptions for drugs with the potential for abuse such as barbiturates, tranquilizers, or amphetamines. The Court unanimously upheld reporting as "a reasonable exercise of the state's broad police powers" (*Whalen v. Roe* 1977). But, perhaps more tellingly, the Court rejected the notion that any chink in the armor of privacy would threaten the clinical relationship. The physicians who joined the patients in bringing the case argued that the law made them reluctant to prescribe Schedule II drugs, representing interference in appropriate medical treatment. These drugs—such as opium and its derivatives, methadone, amphetamines, and methaqualone, which were used to treat conditions like epilepsy, narcolepsy, hyperkinesias, migraine headaches, and schizo-affective disorders—had accepted medical uses but also a high potential for abuse. Although a district court had maintained that "the doctor–patient relationship is one of the zones of privacy accorded constitutional protection" (*Roe v. Ingraham* 1975), the Supreme Court maintained that the New York statute did not represent state interference in medical decision making, for while patients might refuse needed medications based on concerns about potential disclosures, the law did not, in fact, deprive patients from access to Schedule II drugs nor prohibit physicians from prescribing them.

Although *Whalen v. Roe* focused explicitly on surveillance, it was part of a larger demographic challenge that would be framed under the rubric of privacy beginning with *Griswold v. Connecticut* in 1965 and culminating with *Roe v. Wade* and *Doe v. Bolton* in 1973. While initially acknowledging the authority of the physician in the doctor–patient relationship, these landmark Supreme Court privacy decisions involving reproductive rights would ultimately be read as recognizing the autonomy of the patient in medical decision making (Tribe 1988). That patients ultimately lost the battle in *Whalen* is less significant than that they engaged it. Indeed, these first encounters became, by the late twentieth century, a major conflict over patient privacy. In *Whalen,* the notion of paternalistic privacy began to yield to a notion of democratic privacy. The right of the doctor as guardian yielded to the subjective right of privacy based in the patient.

The notion of democratic privacy represented more than the idea that individuals were autonomous. Rather, it involved a new popular engagement in an area that had long been mediated by medicine and the state; for now patients themselves began to seek to define the terms of privacy. In the years after *Whalen,* patients entered into the policy fray regarding the proper limits of the state. The agenda was twofold: to democratize the practice of public-health surveillance and to give voice to those on the sexual, racial, and economic margins of American society.

## Conclusion

The ideal of democratic privacy reached its fullest expression in the battle over HIV reporting, as community groups assaulted the privacy-limiting features of surveillance activities. Despite initial controversy over whether the Centers of Disease Control needed the names of those diagnosed with AIDS, public-health workers and most in the affected communities quickly came to view AIDS case reporting as an epidemiological necessity in the face of a fatal disease with an unknown causal agent (Bayer and Fairchild 2002). But as it became possible to test for the presence of the antibody to HIV in 1985, pressure began to mount to extend surveillance beyond AIDS cases to those with HIV infection. Though consensus on the importance of AIDS-case reporting had been achieved relatively easily, this was not the case for HIV surveillance, where the affected communities resisted the registration of cases by name at the state and local levels. At least one opponent of name-based reporting linked the practice to genocide: "The road to the gas chambers began with a list in Weimar Germany." Others framed the issue in terms of public respect and social exclusion: "The fear, anger, and mistrust felt by me and many other groups," explained one advocate, "reflects our profound belief that the threat to our fundamental human rights posed by the existence of AIDS is an evil of equal strength to the disease itself. . . . To ignore our feelings will only alienate the gay community thereby impeding [the health department's] often legitimate efforts to arrest this serious health problem" (Bayer 1989, 131). With AIDS, patient advocacy and patient preferences became instrumental to the success of public health.

Marking the extent to which individuals acting in solidarity have shaped the practice of HIV surveillance, all but two states that adopted an HIV case-reporting system after 2000 chose to employ codes instead of names, following the path first pioneered by Maryland when it implemented its unique identifier system. When the 1990 Ryan White Care Act was reauthorized, however, it directed that the formulas for the allocation of funds to state and "eligible metropolitan areas"—those with populations of 500,000 or more that had in the past five years recorded 2,000 or more AIDS cases—incorporate data on reported cases of HIV infection. Such data are to be used in allocations soon if the secretary of health and human services determines that they are sufficiently accurate for resource-allocation purposes (Institute of Medicine 2003, 30). States will be provided with technical assistance to assure that case reporting is deemed acceptable. The deadline for attaining the requisite level of proficiency is 2007. In reauthorizing the act, Congress remained silent on whether name reporting was preferred to anonymous coding. With billions of dollars in aid at stake—seventy percent of Ryan White funds, $1.3 billion in fiscal year 2002 alone, were allocated under the act—it is not clear whether coded reporting systems, conceived as a response to the concerns of those living with HIV, will endure. Indeed, whether individuals with HIV will continue to prioritize privacy if the funding terrain shifts remains to be seen. Recent history makes clear that the democratization of privacy does not inevitably mean that individuals will always prize privacy above all else; in some instances, they explicitly reject it as a value trumping all other interests, such as research leading to effective prevention or treatment (Johnson 2004; Bayer and Fairchild 2002).

Nevertheless, we are at a very different place at the beginning of the twenty-first century than we were at the end of the nineteenth. When the modern era of disease surveillance began, doctors protected privacy as an instrumental value, acting on behalf of patients and trusted to do so by public-health officials. Since the 1960s, patient advocates and their constituencies have been actively engaged in defining the benefits and limits of privacy as an individual right. Today, privacy is framed by concerns over the searching eyes of the state in the wake of the terrorist attacks of September 11, 2001 (Bayer and Colgrove 2002). However the new tension between the interests of the state and those of individuals is resolved, one thing is certain: the concept of privacy is neither absolute nor static. While the conflict between individual rights and social protection in the face of disaster will continue, we cannot assume that individual privacy will continue in its present form indefinitely.

## Notes

1. Douglas's dissenting opinion in *Osborne v. United States* also represented a dissent in *Lewis v. United States* and concurrence with Justice Clark in *Hoffa v. United States*.

## References

American Association for Study and Prevention of Infant Mortality. 1919. Ninth Annual Meeting, Chicago, 5–7 December. *New York Medical Journal* 109: 126.

American Medical Association (AMA). 1918. Control of Venereal Disease in Massachusetts. *Journal of the American Medical Association* 70, no. 17: 1234

———. 1924. *Principles of Medical Ethics.* Chicago: American Medical Association.

American Public Health Association, The American Social Health Association, The American Venereal Disease Association, The Association of State and Territorial Health Officers, with the cooperation of the American Medical Association. 1966. Today's VD Problem. February, p. 33. RG 442, Box 318288, File VD Program Informational Materials. Atlanta: NARA.

Assistant Secretary for Planning and Evaluation (ASPE), Secretary of the U.S. Department of Health and Human Services. 1977. Recommendation 10, Personal Privacy in an Information Society, Chapter 7, Record-keeping in the Medical-Care Relationship Portion of the report of the Privacy Protection Study Commission addressing health records. http://aspe.hhs.gov/datacncl/1977privacy/c7.htm.

Baldwin, W. 1906. Compulsory Reports and Registration of Tuberculosis in the United States. *New York Medical Journal* 84: 1122.

Bauer, T. 1962. Assistant Surgeon General to Surgeon and Chief, Bureau of State Services, Letter. Re: Task Force Report on Syphilis Control in the United States, 12 January. RG 442, Box 105232, Folder Task Force Report on Syphilis Control in the United States. Atlanta: NARA.

Baumgartner, L. 1962. Syphilis Eradication—A Plan for Action Now. *Proceedings of World Forum on Syphilis and Other Treponematoses.* 4–8 September. Washington, DC: U.S. Department of Health, Education, and Welfare, Public Health Service.

Bayer, R. 1989. *Private Acts, Social Consequences: AIDS and the Politics of Public Health.* New Brunswick, NJ: Rutgers University Press.

Bayer, R., and J. Colgrove. 2002. Bioterrorism vs. Civil Liberties. *Science* 297: 1811.

Bayer, R., and A. Fairchild. 2002. The Limits of Privacy: Surveillance and the Control of Disease. *Health Care Analysis* 10: 19–35.

Biggs, H. 1894. The Registration of and Preventive Measures against Tuberculosis. *Boston Medical and Surgical Journal* 29 March.

———. 1900. The Registration of Tuberculosis. Read before the Philadelphia County Medical Society, 14 November. Reprinted in the *Philadelphia Medical Journal on Tuberculosis*, 1923, vi.

———. 1913a. *Monthly Bulletin of the Department of Health of the City of New York* 3: 1.

———. 1913b. Venereal Diseases. The Attitude of the Department of Health in Relation Thereto. *New York Medical Journal* (17 May).

———. 1913c. The Public Health. *Monthly Bulletin of the Department of Health of the City of New York* 3: 6.

———. 1912. The Registration and Sanitary Supervision of Pulmonary Tuberculosis in New York City. *Department of Health of the City of New York Monograph Series* 1: 14, 20–22, 60.

Brandt, A. 1987. *No Magic Bullet: A Social History of Venereal Disease in the United States since 1880*. New York: Oxford University Press.

Brenton, M. 1964. *The Privacy Invaders*. New York: Coward-McCann, Inc.

*California State Journal of Medicine*. 1918. New Regulation for Venereal Disease Reports 16: 375.

Clark, W. 1947. Find the 'Missing Million'—and Help Stamp Out Venereal Disease. *Social Hygiene* 33: 8.

Cole, H. 1919. How Physicians of Ohio May Aid in the Campaign Against Venereal Diseases. *Ohio State Journal of Medicine* 15: 69.

Cope, F. 1904. A Model Municipal Department II. *The American Journal of Sociology* 9: 5.

Douglas, W. 1958. *The Right of the People*. New York: Doubleday.

Dublin, L., and Clark, M. 1921. A Program for the Statistics of the Venereal Diseases. *Public Health Reports* 36, no. 50: 3072.

Duffy, J. 1990. *The Sanitarians: A History of American Public Health*. Urbana: University of Illinois Press.

Emerson, H. 1917. *A Monograph on the Epidemic of Poliomyelitis [Infantile Paralysis] in New York City in 1916*. Based on the Official Reports of the Bureaus of the Department of Health. New York: Department of Health.

Faden, R., T. Beauchamp, and N. M. P. King. 1986. *A History and Theory of Informed Consent*. New York: Oxford University Press.

Fee, E. 1987. *Disease and Discovery: A History of the Johns Hopkins School of Hygiene and Public Health, 1916–1939*. Baltimore: The Johns Hopkins University Press.

Fox, D. 1975. Social Policy and City Politics: Tuberculosis Reporting in New York, 1889–1900. *Bulletin of the History of Medicine* 49: 169–195.

*Frank v. Maryland*. 1959. 359 U.S. 360.

Godfrey, E. 1937. The New York State Program for Syphilis Control. *Social Hygiene* 23: 1.

Havlak, R. 2003. E-mail communication to author, 20 March.

*Illinois Medical Journal*. 1904. Peoria Begins a Crusade Against Tuberculosis. 6: 397.

———. 1917. Venereal Diseases A Special Feature. 32: 293.

———. 1918a. Reporting Venereal Diseases. 33: 51–52.

———. 1918b. Venereal Diseases Regulations Explained: Observance Declared Patriotic Duty. 33: 342–343.

Institute of Medicine (IOM). 2003. *Measuring What Matters: Allocation, Planning, and Quality Assessment for the Ryan White CARE Act*. Washington, DC: The National Academies Press.

In the Matter of the Application of William H. Allen, Appellant, to Examine Certain Records on File in the Department of Health in the City of New York, Respondent, Court of Appeals of New York, 205 N.Y. 158; 98 N.E 470; 1912 N.Y. Lexis 1201.

Johnson, B. 1938. State Laws and Regulations of State Boards of Health Which Deal with the Venereal Diseases. *Social Hygiene* 24: 8.

Johnson, P. 2004. CDC Accused of Purposely Undercounting HIV Cases. http://www. 365gay.com/newscon04/05/051004hivNos.htm (posted 10 May).

Journal of the American Medical Association. 1989. The Compulsory Notification of Venereal Diseases. *JAMA* 31: 1119–1120.

Kampmeier, R. H. 1962. Responsibility of a Physician in a Program for Syphilis Eradication. Proceedings of World Forum on Syphilis and Other Treponematoses. 4–8 September. Washington, DC: U.S. Department of Health, Education, and Welfare, Public Health Service.

Katz, J. 1984. *The Silent World of Doctor and Patient*. New York: Free Press.

Kelley, E., and A. Pfeiffer. 1924. Some Special Features of Massachusetts' Program for Venereal Disease Control. *JAMA* 83: 12.

Knopf, S. 1922. *A History of the National Tuberculosis Association*. New York City: National Tuberculosis Association.

Konold, D. 1962. *A History of American Medical Ethics, 1847–1912*. Madison: The State Historical Society of Wisconsin for the Department of History, University of Wisconsin.

Latour, B. 1988. *The Pasteurization of France*. Cambridge, MA: Harvard University Press.

Ludmerer, K. 1985. *Learning to Heal: The Development of American Medical Education*. New York: Basic Books.

Mills, C. 1951. *White Collar: The American Middle Classes*. New York: Oxford University Press.

Moore, H. 1919. Four Million Dollars for the Fight against Venereal Diseases. *Social Hygiene* 5: 15–26.

Morrow, P. 1911. Health Department Control of Venereal Diseases. *New York Medical Journal* 94.

New York City Department of Health. 1895. *Annual Report of the Department of Health of the City of New York for the Calendar Year 1894*. New York: William Bratler, Inc.

———. 1919. *Annual Report of the Department of Health of the City of New York for the Calendar Year 1918*. New York: William Bratler, Inc.

New York Medical Journal. 1894. Tuberculosis and Boards of Health. *New York Medical Journal* 59: 277.

———. 1904. Control of Tuberculosis. *New York State Journal of Medicine*.

*Osborne v. U.S., Lewis v. U.S., Hoffa v. U.S.* 1966. 385 U.S. 323, 87 S. Ct. 439.

Packard, V. 1964. *The Naked Society*. New York: David McKay.

Pernick, M. 1982. The Patient's Role in Medical Decision Making: A Social History of Informed Consent in Medical Therapy. *Making Health Care Decisions* 3.

Public Advisory Committee on Venereal Disease Control: A Follow-Up Report of The Surgeon General's Task Force on Syphilis Control. 1966. 16–17 June (U.S. Department of Health, Education, and Welfare, Public Health Service, 1967): 7. RG 90, Box 334068, Folder Public Advisory Committee on VD Control. Atlanta: NARA.

*Public Health Reports*. 1919. The Notifiable Diseases: Diseases and Conditions Required to be Reported in the Several States (7 February), 233, 238.

Regan, Priscilla M. 1995. *Legislating Privacy: Technology, Social Values, and Public Policy*. Chapel Hill: University of North Carolina Press.

Robertson, W. 1921. *Medical Conduct and Practice: A Guide to the Ethics of Medicine.* London: A&C Black.

*Roe v. Ingraham.* United States District Court for the Southern District of New York Your, 403 F. Supp. 931; 1975 U.S. Dist. LEXIS 16590.

Rosenberg, C. 1979. The Therapeutic Revolution. In *The Therapeutic Revolution,* eds. M. Vogel and C. Rosenberg, 3–25. Philadelphia: University of Pennsylvania Press.

Rothman, D. 1991. *Strangers at the Bedside: A History of How Law and Bioethics Transformed Medical Decision Making.* New York: Basic Books.

Seymour, G. 1919. A Year's Progress in Venereal Disease Control. *Social Hygiene* 5: 61.

Smith, R. 1913. Municipal Control of Tuberculosis. *Northwest Medicine* (March): 75–76.

*Social Hygiene.* 1915. Legislation to Prevent the Spread of Venereal Diseases. 1, no. 4: 636.

————. 1919. Physicians Indorse Campaign. *Social Hygiene* 5: 392

Starr, P. 1982. *The Social Transformation of American Medicine: The Rise of a Sovereign Profession and the Making of a Vast Industry.* New York: Basic Books.

State and Territorial Health Officers with the United States Public Health and Marine-Hospital Service. 1904. Transactions of the Second Annual Conference of State and Territorial Health Officers with the United States Public Health and Marine-Hospital Service. Washington, DC: GPO.

Sunkes, E. 1962. Health Department Responsibilities to Private and Hospital Laboratories. Proceedings of World Forum on Syphilis and Other Treponematoses. 4–8 September. Washington, DC: U.S. Department of Health, Education, and Welfare, Public Health Service.

Trask, J. 1915. Vital Statistics: A Discussion of What They Are and Their Uses in Public Health Administration. *Public Health Reports* 30, no. 12: 2.

Tribe, L. 1988. *American Constitutional Law.* Second ed. Mineola, NY: The Foundation Press.

U.S. Department of Health, Education, and Welfare, Public Health Service (DHEW). 1966. Report of the Venereal Disease Branch Fiscal Year 1966 (CDC: Atlanta, Georgia): 9–10. RG 90, Box 334069, Folder VD Branch Report, FY 1966. Atlanta: NARA.

Venereal Disease Branch, U.S. Department of Health, Education, and Welfare, Public Health Service, Communicable Disease Center. 1962. Field Manual. PMD-6. Atlanta: NARA.

Venereal Disease Branch Chief's Statement, Control of Venereal Diseases. 1963. RG 442, Box 108374, Folder Program Planning Conference. December, Parts I and II. Atlanta: NARA.

Venereal Diseases Branch Chief, Public Health Service, Center for Disease Control and Prevention (CDC). 1964. Memorandum to Assistant Chief, Communicable Disease Center, 27 February and attached California Administrative Code. RG 442, Box 108379, Folder Legal 1964, Proposed Legislation. Atlanta: NARA.

Warner, J. 1986. *The Therapeutic Perspective: Medical Practice, Knowledge, and Identity in America, 1820–1885.* Cambridge, MA: Harvard University Press.

Warren, S., and L. Brandeis. 1890. The Right to Privacy. *Harvard Law Review* 3, no. 5: 214.

Westin, A. 1967. *Privacy and Freedom.* New York: Antheneum.

*Whalen v. Roe.* 1977. 429 U.S. 589.

Whyte, W. 1956. *The Organization Man.* New York: Simon and Schuster.

Winslow, C. 1929. *The Life of Hermann Biggs.* Philadelphia: Lea & Febiger.

# Building a Toxic Environment

## Historical Controversies over the Past and Future of Public Health

On September 5, 2003, the *New York Times* business section announced a startling new problem. Silicosis, an occupational lung disease caused by the inhalation of silica sand and considered in the 1940s and 1950s a "disease of the past," was now rivaling asbestosis as the single most important source of toxic tort litigation in the United States. The *Times* noted that the disease had been a well-documented threat for at least seventy years and the courts were confronting an interesting legal issue (Glater 2003). Liability suits were clearly going to sky-rocket, but since workers' compensation protected employers from liability suits due to exposures on the job, the diseased workers were suing the corporations who manufactured and sold the silica sand and the masks and equipment meant to protect the lungs of the workers.

The *Times* article illustrates what a crucial role history is playing in these lawsuits. Over the course of the past thirty years we have seen a growing list of substances, circumstances, and events in which the historical record and its interpretation has emerged as an important element. One need only recall the public debates over responsibility for damages caused by silicone implants, tobacco, radiation, and a wide range of environmental disasters in Love Canal, New York, and Times Beach, Missouri, among others, in which historical analysis played an important part in ascribing responsibility for harm. Press attention to environmental hazards has elevated what were once limited liability issues into national concerns.

At the core of the legal and policy debates are questions regarding the honesty and integrity of individual corporations and whole industries that are suspected of having knowingly poisoned workers, consumers, and communities alike. An essential part of that knowledge has been the scientific research that was either ignored or manipulated in an effort to create or preserve a market for toxic substances. In this chapter we look at a number of cases in which industries have used a variety of methods to shape the scientific and professional debates over the safety or dangers of its industrial products and byproducts.[1] We are not dealing here with issues of genuine scientific ambiguity. Rather, we are discussing how industry has used its money and power to prevent the debate that might force it to alter its procedures or cease manufacturing its products.

Industries have used a variety of tactics to forestall judgments of legal liability, legislation, and regulations aimed at restricting their use of various substances or products. Some of these tactics have been fairly obvious, even bold. In the face of scientific evidence that documented danger, some industries have sought to hire or provide grants to respected scientists to conduct research to find contrary evidence. When industrial medical departments or research arms have discovered data on the deleterious effect of new substances on workers' health or on the environment, such data were, at times, kept secret, withheld from the public, hidden from the workforce, or denied to the government.

Other tactics have been subtler and quite sophisticated. When results of public scientific studies suggested that danger might exist, industries have sometimes sought to publicize the ambiguity inherent in science. Particularly in the case of environmental hazards, where proof of danger is often difficult to establish, industry creates controversy over the validity of negative data to forestall regulation and combat legal challenges. Industries have also sought to direct public and professional attention away from potential dangers through sophisticated public relations and advertising campaigns. In addition, industries have traditionally downplayed the risks associated with their products through sophisticated uses of scientific ambiguity and claims that risk no longer exists because of self-regulation and modern industrial practices. Finally, in the wake of the establishment in the early 1970s of regulatory agencies such as the Occupational Safety and Health Administration (OSHA), the Mine Safety and Health Administration (MSHA), and the Environmental Protection Agency (EPA), industries have become much more active in finding ways to forestall government from curtailing industry practices or recommending stricter standards and better enforcement. They argue that the relative costs of new environmental regulations are too high given the uncertainties about potential health benefits. Further, the money spent protecting small numbers of workers from relatively rare diseases produced by new toxins could be better used in campaigns to change personal behaviors (such as drinking and smoking) that place a greater burden on the public-health system.

## "A Disease of the Past": Industry's Use of Whig History

Many industries' first defense when accused of using toxic materials or selling toxic products is to argue that they had no way to know that such materials or products were dangerous either to the workforce or the public. After historians document the extent of knowledge in the industry, as they have done in the cases of tobacco, asbestos, silica, and other substances, industry has shifted its argument to one that posits that the hazards were so well known that there was no need to warn either the worker or the consumer. When disease is documented among the workforce, industry has used the historical record to claim that the disease exists because of a legacy of past bad practices—practices that no longer exist because of self-regulation. Government regulation and stronger standards are therefore unnecessary.

The story of silicosis, and specifically its rediscovery as a major problem from the 1970s through the 1990s, is a telling testament to the power and ability of industry to bury troubling scientific information about the dangers of their products and processes. Further, industrial presentations play on popular conceptions of the progressive nature of history, in which science and technology are motored by self-correcting, modernizing, and improving forces. In the 1930s, when silica was identified as perhaps the most serious industrial poison in the nation, the government, industry, and labor unions were all made aware of the national epidemic of silicosis. By the end of the 1940s, however, industry efforts to take silicosis out of public view and to declare the issue dead were wildly effective in allaying professional and public concern about the severity of the epidemic. Silicosis remained a silent, generally ignored issue through the 1960s, until, in the early 1970s, the newly established National Institute of Occupational Safety and Health (NIOSH) sponsored an independent investigation of sand blasting throughout the country and uncovered sloppy industrial practices and inadequate protection that led to outbreaks of silicosis among ship builders, sand blasters, and steel fabricators. In 1974, the agency issued a Criteria Document Recommendation for a crystalline silica standard which called for OSHA to cut in half the existing Permissible Exposure Limit (PEL). The document further recommended that silica be banned in abrasive blasting.

Industry's reaction was swift. In February 1975 the producers of sand joined with equipment manufacturers, painting companies, and sand-blasting contractors to form the Silica Safety Association (SSA), a group dedicated "to represent interested parties in the attempt to assure the continued use of sand in abrasive blasting operations" (Sline 1975). The SSA argued that new federal regulations and standards were unnecessary because sandblasting could be done safely if workers used "proper protective devices" to eliminate excessive silica exposure. The industry claimed that silicosis cases were being reported as a result of past practices in which workers "had no air-fed hoods" (Wright 1977), despite the fact that these hoods had been in use since the 1930s. The SSA was successful in delaying OSHA's adoption of NIOSH's recommendation. In 1980 when Ronald Reagan was elected president, the SSA declared, "with the change in administration, the ever-increasing avalanche of government regulations have been reversed" (Wright 1977). In 1981, the SSA claimed credit for forestalling and delaying the adoption of the proposals: "To date, the efforts of [the SSA] have been the major influence in the continuation of sandblasting in the States" (Wright 1981). By 1982, the antiregulatory and pro-business environment in Washington, combined with the lobbying activities of the SSA, had killed the efforts to lower the silica standard and made further lobbying efforts unnecessary. With its success, SSA found contributions from its member companies drying up. The *Silica Safety Association Newsletter* noted that "it's been a while since our last newsletter [because] Federal regulations have also been few and far between: so, as we say about sleeping dogs . . ." (1982). By June 1983, in a special meeting of the association's board of directors, it was noted that "regulatory activity in and from Washington is at a dormant level . . . no foreseen push on abrasive blasting is seen as long as the present administration is in power, [and] . . . requests to [the SSA] for information from members are rare." The board of directors, therefore, concluded that "the Association should be put on hold" (*Silica Safety Association Newsletter* 1983). The records of the association were placed in storage and the offices closed. As a result, silicosis remained a major problem for workers, only to reemerge as a national issue fifteen years later when the Department of Labor initiated a National Campaign to Eliminate Silicosis in 1997. As of early 2006, however, no new silica standard has been approved.

### Playing on the Ambiguity of Science

Historians of science have long documented the ambiguity inherent in much scientific information. In fact, the lack of definitive proof of a scientific truth is often seen as an intrinsic, even essential, element in the progress and refinement of knowledge. This quality of the scientific and the medical literature on disease and danger is the source of a major public-policy dispute in environmental regulation today. When results of scientific studies suggest that danger might exist, industries have often sought to emphasize the ambiguity inherent in science, claiming that good policy demands proof of danger. Particularly in the case of environmental challenges, where evidence of danger to human populations is often difficult to establish with rigorous statistical or epidemiological tools, industry's emphasis on the ambiguity of the data often plays an important role in creating doubt as to the legitimacy of legal, governmental, and popular challenges.

Industry has helped foster entire new academic disciplines that reinforce the idea that government should refrain from regulation unless it is absolutely clear that it is in the public interest. As Sheldon Krimsky documents, the new science of risk analysis, most directly fostered by the Center for Risk Analysis at Harvard's School of Public Health, has "promoted ideas about regulation that were consonant with many sectors of the corporate community, such as the use of the market more forcefully in lieu of regulation, quantitative risk analysis (which sets a high burden of proof for regulatory action), comparative risk analysis (which conflates voluntary and involuntary risks), and cost-benefit analysis (which ranks human health risks against corporate profits)" (Krimsky 2003, 40).

For the most part, until the late 1990s the critiques of environmentalism focused on local or national disputes. But recently, the arguments have taken on international dimensions, especially during and after the debates over the Kyoto Protocol on Global Warming. The international discussions have significantly raised the stakes in what was once a relatively limited debate about how to respond to particular crises such as in Love Canal or Convent, Louisiana, or specific threats such as lead or vinyl chloride. Issues that were once of concern to particular companies and local communities are now of concern to multinational corporations and the world. The Business Roundtable, an association of 200 of the nation's largest corporations, founded in 1972 to counter the government's growing regulatory role, has now taken an active role in debates concerning environmental pollution. In recent years, the Roundtable has actively opposed the Kyoto Protocol. Roundtable spokespeople argue that to delay implementation for developing countries would put the United States at a special disadvantage economically, that voluntary efforts to stem the release of greenhouse gases should prevail over mandatory requirements, that the development of new technologies rather than conservation and energy efficiency should be the focus of United States efforts. This influential body has argued that there is no imminent crisis and that the long-term nature of global environmental change gives us the opportunity to study the science of global change more closely to be able to arrive at conclusive judgments. "Because climate change is a complex issue which will evolve over many decades," the Business Roundtable asserted in 1996, "no policy commitments should be made until the environmental benefits and economic consequences of global climate change proposals are thoroughly analyzed and reviewed" (Business Roundtable 1996).

Conservative intellectuals have played a prominent role in promulgating this business agenda. For example, Edith Efron, whose research was funded by the Olin and Pepsico Foundations, wrote in her 1984 book *The Apocalyptics: Cancer and the Big Lie* that elite scientists had perpetuated a tremendous hoax on the American people by claiming that cancer was a result of industrial production. She claimed that science itself had demonstrated exactly the opposite: that there was no scientific proof of a link between cancer and exposure to a variety of chemicals, but that ideologically driven radical scientists from elite universities had intimidated other scientists and thus kept them from proclaiming this truth. Conservative intellectuals have even argued that there was no reason for government to act because technological innovation combined with a resilient earth would easily absorb any human-made insult.

Another author, Elizabeth Whelan, the president of the American Council on Science and Health, an organization founded in 1978, published *Toxic Terror* in 1985 (and again in 1993) which made virtually the same argument. Whelan found "an astounding gap between the consensus in the scientific and medical community on environmental issues versus what was being presented in popular publications, on television and radio and in books" for the layman (15). She argued that the "extreme environmentalist movement" had needlessly terrorized the public into believing that chemicals were unduly hazardous and called for "Americans to recognize the severity of the gap between science and popular public thought, and the dramatically unpleasant side-effects that a continued embracing of environmental alarmism will have for our country" (16). Why, she asked "are the media so gullible when it comes to swallowing whole the utterances of the doomsayers" and "why haven't the vast majority of American scientists and physicians come forth publicly in defense of the truth?" (16).[2]

The American Council on Science and Health (ACSH), distinguishing itself from "so-called consumer-advocacy organizations that misrepresent science and distort health priorities," claims to represent "mainstream science, defending the achievements and benefits of responsible technology within America's free-enterprise system."[3] The organization receives financial support from major chemical industries and conservative foundations, and some analysts consider it to be a front for industry (Rampton and Stauber 2001). In

1994 *Consumer Reports* published a critique of the ACSH, "Forefront of Science, or Just a Front?" noting that the organization received "forty percent of its money from industry, particularly manufacturers in the food processing, beverage, chemical, and pharmaceutical industries, and much of the remainder from industry-sponsored foundations" (319). Major contributors included American Cyanamid, Dow, Exxon, Union Carbide, Monsanto, and Uniroyal Chemical Company, the very companies that had fought against the vinyl chloride standard (see below). *Consumer Reports* argued that "sometimes, the council appears more interested in fighting regulation than in promoting good science or health" (319).[4] As Sheldon Rampton and John Stauber have noted, although the organization recognized the dangers of smoking and opposed the tobacco industry, it denied the relationship between asbestos, agent orange, DDT, lead, and chemical food additives and environmental disease (Rampton and Stauber 2001).[5]

## Obscuring Danger
### Public Relations Campaigns

Industries have long maintained that the environmental health issues that emerged in the late twentieth century could not have been anticipated and that the industries themselves bore little or no responsibility for the public's use of toxic products. In fact, industries have often engaged in major public relations campaigns to assuage public and professional fears about the potential dangers of their products when evidence of harm has led physicians and scientists to question their safety. The tobacco industry, of course, is a well-known example of the uses of marketing to counteract threats to their public image. From the 1940s through the 1960s, the use of physicians, nurses, and scientists in their marketing campaigns paralleled the growing attention to the dangerous, health-threatening qualities of their product.

The lead industry is a less well-known case. Over the course of the last century, literally hundreds of millions of pounds of lead in the form of lead carbonate paint have been spread on the walls of the nation's homes. This has created perhaps the biggest public health threat to children, as ingested lead dust and chips can cause neurological and other damage that affect learning and behavior and, at higher levels, can lead to convulsions and death. A number of cities and the state of Rhode Island have instituted lawsuits against several lead companies that produced the vast majority of the lead pigment that was used in paint so as to recover the costs of educating and caring for these children as well as to prevent future cases through lead abatement of older houses. As a result, historians have been engaged in a bitter dispute over the historical record. On the one hand, the industry's historians argue that the lead-pigment manufacturers bore no responsibility for the tragedy because most of the damage caused to children was due to "old paint" which was put on walls before scientific understanding of its dangers existed (English 2000).

Those who have weighed in on behalf of the states and communities, however, have developed a very different analysis of the issue (Markowitz and Rosner 2002). Not only, they argue, was there ample scientific and clinical evidence of lead's dangers to children by the mid-1920s, but the response of the lead industry to reports on these dangers was a thirty-five-year advertising campaign to convince people that lead was safe. The industry marketed to children and their parents. Beginning in 1918, just as studies confirmed that lead paint was a danger to children, the industry undertook a sustained and continuous advertising and promotion campaign designed, in the words of National Lead's trade magazine, *Dutch Boy Painter,* to "cater to the children" (*Dutch Boy Painter* 1918). In addition, National Lead aligned itself with the growing public-health movement that viewed the old clutter of Victorian homes as a potential haven for germs and disease. The themes of order, cleanliness, and purity that were hallmarks of the efforts to reform and sanitize American life were quickly incorporated into the promotional materials developed by the lead-paint industry.

Beginning in the 1950s and 1960s, the public-health community rejected the arguments of industry and progressively lowered the acceptable blood-lead level for children from eighty micrograms per deciliter to ten micrograms per deciliter. At the turn of the new century, independent scientists have concluded that even this relatively low level represents a threat to cognitive functioning and behavior in children, and lead researchers have been putting increasing pressure on the Centers for Disease Control (CDC) to lower the acceptable level still further.

## Politicizing Science

Since the 1970s, the CDC has depended upon independent scientists and policy consultants who are experts in their fields to gather information and provide advice regarding policy initiatives for a variety of toxic materials. These advisors are expected to utilize the most up-to-date information in providing guidance and expert opinion. As technologies improve and more information becomes publicly available, the CDC reshapes and reformulates policy. The Federal Advisory Committee Act that established the advisory structure was passed in 1972, shortly after the burst of federal activity that established OSHA, NIOSH, MSHA, and the EPA. The act "require[s] the membership of the advisory committee to be fairly balanced in terms of the points of view represented and the functions to be performed by the advisory committee" and to "assure that the advice and recommendations of the advisory committee will not be inappropriately influenced by the appointing authority or by any special interest, but will instead be the result of the advisory committee's independent judgment."[6]

One of the most important safeguards of the scientific integrity of governmental policy and research has been the 258 scientific advisory committees to the various branches of the CDC that presently help policy makers decide on the appropriate means of addressing serious scientific issues. These advisory committees, while not themselves possessing the power to reshape policy, are important in their role as the font of expert opinion available to various CDC chiefs. The administration of George W. Bush sought to short-circuit the traditional manner of appointments to these committees and to substitute a politicized process that by and large has reflected its own well-known antiregulatory and anti-environmental agenda. In this chapter, we will look at this recent process, focusing on one important committee that has been responsible for protecting the nation's children from the devastating effects of lead on their neurological well-being: the Lead Advisory Committee.

Members of the Lead Advisory Committee in the past have been the scientific community's leaders. They have pioneered new methodologies for measuring the presence of lead and have conducted epidemiological studies to assess lead's effects on children. They have then sought to apply this research to CDC recommendations. In 2002, the George W. Bush administration announced it was rejecting recommendations of the CDC staff and Lead Advisory Committee members for new appointments to the committee. Longtime lead researcher Ellen Silbergeld stated that "the last time anything like this happened was under Reagan" (Ferber 2002, 1456). Health and Human Services' Secretary Tommy Thompson rejected the recommended reappointment of Dr. Michael Weitzman, a member of the Department of Pediatrics at the University of Rochester and pediatrician-in-chief of the Rochester General Hospital, a member of the Advisory Committee since 1997, and author of many publications on lead poisoning in peer-reviewed journals. Thompson also rejected new nominations of Dr. Bruce Lanphear, the Sloan Professor of Children's Environmental Health in the Department of Pediatrics at the University of Cincinnati, and author of numerous epidemiological studies of lead-contaminated house dust and residential soil which were used by the Environmental Protection Agency to establish federal standards for lead in residential dwellings. He also rejected the nomination of Dr. Susan Klitzman, associate professor of Urban Public Health at the Hunter College School of Health Sciences. She too is the author of numerous peer-reviewed publications on lead poisoning (Markey 2002).

In their stead, the administration nominated individuals whose ideological commitments, past intellectual work, or connections to the lead industry virtually guaranteed that they would not be amenable to lowering the standard for acceptable levels of lead in paint. These nominees may represent the administration's broader approach to reshaping the nation's science. Perhaps the most controversial nomination was William Banner, a physician who presently is an attending at Children's Hospital and St. Francis Clinical Professor of Pediatrics at the University of Oklahoma College of Medicine. Unlike other committee members, he has written few publications on lead poisoning in children but has served as an expert witness on behalf of the lead industry in the landmark lead-poisoning lawsuit brought by Rhode Island's Attorney General Whitehouse against lead pigment manufacturers.[7] Banner's recent depositions for that case and another in Milwaukee are revealing, for they illustrate his belief that lead poisoning in children is an insignificant problem that has been grossly overemphasized. Despite the CDC's lowering of the acceptable blood-lead levels, Banner testified that lead is toxic to the brain only at levels "over seventy and closer to one hundred, probably" (Banner 2002, 115). His views ignore a generation of research on lead poisoning and seem to reflect ideas that prevailed in the decades before the 1970s (Banner 2002, 136).

The impact of the George W. Bush administration's attempts to undermine the purpose and safeguards established under the Federal Advisory Committee Act has not gone unnoticed by the scientific and technical community. Recently, David Michaels, former assistant secretary of the Department of Energy in the Clinton administration; Eula Bingham, former administrator of OSHA under President Carter; Sheldon Krimsky, professor of environmental sciences and a long-time writer on environmental policy; Celeste Montforton, former assistant to the administrator of MSHA; David Ozonoff, professor of public health at Boston University; Anthony Robbins, one of the first chiefs of NIOSH in the 1970s; and others wrote an insightful editorial for *Science* magazine that laid out their concern that the Bush administration's appointments were undermining the "vital role" that the advisory committees play in developing and guiding the federal government's science policy. They cite, for example, Tommy Thompson's efforts to limit the scientific discussion: "to avoid getting advice that is discordant with the administration's policy agenda, [Thompson] disbanded the National Human Research Protections Advisory

Committee and Advisory Committee on Genetic Testing, both of which were attempting to craft solutions to the complex problems accompanying genetic testing and research; solutions that apparently conflicted with the religious views of certain political constituencies." They go on to describe how Secretary Thompson replaced fifteen of the eighteen members of the Advisory Committee and the director of the National Center for Environmental Health with "scientists that have long been associated with the chemical or petroleum industries, often in leadership positions of organizations opposing public health and environmental regulation" (Michaels et al. 2002, 703).

As Michaels and his fellow authors point out, "instead of grappling with scientific ambiguity and shaping public policy using the best available evidence (the fundamental principle underlying public health and environmental regulation), we can now expect these committees to emphasize the uncertainties of health and environmental risks, supporting the administration's anti-regulatory views and in those areas where there are deeply held conflicts and values, we can expect only silence. Regulatory paralysis appears to be the goal here, rather than the application of honest, balanced science" (703).[8]

## Keeping Knowledge Secret

For much of the twentieth century, industrial concerns have engaged in major research efforts as part of product-development programs. At times, these efforts have directly addressed the potential toxicity of new materials and products. In large measure, information gleaned from scientists in labs or from company doctors overseeing the health of the workforce has been seen as proprietary and reserved exclusively for internal use by industry. Regulation of the health of the workforce and the safety of consumer products, industrial leaders have argued, should remain largely an industry responsibility, immune from external regulation or oversight. This commitment to self-regulation and opposition to governmental intervention has sometimes come into conflict with a growing societal impulse to increase openness and access to information. Workers' Right to Know legislation, the Freedom of Information Act and federal agencies such as OSHA, NIOSH, and the EPA seek to provide workers and the public with alternative sources of information, research, and protection.

In the early 1970s, as public policy reflected a broader call for openness and rejected the argument for preserving industry "trade secrets," a drama played out in the chemical industry. Plastics had emerged in the 1950s as a mainstay of the petrochemical industry. Polyethylene, polypropylene, polystyrene, and polyvinyl chloride among others were all synthetic materials that began to permeate American life. But, some, particularly polyvinyl chloride, were unusual in that they were created from chemical combinations that did not exist naturally, such as chlorine-carbon molecules, and therefore their impact on the environment and on human health was completely untested. Through the 1950s and 1960s, and even into the early 1970s, the chemical industry's trade association, the Manufacturing Chemists Association (MCA), wrote that vinyl chloride presented "no very serious problem in general handling aside from the risk of fire and explosion" (MCA 1953). In 1954 the MCA set the upper limit of safety for workers exposed to vinyl chloride monomer at 500 parts per million, a figure that would stand as a measure of safety for the next two decades.

In 1970, the industry learned that rats exposed to 30,000 ppm of vinyl chloride monomer gas developed tumors of the skin, lungs, and bones (Harris 1976). A few months later the MCA learned that another study had found tumors in ten to fifteen percent of rats at 5,000 ppm (Union Carbide 1971).[9] Then, in 1972, an Italian researcher found that rats exposed to as little as 250 ppm of vinyl chloride, one-half the recommended exposure limit for workers, developed cancers in their livers and kidneys.[10] The European and American vinyl manufacturers signed secrecy agreements prohibiting any disclosure of these results outside of the industry, including their workforces and their respective governments.

The chemical industry's commitment to objective science and public access to information was tested in January 1973 when NIOSH published a "Request for Information" on the potential hazards of vinyl chloride in the *Federal Register*. NIOSH was preparing a document on the appropriate and safe exposure levels to vinyl chloride and sought information about the potential health hazards of this product from all quarters—scientists, corporations, public health officials, and others. This request for information put tremendous pressure on MCA members as they sought to develop a common position concerning the health risks of vinyl chloride. NIOSH was a relatively new government agency, and its mandate to establish "Criteria Documents" that would guarantee a safe work environment meant that safety and health standards, previously a private matter for individual companies and their trade associations, were now in the public sphere. Industry faced a serious problem. In order to maintain its influence with the agencies that regulated it, industry would need to comply with NIOSH's request, but this would provide NIOSH with information that would lead to regulations that were anathema to industry (Williams 1973). In a detailed memo to all its management contacts on March 26, 1973, MCA acknowledged that it had a "moral obligation not to withhold from the government significant information having occupational and environmental relevance." It also recognized that by taking the initiative it could forestall embarrassment if the information eventually became public and caused a scandal (Best 1973a).

But MCA also acknowledged that their confidentiality agreement with the Europeans inhibited any free interchange of scientific findings with government. This posed a moral and political dilemma for the industry. Would they be willing to fulfill what they considered to be their moral obligation by revealing their findings to the United States government, even if it meant violating the trust between the American chemical companies and their European brethren? Or would it keep vital information secret from the government and the public, and thus prevent public health authorities from having the information they needed to pursue a rational public policy?[11]

In the spring of 1973, MCA agreed on a plan that would both maintain their secrecy agreement with the Europeans and, at the same time, give the appearance of responding to NIOSH's request for information. Rather than waiting for NIOSH to contact the organization, MCA called to set up a meeting with Marcus Key, NIOSH's new administrator, whose role was to provide OSHA with state-of-the-art scientific information that could be used to establish regulations to ensure safe and healthy working conditions (Sourwine 1973; Vinyl Chloride Research Coordinators 1973).

Perhaps most troubling to the MCA representatives was the realization that the March 26 MCA letter "to Company Contacts," which acknowledged "a moral obligation" to inform NIOSH about the European's studies, was a legal minefield. They feared the letter could be interpreted to indicate that the industry was planning to mislead the government. According to Union Carbide's representative to MCA, the memo "could be construed as evidence of an illegal conspiracy by industry if the information were not made public or at least made available to the government" (Wheeler 1973b).

Throughout the early summer of 1973, the Americans continued to meet among themselves and with the Europeans to plan the presentation to NIOSH, scheduled for July 17 (Duffield 1973). The Europeans and Americans decided on a pragmatic plan for protecting the industry. They would "comply" with NIOSH's request for information but in a way that was less than thorough and diverted attention from the seriousness of the facts (Kuznets 1973). The goal of the meeting was to make sure that the agency would "take no precipitous action now." Furthermore, "We should recommend no shift in priorities" and at the meeting "our people [should] get off the topic of animal work as quickly as possible" (Kuznets 1973).

The July 17 meeting took place at 1 pm at the NIOSH offices in Rockville, Maryland. Five industry representatives met across the table from five government scientists. Dr. V. K. Rowe of Dow, Dr. William E. Rinehart of Ethyl, Robert N. Wheeler of Union Carbide, and George E. Best of the MCA represented the United States industry. Dr. David P. Duffield of ICI represented the Europeans (Dr. Tiziano Garlanda of Montedison, the Italian vinyl producer, was unable to attend). Dr. Marcus M. Key, the director of NIOSH, and members of his staff, Dr. Keith Jacobson, Richard B. James, Dr. Donald Lassiter, and Dr. Frank Mitchell, represented the U.S. government. The meeting was polite, collegial, and seemingly open. The American and European vinyl producers presented an apparently complete and forthright description of the industry and any potential problems. In fact, only the industry knew the presentation was skewed, deceptive, and distorted. Dr. Rowe made the formal presentation, speaking from penciled notes. He began by emphasizing the size and scope of the vinyl-chloride industry and described the industry's efforts to address the health concerns about acroosteolysis and cancer. Dr. Duffield went on to describe the "exhaustive" studies of vinyl chloride and polyvinyl chloride workers at ICI's European plants that revealed no "indication of hazard." No mention was made of kidney or liver cancers (Best 1973c; Wheeler 1973a).

True to their earlier plan, the companies gave the NIOSH representatives only previously published or reported materials (Best 1973c). NIOSH asked "to be kept fully appraised of the on-going work both the U.S. and the European industries have in progress," believing that they had been brought up-to-date on the status of knowledge up to that point (Kennedy 1973).

At the end of the day, MCA and its various companies were pleased with the meeting and reported that "the chances of precipitous action by NIOSH on vinyl chloride were materially lessened" (Wheeler 1973a). The word that spread to member companies whose representatives had not attended the meeting was that "no problems were encountered" and the "presentation was well received and appreciated" (Kennedy 1973; Best 1973b). Leaving the government with the impression that the companies were on top of the issue and that research up to that point had not indicated any serious problem with cancers among workers, the industry had accomplished its most difficult objective. It had appeared forthcoming and responsible to NIOSH officials without violating the agreement of secrecy with their European counterparts. The industry had avoided the issue of environmental danger in consumer products, remained silent on the primary liver and kidney cancers observed in the European experiments, and not mentioned the industry's own concern that the 200 ppm threshold limit for vinyl chloride exposure was not adequate.[12] In short, the industry had reassured NIOSH regarding the dangers to workers and consumers alike from vinyl chloride, maintaining what they saw as their prerogative to keep information secret. It was not until January of 1974, when four workers at a single polyvinyl chloride plant in Louisville, Kentucky, had been diagnosed with angiosarcoma of the liver—the same kind of cancer found by Maltoni in rats—that the dangers of vinyl chloride monomer to workers became public. As a result, and over the objections of industry, OSHA reduced the maximum exposure to vinyl chloride monomer to 1 ppm.

## The Uses of Economic Power

For much of the twentieth century, industry portrayed pollution as a necessary price that communities and the nation must pay for progress and economic growth. The chemical industry specifically argued that the pollution from its plants constituted a nuisance, not a health hazard. Following World War II, the chemical industry proclaimed for itself a special role in America's new-found affluence. DuPont announced that the American century was made possible by "Better Things for Better Living . . . Through Chemistry." For over fifteen years, despite localized environmental crises and increased concern about pollution among scientists, Americans, hypnotized by a parade of technological advances, remained largely unaware of the ecological and health costs of progress. Most were eagerly incorporating the products of the chemical industry into their lives, never thinking for a moment that the synthetic chemicals in these products could possibly pose a danger.

By the 1960s, however, the publication of Rachel Carson's *Silent Spring* and a growing environmental movement undermined the argument that pollution was inevitable and necessarily linked to progress. During the 1980s and 1990s, this growing distance between the views of industry that saw pollution as a necessary evil and communities that saw it as a threat was played out in two tiny communities in Louisiana.

In the post–World War II era the chemical industry built massive plants along the Mississippi River corridor between Baton Rouge and New Orleans, in a poor state with weak environmental regulations and a government eager to attract modern industry. In the 1980s and 1990s, two communities discovered that a growing number of their wells were polluted with various chemicals used in the production process of vinyl chloride. Morrisonville, Louisiana, a largely African American community situated on the river bordering a Dow Chemical company plant, had been founded in the 1870s by slaves freed from the Australia Plantation, just north of Plaquemine (O'Byrne 1991). Dow, fearing potential lawsuits from residents for damages resulting from explosions, pollution of water tables, or diseases resulting from air pollution, tested a new strategy to deal with the local consequences of environmental pollution: they would buy the town and all the homes in it, move the residents away and create a buffer between the plant and the surrounding population (Bowermaster 1993). In 1989, just before damaging federal data was revealed about toxic releases from the plant, Dow let it be known to the residents of Morrisonville that it was the only buyer in town, and if they didn't sell to Dow, their property would later be worthless (Bowermaster 1993). One of the last to leave, G. Jack Martin, a deacon at the Nazarene Baptist Church, the historic heart of Morrisonville, summarized his experience: "Dow didn't exactly ask for our input. They just came in and told us what they were going to do. I guess Dow is the plantation now" (Bowermaster 1993, 48). The town's "big mistake," according to Martin, was that it "sold Dow some land in 1959." Before that, there had been a green belt between the town and the plant, but the company "built on it right out to the fence until they were on top of us" (O'Byrne 1991). While most of the residents accepted Dow's offer to buy out their homes and land, about twenty Morrisonville families refused: "Dow doesn't pay for attachment to land, for the inheritance that is in this community," said Rosa Martin, Jack's wife and the town's informal historian, who owned a house so close to the plant's property that the plant's loudspeakers could be heard inside her living room (Schneider 1990, A-1). In the end the town of Morrisonville was abandoned.

A similar drama took place in the town of Reveilletown, just south of Plaquemine center where there was a Georgia Gulf plant. Residents of this primarily African American community had complained about the fumes and emissions from the plant and argued that "the entire community was poisoned by vinyl chloride emissions loosed from Georgia Gulf's manufacture of plastics." One of the residents of Reveilletown, Janice Dickerson, became active in the environmental-justice movement and helped organize a candlelight vigil in 1989 "in which black and white environmentalists mourned the death" of the community (Bryant 1990, 28). The Georgia Gulf Company, realizing that the growing protest among residents might result in lawsuits, literally razed the town and constructed new homes for residents elsewhere (Harden 1997).

The companies considered the buyout an effective way to protect local residents from possible harm from dangerous explosions and toxins released into the air. "It makes sense in putting a [buyout] program together instead of waiting for an accident," remarked Michael Lythcott, a consultant who helped design similar efforts for other companies (Schneider 1990, A-1).

Environmental activists saw the issue differently. Mary Lee Orr, the executive director of the Louisiana Environmental Action Network (LEAN), stated that "companies are reducing their problems by moving people instead of reducing accidents and pollution" (Schneider 1990, A-1). The approach was not specific to Dow or Louisiana. As the *New York Times* noted in 1990, "Prodded by lawsuits over pollution and damage claims from a number of explosions, several of the nation's largest oil and chemical companies are spending millions of dollars to create safety zones by buying up the homes around the plants" (Schneider 1990, A-1). All that is left to mark the sites of Morrisonville and Reivelletown today are a signpost and a fence in the shadow of giant chemical plants, the graveyard of Morrisonville's Nazarene Baptist Church, and an open-sided wooden prayer site, built by Dow, for family members returning to visit the graves.

Businesses often portray the act of buying out communities as a responsible act in which industries are protecting communities from possible danger. In Love Canal and Times Beach, for example, entire communities were emptied out after the discovery of polluted basements, roads, and school yards. Yet, when looking at the dynamics of destruction historically, the seemingly benevolent acts of industries to remedy environmental damage looks self-serving. It allows the plants to go on creating environmental hazards that threaten their workforces and can potentially affect a much broader population (polluted air and water do not remain localized). Industry also uses the fact that they are polluting as a weapon to force people to move, even unwillingly. It is only because of the pollution that the residents' property is worthless to anyone but the company.

## Conclusions and Policy Recommendations

Without open information or a public scrutiny of industry activities there is little way to make rational decisions rationally about the introduction of thousands of potentially toxic substances and products into the environment. Ultimately, there has been a conflict between the principles of prevention and precaution and the stark world of economic competition, power, and trade secrets. Under the rubric of "progress" being "our most important product," we have seen numerous assaults on the principles of public-health policy. In some instances, industries have sought to shape scientific debates by producing their own studies. In other instances, industries have funded research in prestigious universities, leading to questions about possible conflicts of interest for researchers and the integrity of the research conclusions. In recent years academic centers, often supported by industries and various trade associations, have developed extensive programs in risk- and cost-benefit analysis, even in schools of public health. Skeptics see these new economic and ostensibly objective scholarly tools as another method by which industrial interests undermine the academy and institutions of science.[13] In light of the abuses that have been described in this chapter and are regularly documented in the professional literature and popular press, we must more fully embrace policies that emphasize precautionary principles, particularly when scientific data and general evidence of danger are ambiguous or incomplete.

While many environmentalists and public-health professionals have called for a concerted effort to develop better data on the relationship between industrial pollution and disease, some also argue that, in the absence of final proof, the government must step in to protect people and a fragile environment from a host of human-made insults. As the signers of the Wingspread Statement on the Precautionary Principle put it in January 1998, the principle of precaution should be the overriding policy in environmental and health matters. Rather than await definitive proof, society must require a certain degree of confidence in a material's safety before allowing it into the human environment and continuously seek the safest means to achieve particular goals. Perhaps we should consider the admonition of the National Research Council in 1991: "Until better evidence is developed prudent public policy demands that a margin of safety be provided regarding potential health risks. . . . We do no less in designing bridges and buildings. We do no less in establishing criteria for scientific credibility. We must surely do no less when the health and quality of life of Americans are at stake" (National Research Council 1991, 270). The precautionary principle that is now regularly discussed among environmentalists is a new iteration of the age-old values that underlie public health as a preventive discipline.

Certainly, historians also have an obligation in this ongoing debate about the place of industry in science and society. Their responsibilities are both to the accuracy and honesty of the scientific record as well as to the society that will ultimately depend on that record to create well-grounded and meaningful social policies. Historians have a special role to play in reminding professionals and the population at large of the complex relationship that has existed between industry and public-health advocates over the last century. Historians are able to gain access to archival materials, public documents, and, increasingly as lawsuits over toxic torts evolve, internal industry memoranda, minutes, and letters. This, combined with their analytic expertise and training, provides them with a special opportunity to be engaged in contemporary policy disputes.

## Notes

1. For an extended discussion, see Markowitz and Rosner 2002.

2. See also, a later edition of this book, *Toxic Terror, The Truth Behind the Cancer Scares,* (Buffalo: Prometheus Books, 1993), 35.

3. See the American Council on Science and Health's web site for this description, "About ACSH," http://www.acsh.org/about/index.html.

4. See also Ernest W. Lefever, Raymond English and Robert L. Schuettinger, *Scholars, Dollars and Public Policy: New Frontiers in Corporate Giving* (Washington: Ethics and Public Policy Center, 1983), 55.

5. Michael Fumento, in *Science Under Siege*, also focuses on the need to base policy on sound science, not on political considerations, but then goes on to equate the alarm sounded by environmentalists with the Reign of Terror during the French Revolution. "What is needed is to end our reign of terror, to restore sanity and sound principles to our revolution . . . it is time to begin shaping policies on the basis of science, rather than shaping science to fit policies." Michael Fumento, *Science Under Siege: Balancing Technology and the Environment* (New York: William Morrow and Co., 1993), 372.

6. See http://www.archives.gov/federal_register/public_laws/federal_advisory_committee_act/05.html. (accessed 7 January 2003).

7. This suit has galvanized the attention of the industry and the nation's attorneys general because of its scope and implications for the future. In brief, Rhode Island is suing for compensation for the millions of dollars it has been forced to pay for Medicaid and other medical expenses for upwards of 35,000 children poisoned over the past few years. It is also asking for recovery of the costs for special education programs for these children and, most importantly, money for abating the lead hazard in as much as eighty percent of Rhode Island's housing stock.

8. Others have pointed out the ways that traditional review procedures are being attacked by the Secretary and the administration. See, for example, Dana Loomis, "Unpopular Opinions Need Not Apply," *Science,* 298 (15 November 2002), 1335–1336.

9. See also S. F. Pits to D. O. Popovac, CONOCO Interoffice Communication, "On MCA VCM Toxicity Subcommittee," 18 November 1971, MCA Papers.

10. It is unclear from the documentation whether or not Dr. Viola actually delivered this paper. See George Roush to Richard Henderson, June 24, 1970, MCA Papers.

11. In April, 1973 Cesare Maltoni gave a paper at the Second International Cancer Conference in Bologna on occupational carcinogenesis, which, according to Sir Richard Doll, included information on the carcinogenic properties of vinyl chloride (Deposition of William Richard Shaboe Doll, 26 January 2000, London, England, in *Carlin David Staples et. al. v. Dow Chemical,* p. 27). The data seemed to have little impact on an audience unaware of the significance of the information that low-level exposures could cause cancer. Surprisingly, with the exception of Sir Richard Doll, it appears that no one remembers hearing this information, including one American representing the National Cancer Institute. Indeed, at the time, the MCA never remarked on the incident, and subsequent events indicate that they believed that the information was still secret in the United States. Testimony of Cesare Maltoni, 1999, Venice, Italy, Tape 1067, p. 2, Transcript courtesy of Judith Helfand. Doll Deposition, 1999, Scafiati Deposition, 1999.

12. A nongovernmental organization, The American Conference of Governmental Industrial Hygienists, had set this limit in 1972.

13. See, for example, Philip Mirowski and Esher-Mirjam Sent, *Science Bought and Sold: Essays in the Economics of Science* (Chicago: University of Chicago Press, 2002); Daniel S. Greenberg, *Science, Money, and Politics: Political Triumph and Ethical Erosion* (Chicago: University of Chicago Press, 2001); Daniel S. Greenberg, *The Politics of Pure Science* (Chicago: University of Chicago Press, 1999); Gerald Markowitz and David Rosner, *Deceit and Denial: The Deadly Politics of Industrial Pollution* (Berkeley: Milbank/University of California Press, 2002); Sheldon Krimsky, *Science in the Private Interest: Has the Lure of Profits Corrupted Biomedical Research?* (Lanham: Rowman & Littlefield, 2003).

## References

Banner, W., Jr. 2002. Deposition, June 13.

Best, G. 1973a. Leter to J. D. Bryan. MCA Papers, 26 March.

Best, G. 1973b. Letter to Management Contacts of Companies. MCA Papers, 20 July.

Best. G. 1973c. Notes on Meeting Between Representatives of MCA Technical Task Group on Vinyl Chloride Research and NIOSH. MCA Papers, 17 July.

Bowermaster, J. 1993. A Town Called Morrisonville. *Audubon* 95: 42–51.

Bryant, P. 1990. A Lily-white Achilles Heel. *Environmental Action* 21: 28–29.

Business Roundtable. 1996. Rush to Judgment: A Primer on Global Climate Change. 11 September. www.brtable.org/document.cfm/30.

*Consumer Reports.* 1994. The ACSH: Forefront of Science, or Just a Front? May.

Duffield, D. P. 1973. Vinyl Chloride Toxicity—Meetings Held at MCA Headquarters, Washington, DC and National Institute of Occupational Safety and Health, Rockville, MD. 16 and 17 July. MCA Papers, 20 July.

*Dutch Boy Painter.* 1918. Cater to the Children. January/February: advertising section.

Efron, E. 1984. *The Apocalyptics: Cancer and the Big Lie.* New York: Simon and Schuster.

English, P. 2000. *Old Paint: A Medical History of Childhood Lead Poisoning.* New Brunswick, NJ: Rutgers University Press.

Ferber, D. 2002. Environmental Health. Critics See a Tilt in a CDC Science Panel. *Science* 297: 1456.

Glater, J. D. 2003. Suits on Silica Being Compared to Asbestos Cases. *New York Times,* 6 September: C-1.

Harden, M. 1997. Letter to editor. *The [Baton Rouge] Advocate,* 21 July, 8B.

Harris, W. D. 1976. Handwritten Notes. Given to R.J.O. MCA Papers, 17 May.

Kennedy, F. 1973. Letter to R.W.G. et al. VCM. MCA Papers, 19 July.

Krimsky, S. 2003. *Science in the Private Interest: Has the Lure of Profits Corrupted Biomedical Research?* Lanham, MD: Rowman & Littlefield Publishers, Inc.

Kuznets, H. L. 1973. To Files. Private and Confidential. MCA Papers, 17 July.

Markey, E. 2002. Lead Poisoning Advisory Panel Weighed Down by Lead Industry's Friends. U.S. Congress, Massachusetts 7th District, News from Ed Markey, 8 October.

Markowitz, G. and D. Rosner. 2002. *Deceit and Denial: The Deadly Politics of Industrial Pollution.* Berkeley: Milbank/University of California Press.

Michaels, D., E. Biingham, L. Boden, R. Clapp, L. R. Goldman, P. Hoppin, S. Krimsky, et al. 2002. Advice without Dissent. *Science* 298: 703.

National Institute for Occupational Safety and Health. 1973. Request for Information. *Federal Register,* 30 January.

National Research Council. 1991. Committee on Environmental Epidemiology. *Environmental Epidemiology* Vol. 1, Public Health and Hazardous Wastes. Washington, DC: National Academy Press.

O'Byrne, J. 1991. The Death of a Town: A Chemical Plant Closes In. *New Orleans Times-Picayune,* 20 February, A-12.

Rampton, S., and J. Stauber. 2001. *Trust Us, We're Experts! How Industry Manipulates Science and Gambles with Your Future.* New York: Jeremy P. Tarcher/Putnam.

Schneider, K. 1990. Chemical Plants Buy Up Neighbors for Safety Zone. *New York Times,* 28 November, A1.

*Silica Safety Association Newsletter.* 1982. SSA Papers, 22 February.

————. 1983. SSA Papers, 22 June.

Sline, L. 1975. Letter to Dear Sir. Silica Safety Association, Volume 1, 21 March.

Union Carbide. 1971. Memo on the Manufacturers Chemists Association Occupational Health Committee VC Conference. MCA Papers, 23 November.

Vinyl Chloride Research Coordinators. 1973. Minutes of Meeting. MCA Papers, 4 April.

Wheeler, R. N. 1973a. Letter to Carvajal, et al. MCA Papers, 19 July.

Wheeler, R. N. 1973b. Letter to Eisenhour. MCA Papers, 31 May.

Whelan, E. M. 1985. *Toxic Terror.* Ottawa, IL: Jameson Books.

Williams, G. J. 1973. Letter to C. A. Gerstacker. DOW. MCA Papers, 5 March.

Wright, B. C. 1977. Future of Abrasive Blasting. *Proceedings of the Regional Meeting of the National Association of Corrosion Engineers.* SSA Papers, 5 October.

Wright, B. C. 1981. Silica Safety Update—History—Current Endeavors—Future Plans. SSA Papers, 26 May.

# Part III

# Priorities
and Politics

# Situating Health Risks

## An Opportunity for Disease-Prevention Policy

The health care issues that capture significant public and professional attention are not necessarily the most important. As potential points of policy intervention, some intellectual assumptions, clinical practices, and structural relationships are so tightly woven into social, economic, and scientific life that they are in some sense invisible. Take, for example, one of the most contentious American health-policy controversies in recent years—Medicare coverage for prescription medications. Participants in this controversy have focused almost exclusively on financial and administrative issues such as cost, the scope of benefits, and the role of private insurers. Seemingly—and strangely— absent from political and policy debates is any mention of which drugs seniors take and why. But consider that twenty of the forty-six drugs most widely used by the elderly in 2000 were drugs prescribed to treat asymptomatic "risk factors" such as osteoporosis and hypertension.[1]

The definition, scope, and significance of many of these health risks, such as the treatment of high serum cholesterol levels in the elderly, have been widely contested (Alibhai and Rochon 1998; Aronow 2002; Eisenberg 1991; Froom 1991; LaRosa 2002; Oliver 1997; Wenger 2002). In addition, the demand for risk-reducing medications has been heavily influenced by direct marketing to consumers, the sometimes exaggerated claims of self-interested parties, and problematic assumptions used in the extrapolation of aggregate data to individual decisions. I want to argue here that developments leading to this state of affairs represent missed opportunities for policy analysis and intervention. Understanding them as policy issues has the potential to significantly impact both population health and our economic well-being.

## The Limitations of Current Disease-Prevention Policy

The elderly's high use of risk-reducing drugs is but one aspect of a disease-prevention landscape that in recent decades has been transformed by social, demographic, economic, intellectual, and technological forces. Yet our traditional mode of making health policy—from FDA regulation of new drugs to expert consensus review of existing clinical practices—is not designed for the challenge posed by the radically changed character, magnitude, and mix of current and future risks and prevention practices. Policymakers have generally responded to the increasing number of newly defined and controversial health risks, screening tests, and risk-reducing drugs long after most have found a secure niche in medical and/or popular ideas and practices. They have not understood developments that occur "upstream" from the time when these prevention ideas and practices take root as potential points of policy intervention. Nor have they adequately grappled with the questions and challenges raised by the nonarbitrary ways that health risks emerge and are responded to. Notably, why have we embraced these risks, drugs, and practices rather than others? Should insurers, purchasers, and regulators intervene to regulate health-risk research and scientific and marketplace developments that contribute to the success or failure of new health risks and prevention practices?

Disease-prevention policies have generally been based on the critical evaluation of medical evidence about the efficacy and safety of particular screening tests, preventive medications, and calls for behavioral change. Although there has been a great deal of careful evidence-based appraisal of specific preventive policies, and although the ongoing policy response by government and professional groups is in many ways more extensive than the regulation of existing diagnostic and therapeutic practices and technologies, disease-prevention policies have generally been reactive and after-the-fact.

The changed disease-prevention landscape is a present concern. Insights derived from the sequencing of the human genome, for example, are already leading to many newly defined genetic "risks" as statistical correlations are made between bits of genomic variation and disease (e.g., breast cancer genes or Alzheimer genes). Such knowledge will inevitably result in new screening tests, disease classifications, and points of intervention. The pace, shape, and use of these insights and developments are substantially influenced by organizations that finance research, seek patents, and market or franchise genetic tests and preventive measures. It seems myopic to bring the considerable analytic powers of evidence-based medicine to each newly established genetic risk and test without also examining the upstream processes that systematically create these particular risks and tests.

A recent experience reminded me of the increasingly important role that the search for profits and markets plays in shaping the definition of health risks and the demand for prevention. After I gave a talk on the history of symptoms, I was surprised to find several pharmaceutical company representatives waiting to ask me a series of "prediction" questions. I learned that they had attended my talk because they were trying to understand what common symptoms and risks might be the next target for medical interventions—the next Viagra or Premarin. New symptom complexes and health risks are an extremely important frontier for pharmaceutical companies because drugs directed at them have potential markets in the tens of millions and the duration of treatment is often life-long.

We need to find upstream points of policy intervention not just because narrow interests play powerful roles in shaping and responding to health risks or because disease-prevention policy is in danger of resembling a complex group process about the best way to close the barn door after the horse has left. We also presumably want our limited research and health-care resources to be deployed in ways that reflect significant health problems and the interests of a diverse society. So we need to understand the processes through which we come to recognize and agree about the importance of some health risks and not others.

Take, for example, the political decisions that determine the regulatory options for environmental health risks, such as novel workplace exposures or industrial pollutants. These options are self-evidently a function of prior funding for research and surveillance activity by agencies such as the Environmental Protection Agency. We can only regulate dangerous substances and practices that have been previously recognized and investigated. As a result, the very terms of a political and social debate about environmental activism and regulation are often directed by decisions that in themselves are not directly the subject of self-conscious health-policy concern.

For example, debates about the federal regulation of putative environmental carcinogens necessarily depend on earlier surveillance that might identify the cancer-causing agents. Consider that local public-health officials are often reluctant to investigate reports of unusual clustering of cancer cases in specific geographic areas because such investigations rarely produce solid evidence of specific causal factors (Gawande 1999). The aggregate effect of many local decisions not to investigate cancer clusters may be that a smaller number of chemicals will be subject to future surveillance and regulation. For example, it took a great deal of community pressure and political action to push state health officials to investigate a recent cancer cluster in New Jersey. This study resulted in the discovery of a new putative environmental carcinogen (New Jersey Department of Health 2003). Despite the importance of the political and social processes by which knowledge about environmental health risks is or is not constructed, such processes are not generally deemed relevant to policy.[2]

Does it matter that our current health policies have not adequately come to terms with the complex interactions among social factors and biomedical insights that shape our recognition and understanding of health risks and disease-prevention practices? I would argue that it does. In the sections below, I will present both a rationale for this view and a preliminary sketch of some new areas for disease-prevention policy and policy analysis. This type of thought experiment necessarily involves stretching the typical meaning and context of the term *health policy,* which is generally limited to existing means of resource allocation, legislation, regulation, and large-scale decision making. I will begin with some brief observations about and comparisons among the history of a few late twentieth-century health risks in order to suggest a policy-relevant analytic framework for comparing how different health risks are discovered, made visible, and become objects of interventions. I will then use the recent rise and fall of sex-hormone use to prevent osteoporosis and coronary heart disease to suggest the relevance of the social history of health risks for disease-prevention policy. I will end with a few thoughts about the implications for changing the scope of disease-prevention policy.

## The Natural History of a Health Risk

It is not self-evident why certain health risks attract significant societal and medical attention and become objects of specific prevention practices. It was neither inevitable nor solely determined by biomedical developments, for example, that individuals and groups would search for cancer blood tests in the 1940s (Blood Tests for Cancer 1947), launch large epidemiological studies of "risk factors" for coronary heart disease in the 1950s (Aronowitz 1998), abort efforts to screen smokers for cancer in the 1960s (Evanoff et al. 1993), conceptualize posttraumatic stress disorder in the 1970s (Young 1995), launch national cholesterol guidelines in the 1980s (Cleeman and Lenfant 1987), or develop Lyme-disease vaccines in the 1990s (Rahn 2001). We might find more successful policy leverage upstream from the typical ways we make disease-prevention policy if we understood the generation-specific and contingent influences on the appearance and identity of risks, diagnoses, and prevention practices.

One way to find and understand both the shared and varying influences is to posit the existence of three stages prior to the widespread diffusion of specific drugs, screening tests, or calls for behavioral change: the "discovery" of health risks, making health risks visible to others, and creating demand for specific interventions. While there are no clear boundaries between these stages and many risks and prevention practices have not gone through them in a step-wise manner, this framework can help identify the common elements in the trajectories of disparate health risks as they do or do not elicit specific disease-prevention responses.

In the *discovery* stage, the most important historical problem is to understand the processes by which individuals and groups first recognize new associations among clinical, behavioral, environmental, and laboratory factors and ill health. How does the political and social context in which individuals and groups live affect which risks they identify? How have technological changes and the structure of health systems and markets shaped the discovery of health risks?

Elizabeth Armstrong's study of fetal alcohol syndrome (FAS) illustrates some important features of the discovery stage of health risks (Armstrong 1998). In the early 1970s, activist researchers rediscovered and repackaged older concerns about women, pregnancy, fetuses, and alcohol to construct FAS.[3] Armstrong depicted these activist researchers as "moral entrepreneurs," emphasizing the way they tended to subordinate their own and others' scientific data toward an end about which they had a passionate moral commitment. These moral entrepreneurs took advantage of, and were influenced by, increased medical interest and progress in classifying birth defects. Armstrong's major concern (and that of much of the historical and sociological literature on health-risk discovery) is the way promoters of many twentieth-century health risks (such as fetal alcohol syndrome) reconfigured moral questions—what behaviors are right and wrong, who is and is not responsible for disease—as *seemingly* empirical, value-free questions about health risks.

A characteristic feature of this discovery stage has been the way new clinical and pathological insights, frequently driven by new diagnostic technologies or older ones applied in new circumstances, result in the appearance of novel health risks. The seemingly specific and legitimate associations are often driven by technologies whose reach and limitations are not yet clear (such as ultrasound abnormalities cited in the early FAS papers) and can thus potentially gain, as I have argued, a good deal of scientific and public traction without (at least in retrospect) adequate scientific review (Aronowitz 1992). It often takes a considerable amount of time and tinkering before there are enough data and experiences to evaluate the justification for and strength of initial claims about a new health risk. This is especially true when health-risk research involves new technologies, small numbers of study subjects, and inadequate control groups.

Something akin to this pattern of health-risk discovery occurred when mid-twentieth century American pathologists discovered and promoted new pathological entities, the "in situ" cancers, especially of the breast and cervix, whose definition and meaning straddles the border of risk and disease. Technological innovations such as Pap smears and later screening mammography played important ancillary roles as they led to many women receiving these "pre-cancer" diagnoses. We are still sorting out the significance and implications of these new entities, about which there remains a good deal of uncertainty.

For example, women who received the diagnosis of lobular carcinoma in-situ of the breast (LCIS) in the 1950s were often told that they had a kind of menacing, early cancer and were frequently encouraged to have "prophylactic" surgery. Later in the century, researchers and clinicians became more aware of the problematic and varied natural history of LCIS. By the end of the century, many clinicians and investigators were thinking of the LCIS diagnosis not so much as an early stage of cancer but as a marker of risk whose magnitude and meaning was uncertain and contested. At the same time, many patients have continued to believe they were suffering from a kind of early cancer and that surgical removal of a small area of LCIS cured them of cancer. Similar problems have been posed by the discoveries of the health risks of being a sickle-cell-disease carrier and of mitral valve prolapse syndrome, which were with time found to be overstated, yet for a brief, initial period enjoyed widespread medical credibility (Wailoo 1997; Quill, Lipin, and Greenland 1988).[4] The complex interaction of lay and medical activism, technological change, and other social influences has often led to the rapid—almost instant—construction of health risks, which were, in turn, responded to in ways that would seem, in retrospect, unnecessarily aggressive and/or stigmatizing and whose ontological status would eventually be questioned.

Once discovered, health risks gain *visibility* among different groups. There is often a protracted time period after the initial discovery or promotion of a health risk during which clinicians, researchers, policymakers, and the larger public become—or fail to become—concerned with the putative links among a particular behavior, environmental feature, or biological marker, and ill health. Policymakers might learn a great deal from comparing and contrasting highly visible health risks with two other categories of risk: those which have not been well accepted and diffused beyond a small group of researchers or advocates and those which have had a very long time period between discovery and widespread acceptance and diffusion.

For example, why did decades elapse between clinical and epidemiological observations about tobacco use, lung cancer, and the enlarged visibility of smoking as a major social and public-health problem? Historians and others have suggested that diverse interests and values explain this gap: the smoking habits of investigators and opinion leaders, active obfuscation by tobacco growers and cigarette makers, ignorance of and/or resistance to population-based research and its findings, the desire not to blame victims, and fears that the tobacco-cancer association would diminish concern about environmental causes of cancer (Wydner 1997). Understanding the pattern of structured and contingent influences in the extended time period in which some health risks are contested might very well yield insights into new types of health policies aimed at influencing the processes by which health risks gain or do not gain wide public and scientific visibility.

Finally, how is significant *demand* for particular prevention practices and products created? I mean to call attention here to the multi-faceted ways that prevention products and practices become used and useable. Policy responses—drug regulation, licensing of screening tests, practice guidelines, etc.—to a new preventive practice are ideally based on critical appraisal of rigorous scientific investigations of particular prevention products and practices. But many products and practices are widely assimilated prior to, or independently of, the creation or assessment of medical evidence about prevention.

Prevention products and practices often develop and diffuse in a piecemeal fashion. They often arise within a context removed from disease prevention, such as the consumer market or behaviors not initially rationalized or understood in terms of their impact on health. For example, many technologies ultimately used as screening tests were not developed for screening or other prevention purposes. Instead they had existing or potential uses for etiologic research (e.g., as a way to determine whether a particular virus might cause a clinical syndrome) as well as diagnosis of disease in clinical practice. So it is often difficult to even locate the moment in time at which certain technologies evolved into screening tests. Some of the most important and contested contemporary examples of these mixed-use technologies are the PSA screening test for prostate cancer and mammography for breast cancer. Factors which influenced the transformation to screening tests include heightened fears of cancer, the failure of other screening modalities and educational campaigns, and the interests of specialists and test manufacturers.

The role played by lay advocates in shaping demand for particular prevention practices represents another underappreciated, potential point of policy analysis and intervention.[5] It is also important to consider the ways that
different characteristics of target populations have shaped medical and popular demand for prevention practices.

Consider, for example, the different histories of screening mammography
for breast cancer and screening chest radiographs and sputum cytology for lung
cancer. Although the basic technology for diagnostic and screening mammography had been potentially available since 1910, it was not until the early
1960s that there was a concerted effort on the part of federal cancer control officials, clinical investigators, and leading medical professionals to incorporate
screening mammography into routine clinical practice. The sudden rise in
demand for mammography in the late 1950s suggests that changing attitudes,
values, and professional roles lie at the heart of this change much more than
technological innovations: for example, growing frustration with ineffective
cancer surgery, and public education campaigns (Aronowitz 2001).[6] In other
words, the beginnings of screening mammography were as much or more the
result of changes in the demand for this technology than in the technology
itself.

In contrast to mammography, there has never been much demand—until
very recently—for screening x-rays and sputum cytology to detect lung cancer
among smokers. A limited set of studies beginning in the 1950s suggested that
screening did not save lives and that any apparent benefit was due to lead time
and other biases. But these studies had major flaws and were not designed to
test screening against no screening.[7]

Why was there so little demand to improve upon these studies—and effectively screen smokers for lung cancer—until the 1990s? The answer cannot
reside solely in differences in the effectiveness of lung cancer and breast cancer screening. Ever since the first randomized trial of mammography in the
1960s there has been evidence that screening women under fifty is of limited
value, but such findings have only fueled controversies and stimulated additional studies. This is in marked contrast with the absence of any widespread
research, visibility, and agitation for lung cancer screening in response to early
empiric data on the value of such tests. To understand the differences in
demand between mammography and lung cancer screening, we need to recognize the powerful role of beliefs—for example, smokers are generally considered to be responsible for their cancer and able to prevent cancer by quitting,
while women who develop breast cancer are often seen as innocent victims of
unknown, random influences.

We might also find new sorts of policy leverage from a closer examination of the many incremental bits of tinkering with the social and economic context in which new preventive practices and products are developed and used. Examination of the chronology of developments in screening for hyperlipidemia (such as serum cholesterol tests), for example, makes it clear that the many small innovations in the way lipid-lowering drugs (such as the statins) were promoted, marketed, and used had a profound effect on clinicians' attitudes and behavior. Before these innovations, clinicians had largely ignored this health risk in actual practice despite its acceptance by many researchers and public-health workers as an etiological factor in coronary heart disease (CHD). The change in clinician practice and beliefs did not simply follow from demonstrations of the efficacy of drug therapy. In the 1980s, the ability to quantitatively measure serum lipids, the elaboration of precise cut-offs for different types of interventions, and the ability to treat hyperlipidemia with specific drugs led to a transformation of the CHD-prevention model into something that resembled the diagnosis and treatment of "real" disease, thus overcoming traditional physician lack of interest in and suspicion of prevention (Aronowitz 1998). The complex and incremental construction of a set of prevention routines, norms, and procedures, as much or more than novel data about the efficacy of a new class of drugs, thus contributed greatly to important changes in the way this health risk was routinely understood and managed. Health-policy analysis might profitably focus on such contextual shifts in addition to data on the risks and benefits of new prevention practices.

## The Social History of Sex Hormones

The recent history of sex hormones (that is, estrogen preparations, sometimes in combination with progesterone, that have most frequently, if misleadingly, been labeled as hormone replacement therapy, or HRT) to prevent chronic disease among postmenopausal women suggests that the social history of health risks can be a tool for evaluating existing disease-prevention policies and imagining new ones.[8] In 1941, medical scientists first suggested that estrogen therapy might prevent osteoporosis in postmenopausal women. Additional studies appeared in the 1960s that further supported this proposition. In 1979 the results of a ten-year prospective study on the relationship between estrogen replacement therapy and osteoporosis were published, confirming that estrogen slowed or even reversed bone loss in postmenopausal women (see Albright et al. 1941; Davis et al. 1966; Gordon 1961; Meema and Meema 1968; Natchigall et al. 1979; Alibhai and Rochon 1998). The possible benefits of estrogen in preventing heart disease have perhaps an even longer history, often serving to explain the once widely perceived difference in cardiovascular mortality between men and women.

Sex hormone use for osteoporosis and other types of disease prevention has been controversial over this entire period, but recent analyses of large-scale, placebo-controlled, randomized clinical trials have seemingly resolved the controversy in favor of the skeptics (Rossouw et al. 2002). The most relevant historical observation about the shaping of demand for sex hormones to prevent disease is that this class of drugs has long had other uses—as contraceptives, to combat infertility, to treat menopausal symptoms, to maintain "femininity"—so that the evaluation of how, when, and among whom these medications were taken for prevention of osteoporosis and heart disease is difficult. For many individuals in different eras and settings, chronic disease prevention was just one of many goals.

Claims about maintaining femininity in the 1960s and 1970s were later eclipsed by others focused on preventing osteoporosis and even later CHD. Watkins (2001) describes how the rationale for prescribing HRT to menopausal and postmenopausal women has changed over the past four decades. From the 1960s through the mid-1970s, the pharmaceutical industry (and indeed, physicians) marketed HRT for its putative slowing of the aging process and amelioration of the emotional instability brought on by menopause. However, when studies revealed an association between estrogen use and endometrial cancer, faith in HRT declined and the rationale shifted to the rhetoric of preventing osteoporosis and later cardiovascular disease. MacPherson (1993) cites three sequential rationales for HRT use: 1966–1975, eternal beauty and femininity; 1975–1981, safer, symptom-free menopause; 1981–present, escape from chronic disease. These shifting rationales and blurred boundaries have been fundamental in maintaining and even enlarging demand for the drugs.

Regulators have been hard-pressed to evaluate and keep up with these shifts and changes. For example, it was only in 1989 that the FDA officially evaluated and endorsed HRT use for the prevention of osteoporosis. This was years after osteoporosis prevention (and combination therapy with progesterone) re-energized HRT use in the wake of the downturn caused by the discovery that estrogen increased the risk of endometrial cancer (Worcester and Whatley 1992).

Many observers have noted that another driving force behind the creation and maintenance of demand for sex hormones has been an alliance between pharmaceutical companies and moral entrepreneurs. Supported by pharmaceutical industry, Robert Wilson's book *Feminine Forever* (1966) is frequently credited with jump-starting estrogen use for menopausal symptoms in the

1960s (Worcester and Whatley 1992). Pharmaceutical companies have long recognized that a drug used by every American female over long time periods would create a great market, and they have energetically promoted these drugs through advertising and physician detailing, in addition to sponsoring research, awareness programs, and professional organizations.

Many other investigators and clinicians besides Wilson have received financial support from pharmaceutical companies and pushed for greater HRT use.[9] While I would not claim that the conduct or interpretation of the clinical trials of sex hormones for chronic disease prevention were tainted by the financial support of investigators or by the participation of HRT enthusiasts, such sponsorship or stewardship may very well have affected the content and strength of scientific consensus, as well as kept the use of these drugs on medical and public radar screens.

For example, observational studies have inherent limitations that probably explain the repeated finding of a positive association between HRT and different measures of good health. It is difficult in these trials to fully adjust for the fact that women who take HRT in the real world (as opposed to being assigned randomly) generally have healthier attitudes and lifestyles than those who do not take HRT. It is possible, but I know of no supporting evidence, that some sponsors of studies or HRT enthusiasts anticipated and consciously exploited this weakness. A more reasonable but no less troubling inference is that once there was initial evidence for preventive health benefits in observational trials, drug companies could support many different studies, which in turn reported a large number of weakly positive results. (While replication of research results usually strengthens our belief in their reality, repeated studies that share the same inherent biases should not.) Each study has been judged on its scientific merits, but the net effect of so many of these weakly positive studies was to increase confidence in the reality of the association and to keep it visible among the general public and medical communities.

At the same time, there have been many persistent, skeptical voices about HRT for chronic disease prevention (as well as treatment of menopausal symptoms) within and outside of medicine. "The increased administration of [HRT]," two feminist critics asserted in 1994, was "yet another form of medical violence against women" (Klein and Dumble 1994, 339). Such critics have pointed out the sexist assumptions in constructing menopause as a pathological state: the reductionism inherent in framing menopause as a state of hormone depletion, the cultural myopia and biological determinism in assuming menopausal symptoms are universal, the "heterosexist" assumptions about women's goals and needs, the exploitation of women's fears of aging, and the way that the focus on hormone depletion reflected sexist notions of female frailty and non-normality (Hunt 1994; Worcester and Whatley 1992).

Despite this opposition, the preventive rationale for HRT use in the 1980s and 1990s became medical and public-health wisdom. There was a good deal of research into medical and lay "noncompliance" as well as educational campaigns by medical associations and public-health groups to encourage the preventive use of HRT. But given persistent scientific uncertainty and controversy, the difficulty of weighing small health benefits against health risks like endometrial and breast cancer, and the nuisance and cost of medications, many policy-setting groups ultimately recommended that women become informed consumers and make decisions for themselves (American College of Physicians 1992; AGS Clinical Practice Committee 1996; Nawaz and Katz 1999).[10]

Despite the determined efforts of some medical groups, health activists, and pharmaceutical companies to increase compliance, evidence on actual HRT use has generally shown that only a minority of eligible women were ever prescribed these medications, that only a fraction of women prescribed HRT filled these prescriptions, and that only a smaller fraction actually took the medications for a prolonged period (Nawaz and Katz 1999; Oddens and Boulet 1997). This pattern of use is important because the putative benefits of these drugs to prevent osteoporosis rested on the assumption that women would maintain their high estrogenic state from menopause through the rest of their lives.

Starting in 2000 analysis of data from the Women's Health Initiative (WHI) suggested no benefit in terms of heart disease, stroke, or dementia and a slight risk of breast cancer in the treatment group, eventually resulting in a premature ending of the trial in July 2002 (Rossouw et al. 2002).[11] Along with the coincident reporting of data from other randomized clinical trials, the results of the WHI led to policy statements recommending caution or discontinuation of HRT use to prevent chronic disease. Not surprisingly, this led to a very rapid decline in its use, not only for chronic disease prevention but also for treatment of menopausal symptoms, since in practice the two purposes were often combined.

This history implies the need for greater public and professional skepticism toward attempts to (1) classify as noncompliant patients and doctors who do not follow national consensus recommendations and (2) bring uniformity through research and educational campaigns (Lomranz 2000; Clinkingbeard et al. 1999; Berman, Epstein, and Lydick 1997; Mattsson, Stadberg, and Milson 1996; Limouzin-Lamothe 1996; Stumpf and Trolice 1994; Pitkin 2002;

Lachowsky 2002). The lesson here is to recognize that there may be much latent wisdom among skeptical individuals and groups that is either missing or not accurately accounted for in the ways that prevention policies are ordinarily evaluated and formulated.

Some of the many prescient physicians and women who were skeptical of HRT use in the 1980s and 1990s may have understood the ability of narrow interests to set the agenda and timing of the prevention landscape. Some skeptics may also have been intuitively repelled by the hubris of conceptualizing women's bodies as needing replacement hormones. Others may have discounted the presumed benefits of HRT because they knew that most people were unlikely to take any medicine daily for the rest of their lives. Certainly these factors contributed to my own reluctance to initiate discussions of the preventive use of HRT with my patients during this period. Many physicians and consumers have also worried about the dangers of new putative risk-reducing drugs because of the fate of other highly promoted medications in the recent past, from the 1950s campaigns to promote DES as a fertility drug to the more recent promotion of phen-fen medications for weight loss, as well as the earlier discovery of the risk of endometrial cancer from HRT. A related policy implication, then, is to understand diversity of opinion and practice as a positive factor—and possible source of leverage—in the complex social negotiations over and response to health risks.

We might also more carefully scrutinize those actions of researchers, activists, and clinicians that blur the boundaries between treatment and prevention, and between the relief of symptoms and the promise of continued health. Many women and physicians accepted the risks of sex hormones in treating menopausal symptoms prior to widespread use of these drugs for prevention. This chronology may have contributed to what seems, in retrospect, to have been an overly low threshold for prescribing and using these drugs to prevent chronic disease. This may have resulted from the fact that they were often prescribed for their presumed double effect (treating menopausal symptoms and reducing risk of CHD and osteoporosis).[12]

We might also scrutinize more carefully the increasingly popular resolution of prevention controversies: if the evidence cannot lead to blanket recommendations, decisions should be left to the individual doctor and patient. While this conclusion is perhaps the only way to reach a consensus, it is important to bear in mind that it is not market-neutral. The mid-1990s consensus that the decision to initiate HRT to prevent osteoporosis and CHD was best made by women themselves, in consultation with their doctors, translated directly to advertising campaigns aimed at prospective users and to large profits for drug companies. Even a small share of the potential market of all eligible post- or perimenopausal women is very large in absolute terms.

Policy-making groups might be better off taking more decisive stands than leaving prevention decisions to the individual doctor and patient. Uncertainty is not the same as free choice. If expert policy groups cannot come to an informed judgment, why expect the average American to exercise judgment by default? The equation of uncertainty with choice might be more actively resisted in many policy decisions (for example, federally sponsored consensus groups could be urged to acknowledge no consensus rather than calling for shared decision making).[13]

The fact that pharmaceutical companies and other groups can potentially manage the flow of scientific data by the timing and intensity of funding, by defining the questions they are willing to fund, and by taking advantage of or manipulating the inherent limitations of studies suggests the need for some oversight over how health risks are *discovered* and made *visible*. A similar policy response also follows from the fact that much of the *demand* for HRT use was generated by women's groups and interested health-care workers who genuinely wanted to make women live longer and healthier lives and who felt that they were redressing a historical neglect of older women's health issues. These groups and individuals drew credibility and power from the resonance of this message throughout the medical and lay community, as well as its obvious appeal to pharmaceutical concerns. Thus we are in need of policy activity that provides some counterweight to the power and influence of moral entrepreneurs with a financial or professional stake in the success of particular health risks and disease-prevention practices. Good intentions do not immunize them from advocating bad policies. The moral and material synergy among these different actors requires careful analysis and a strategic response.

At the same time, other individuals and groups were marginalized in the clinical and policy response to the putative health risks posed by "hormone deficiency." Critical commentary on the dangers of medicalizing normal aging and the hegemony, narrow perspective, economic bias, and sexism of medical and pharmaceutical promoters of HRT largely occurred on different turf from the medical controversy over efficacy and risk that played out in medical journals and consensus conferences.

Taken together, these historical observations represent an argument for policy mechanisms that make visible and better incorporate the perspectives of the many social critics who have pointed out the limitations in how knowledge of health risks is generated, legitimated, and used as the basis for action. We may need to develop or encourage new activist, lay constituencies that would balance the message of powerful and appealing coalitions with a compelling message about caution, iatrogenic risk, and medical hubris. We have not tapped the potential of the unorganized but numerous individuals who are unhappily medicalized, suffer side effects of screening or prevention practices, and pay the economic costs of expensive but useless or marginally beneficial prevention practices (Schwartz et al. 2004).[14] These voices ought to be heard more clearly in prevention debates and might constitute a force with wide societal credibility. Adding these voices to policy-making processes would allow simultaneous consideration of the apples and oranges of cultural criticism and medical data. For example, such groups might have weighed the advantages and disadvantages of medicalizing menopause, conceptualizing women's bodies as hormone deficient, or viewing osteoporosis as a female disease, at the same time that there was a critical appraisal of medical and epidemiological data.

This new kind of prevention oversight body might work under the auspices of a prestigious scientific body like the Institute of Medicine. A dose of realism is needed here, however. Policy change will only occur if the rationale is made visible and compelling to actors in the political process—and there has been little societal or medical awareness of the need for such upstream prevention policy interventions.

Lastly, the social history of HRT use in American society reminds us that other approaches to improving the health of the elderly have been neglected by the way the problem was conceptualized and evaluated in the *discovery* stage. Conceptualizing osteoporosis as a latent condition emanating from hormonal loss in menopause, to be cured by a pill, has narrowed policy options. A self-evident consequence has been the myopic lack of interest in male bone weakness. The focus on maintaining bone density through drugs also shifted attention away from the problem of older women breaking hips or knees, whether from "thin" bones, losing their balance or ability to walk, or neglecting their diet or exercise. More generally, the construction of these risks as individual medical problems to be solved by drugs discourages a population approach. Defining the policy debate as weighing evidence about HRT use and demineralization, for example, obscured the formulation of the problem as one of injury prevention. Compared to the considerable societal angst over HRT use, there has been little interest in a population approach to injury prevention through better housing, reduced poverty, less social isolation, and greater social services.

## Conclusion

I have suggested that we need new sorts of oversight, debate, and influence over how risks are discovered, promoted, and made objects of disease prevention. Such policies might include changing priorities for risk-related research that attempts to find some balance between the potential downstream benefits and the costs of such research. We might begin with new types of regulatory bodies with purview over publicly and privately financed health research, which would more closely scrutinize the research and development of screening technologies that have no proven means of effective treatment or evasion (for example, some screening tests for genetic risk of common diseases, such as Alzheimer's).[15]

Just raising the issue of constraining research necessarily and rightfully invites a broad debate. The policy response to this problem is complex, in part because unconstrained scientific inquiry, technological innovation, and market freedom are highly valued. It is also difficult to know what kinds of knowledge will eventually prove useful. On the other hand, the sheer magnitude of the health risks that can be forged from associations between genetic and other health outcomes forces us to ask whether certain types of health-risk research need regulation at the early stages of their development. This complex political, ethical, and scientific debate is unavoidable because different individuals and groups stand to gain or lose depending on which risks and practices are accepted. Historical analysis can contribute to this debate by identifying developments which were not inevitable and which might have been subject to more explicit debate and policy intervention.

Existing forms of practice regulation, such as our shortsighted regulatory focus on new drugs with limited indications, may need to be reevaluated. We need to do a better job of monitoring and regulating the efficacy and safety of prevention technologies, drugs, and practices in the shifting and ambiguous contexts in which they are actually used. We may want to examine and regulate tests and drugs whose context of use has shifted (not merely when manufacturers request a change in product indication and labeling) as if they were entirely new tests and drugs.

We might also want to better scrutinize how health risks are promoted and publicized. Commercial sponsorship of research may need greater checks than our current protections, such as disclosure of funding and peer review in scientific publications. I have suggested that our public-health goals might be expanded to include educational campaigns intended to influence medical and consumer risk-related attitudes and behaviors, such as those aimed at recognizing and preventing medicalization and iatrogenesis as much as putative health risks.[16]

Other relatively unexplored policy responses might be considered. Can we better integrate the cultural and political critique often passionately advanced by lay activists with the processes and outcomes of evidence-based scientific review? Can we find better ways to empower and make visible the interests of the many individuals who are affected by the overselling of health risks because of increased cost and inconvenience, iatrogenic mishaps, or unwelcome messages about their health and lifestyle choices? While these and other questions raised by situating health risks in their social and historical context are difficult to answer, we have ample reasons to begin asking them.

## Notes

1. Compiled by the Pharmaceutical Research in Management and Economics Institute (PRIME), University of Minnesota, for Families USA from data published by the Pennsylvania Pharmaceutical Assistance Contract for the Elderly (PACE) and data found in the Price-Chek PC published by Medi-Span (Facts and Comparisons, Indianapolis), May 2002. I cite forty-six, rather than the fifty drugs listed, because four were different dosages of the same drug (Families USA Foundation 2002).

2. While there are democratizing trends in environmental policy, they mostly concern extremely important yet necessarily "downstream" regulatory processes. In a report on the lax industry-centered attitude of the Reagan administration toward carcinogen regulation and cancer policy, Wines (1983) reported that the Reagan administration's "soft" approach to cancer policy and carcinogen regulation, "usually with an eye toward easing the burdens on the makers and users of chemicals," was hampered by media attention and political response to scandals and mismanagement at EPA. Activists have also been able to use knowledge about environmental health risks (e.g. associations between environmental exposures and cancer and birth defects) as a rallying cry for political action to deal with the environment (Burger 1990). It is also worth noting here that the scientific consensus about the reality and magnitude of environmental dangers is often so contested that the democratizing impulse in policy making has shifted to the credibility of the processes by which regulations and knowledge get produced rather than the scientific basis of policies or knowledge. Jasanoff (1992) argued that the Environmental Protection Agency in the 1970s epitomized a new kind of public science, one in which scientific research and analysis was carried out, in an open forum, for the regulation of risks to health, safety, and the environment. A central development was the EPA's shift from an emphasis on testable knowledge claims to a preoccupation with the process of knowledge production. In other words, the credibility of an important policy making body now derives more from the open and balanced ways that its policies are produced rather than confidence in the evidentiary basis of those policies. Given the difficulty of ever achieving closure on conflicting interpretations of data on health risks, a similarly ambivalent conclusion might be the best we could hope for if disease-prevention policy were to become a more centralized, federal activity.

3. Armstrong's argument is not that alcohol is safe for the developing fetus, but that the appearance of the new diagnosis *fetal alcohol syndrome* at a particular time as

well as the reach and implications of this new diagnosis were much more heavily shaped by social influences than directly determined by research results.

4. What has been controversial is not the existence of prolapsed valve itself or its association with later clinical problems such as valve infection, but the attribution of different cardiac and especially "constitutional" symptoms to the prolapsed valve.

5. There is a growing literature and debate about the role of lay advocacy in a wide range of health policies. Steven Epstein's (1996) analysis of AIDS activists emphasizes the changing, innovative, and, in his view, generally constructive engagement between them and clinicians, investigators, and policymakers in the context of drug development, clinical research, and policy making. In contrast, Marcia Angell's (1997) analysis of the role of lay activists in the visibility of the idea that silicone breast implants cause connective tissue disease stresses the problematic alliance between these groups and personal injury lawyers, their antagonism to mainstream medical researchers and publications, and their undue power to influence federal regulators.

6. Public-health campaigns to get women to see doctors early promoted surgery, yet age-specific death rates did not budge. A growing minority of physicians questioned both the wisdom of the educational campaign and the efficacy of surgery. One solution was to detect cancer even earlier, via mammography.

7. At least ten prospective trials evaluating radiograph screening and/or sputum cytology were begun in the 1951–1975 period. The studies had heterogeneous designs and goals. While some but not all studies reported significant advantages among those screened in terms of "half-way" endpoints such as greater numbers of cancers found, earlier cancer stage at diagnosis, and duration of survival from time of diagnosis, there was no consistent and clear evidence of decreased lung cancer mortality. However, the methodological weaknesses in these studies were comparable to problems in screening research in other diseases in which demand for prevention interventions continued to run high. In these other situations, e.g., mammography for women younger than fifty, weak or negative research findings in studies with methodological problems did not lead to closure of debate and falling off of medical and lay interest. In lung cancer screening, there have been only a few, isolated voices who have argued against the conventional wisdom that screening confers no mortality benefit (see the challenge to the prior consensus posed in Strauss 2000; 1999). In the 1990s, there was renewed interest in lung cancer screening using new technology (e.g., spiral CAT scans) but there continues to be much less public or medical interest in this research than in breast cancer screening.

8. This selective and schematic review of HRT use is based on my own clinical experiences as well as a sampling of the clinical, policy, and social science literature in this highly contentious area. Given how visible this controversy has been, I want to anticipate two a priori objections to finding heuristic value for health policy in this history. First, it might seem implausible to suggest that there might have been even more societal oversight of, and debate about, these practices than that which occurred over the last twenty-plus years. This oversight and debate, however, did not prevent millions of women from taking these hormones to reduce their risk of chronic disease. In retrospect at least, there may have been room for more effective and timely types of societal scrutiny. Second, it could be argued that the success of the Women's Health Initiative (WHI, discussed below) in resolving this controversy proves that current policy mechanisms, especially the use of the placebo-controlled, randomized clinical trial (RCT) as the ultimate mediator, need no improvement.

Despite the remarkable success of the WHI in resolving many aspects of the HRT controversy, we cannot rely on RCTs to settle every prevention controversy in a timely manner. Even in the case of HRT, the WHI's results appeared over twenty years after observational data were first used to suggest a rationale for prescribing female hormones to prevent osteoporosis and heart disease. There are also significant methodological, economic, interpretive, and ethical problems associated with RCTs that make it impossible to deploy in the study of many other preventive practices, e.g., how could one test the effectiveness of PAP smear by an RCT with a "no testing" arm given medical and popular beliefs about the tests effectiveness as a screening tool?

9. For examples of such pharmaceutical sponsorship of research and researchers, see de Aloysio et al. (1999), Pickar et al. (1998), Rossouw et al. (2002), Varas-Lorenzo et al. (1998 and 2000). It is difficult to gauge the extent of this influence, in part because full disclosure of possible financial conflict of interest has been a requirement of journal editors only in recent years. For a good discussion of these issues in the context of HRT use, see Palmlund (1997).

10. Given realities such as the complexity of the data on HRT and the physician's role in prescribing and framing information about risks and benefits, the exact meaning and contours of this autonomy was and remains unclear.

11. The trial was stopped as a result of a complex scientific and ethical judgment about the strength and meaning of the data at a particular point in time. Although the data was by no means unambiguous, the premature ending of the trial made it very difficult, for example, to see and therefore weigh the expected benefit in preventing osteoporosis, the study seems to have been the death knell for the preventive use of these drugs and perhaps even for the wide-scale use of these drugs for the treatment of menopausal symptoms.

12. In addition to the conflation of prevention and treatment, HRT was also marketed as preventing and treating multiple risks such as heart disease, osteoporosis, depression. This was part of a larger appeal that allowed promoters of these drugs to claim highly specific benefits/risk reduction yet having the appeal of setting the body back to normality by working at multiple levels. This is clear in the phrase ultimately most popular for these drugs when used as preventives—*hormone replacement therapy*. These drugs served to fill a gap in the average women who "lost" hormones. We need to be very careful about the emotional and pre-logical appeal of returning the body to some hypothesized normal and natural state via unnatural interventions, especially when supported by such semantic sleight of hands. Eventually, even the official organs of scientific research (NIH) recognized these problems, renaming, in October 2002, HRT as "menopausal hormone therapy" (Kolata 2002).

13. Some observers have pointed out that modern norms and ideals about patient autonomy and informed consent arose in situations like HRT, where a modest and future benefit had to be weighed against small but highly feared risks like endometrial cancer (Kaufert and McKinlay 1985).

14. A recent survey about cancer-screening attitudes and experience found that 38% of the sample of 500 U.S. adults reported they had experienced at least one false positive result on one of three cancer-screening tests (11% for Prostatic Specific Antigen tests, 30% for Pap smears, 35% for mammography). Many of those subjects with false positives waited over a month before finding out they did not have cancer, and reported that this was "very scary" or the "scariest time" of their lives. But before

we jump to the conclusion that such data suggest that all we need is some "tipping point" agitation to create a mass movement of cancer detection skeptics, some 98% of this sample reported that they were glad they had been screened (Schwartz et al. 2004).

15. Regulation of privately financed research raises many complex legal and ethical issues but it is worth noting examples in which shifting medical and popular opinion has rapidly changed the way privately financed research is carried out. I am thinking of the recent rush of announcements from pharmaceutical firms that all research, including negative studies, would be made public and centrally registered.

16. It is not clear who has the credibility and authority to make such judgments—especially given uncertain evidence and the fact that different groups stand to win or lose as a result of particular policies. However, the situation is no different from our current disease-prevention landscape, which is to say we are in need of more transparency and greater representation of different interests in prevention policy formulation.

## References

AGS Clinical Practice Committee. 1996. Counseling Postmenopausal Women about Preventive Hormone Therapy. *Journal of the American Geriatrics Society* 44: 1120–1122.

Albright, F., and P. H. Smith, et al. 1941. Postmenopausal Osteoporosis. *Journal of the American Medical Association* 116: 2465–2474.

Alibhai, S. M., and P. A. Rochon. 1998. The Controversy Surrounding Cholesterol Treatment in Older People. *Geriatric Nephrology and Urology* 8, no. 1: 11–14.

American College of Physicians. 1992. Guidelines for Counseling Postmenopausal Women about Preventive Hormone Therapy. *Annals of Internal Medicine* 117, no. 12: 1038–1041.

Angell, M. 1997. *Science on Trial: The Clash of Medical Evidence and the Law in the Breast Implant Case.* New York: W. W. Norton.

Armstrong, E. M. 1998. Diagnosing Moral Disorder: Why Fetal Alcohol Syndrome Appeared in 1973. *Social Science and Medicine* 47, no. 12: 2025–2042.

Aronow, W. S. 2002. Should Hypercholesterolemia in Older Persons Be Treated to Reduce Cardiovascular Events? *The Journals of Gerontology,* Series A: *Biological Sciences and Medical Sciences* 57, no. 7: M411–413.

Aronowitz, R. A. 1992. From Mylalgic Encephalitis to Yuppie Flu: A History of Chronic Fatigue Syndromes. In *Framing Disease,* eds. C. Rosenberg and J. Golden, 155–184. New Brunswick, NJ: Rutgers University Press.

———. 1998. The Social Construction of Coronary Heart Disease Risk Factors. In *Making Sense of Illness: Science, Society, and Disease,* ed. R. A. Aronowitz, 111–144. Cambridge: Cambridge University Press.

———. 2001. Do Not Delay: Breast Cancer and Time, 1900–1970. *Milbank Quarterly* 79, no. 3: 355–386.

Berman, R. S., R. S. Epstein and E. Lydick. 1997. Risk Factors Associate with Women's Compliance with Estrogen Replacement Therapy. *Journal of Women's Health* 6, no. 2: 219–226.

Blood Tests for Cancer. 1947. *Science News Letter* 13 September: 163.

Burger, E. J., Jr. 1990. Health as a Surrogate for the Environment. *Daedalus* 119, no. 4: 133–153.

Cleeman, J. I., and C. Lenfant. 1987. New Guidelines for the Treatment of High Blood Cholesterol in Adults from the National Cholesterol Education Program. From Controversy to Consensus. *Arteriosclerosis* 7, no. 6: 649–650.

Clinkingbeard, C., B. A. Minton, J. Davis, K. McDermott. 1999. Women's Knowledge about Menopause, Hormone Replacement Therapy, and Interactions with Healthcare Providers: An Exploratory Study. *Journal of Women's Health and Gender Based Medicine* 8, no. 8: 1097–1102.

Davis, E., N. M. Strandjord, and L. H. Lanzl. 1966. Estrogens and the Aging Process. *Journal of the American Medical Association* 196, no. 3: 129–134.

de Aloysio, D., M. Gambacciani, M. Meschia, F. Pansini, A. B. Modena, P. F. Bolis, M. Massobrio, G. Aiocchi, and E. Perizzi. 1999. The Effect of Menopause on Blood Lipid and Lipoprotein Levels. The Icarus Study Group. *Atherosclerosis* 147, no. 1: 147–153.

Eisenberg, J. M. 1991. Should the Elderly Be Screened for Hypercholesterolemia? *Archives of Internal Medicine* 151, no. 6: 1063–1065.

Epstein, S. 1996. *Impure Science: AIDS, Activism, and the Politics of Knowledge.* Berkeley: University of California Press.

Evanoff, H., N. Checkowat, N. Weiss, and L. Rosenstock. 1993. Periodic Chest X-Ray for Lung Cancer Screening: Do We Really Know It's Useless? Abstract, presented to the Annual Meeting of the Robert Wood Johnson Foundation Clinical Scholars Meeting, Ft. Lauderdale, Fla.

Families USA Foundation. 2002. *Bitter Pill: The Rising Prices of Prescription Drugs for Older Americans.* Families USA Publication No. 02–104. Washington, DC: Families USA. Also available at <http://www.familiesusa.org/site/DocServer/BitterPillreport .pdf?docID=261> (accessed 26 May 2004).

Froom, J. 1991. Blood Cholesterol Lowering in Elderly Patients. *Journal of the American Board of Family Practice* 4, no. 1: 61–62.

Gawande, A. 1999. The Cancer-Cluster Myth. *The New Yorker* 8 February, 34–37.

Gordon, G. S. 1961. Osteoporosis Diagnosis and Treatment. *Texas State Journal of Medicine,* 740–747.

Hunt, K. 1994. A Cure for All Ills? Constructions of the Menopause and the Chequered Fortunes of Hormone Replacement Therapy. In *Women and Health: Feminist Perspectives,* eds. S. Wilkinson and C. Kitzinger, 141–165. London: Taylor and Francis.

Jasanoff, S. 1986. *Risk Management and Political Culture.* New York: Russell Sage Foundation.

———. 1992. Science, Politics, and the Recognition of Expertise at EPA. *Osiris* 7: 192–217.

Kaufert, P. A., and S. M. McKinlay. 1985. Estrogen-Replacement Therapy: The Production of Medical Knowledge and the Emergence of Policy. In *Women, Health, and Healing: Toward a New Perspective,* eds. E. Lewin and V. Olesen, 113–138. New York: Travistock Publications.

Klein, R., and L. J. Dumble. 1994. Disempowering Midlife Women: The Science and Politics of Hormone Replacement Therapy. *Women's Studies International Forum* 17, no. 4: 327–344.

Kolata, G. 2002. Replacing replacement therapy. *New York Times,* 27 October, WK2.

Lachowsky, M. 2002. Estrogen Therapy: From Women's Choice to Women's Preference. *Climacteric* 5: 246–249.

LaRosa, J. C. 2002. Justifying Lipid-lowering Therapy in Persons > /=65 Years of Age. *American Journal of Cardiology* 90, no. 12: 1330–1332.

Limouzin-Lamothe, M. A. 1996. What Women Want from Hormone Replacement Therapy: Results of an International Survey. *European Journal of Obstetrics and Gynecology and Reproductive Biology* 64: S21–24.

Lomranz J., D. Becker, N. Eyal, A. Pines, and R. Mester. 2000. Attitudes Towards Hormone Replacement Therapy Among Middle-Aged Men and Women. *European Journal of Obstetrics and Gynecology and Reproductive Biology* 93, no. 2: 199–203.

MacPherson, K. I. 1993. The False Promises of Hormone Replacement Therapy and Current Dilemmas. In *Menopause: A Midlife Passage*, ed. J. Callahan, 145–159. Bloomington, IN: Indiana University Press.

Mattsson, L. A., E. Stadberg, and I. Milsom. 1996. Management of Hormone Replacement Therapy: The Swedish Experience. *European Journal of Obstetrics and Gynecology and Reproductive Biology* 64: S3–5.

Meema, E., and S. Meema. 1968. Prevention of Postmenopausal Osteoporosis by Hormone Treatment of the Menopause. *Canadian Medical Association Journal* 99, no. 6: 248–251.

Natchigall, L. E., R. H. Natchigall, R. D. Natchigall, and R. M. Beckman. 1979. Estrogen Replacement Therapy I: A 10-Year Prospective Study in the Relationship to Osteoporosis. *Obstetrics and Gynecology* 53, no. 3: 277–281.

Nawaz, H., and D. L. Katz. 1999. American College of Preventive Medicine Practice Policy Statement. Perimenopausal and Postmenopausal Hormone Replacement Therapy. *American Journal of Preventive Medicine* 17, no. 3: 250–254.

New Jersey Department of Health. 2003. *Case Control Study of Childhood Cancers in Dover Township (Ocean County), NJ Vol. 1, Summary of the Final Technical Report.* http://www.state.nj.us/health/eoh/hhazweb/case-control_pdf/Volume_I/vol_i.pdf (accessed 15 September 2004).

Oddens, B. J., and M. J. Boulet. 1997. Hormone Replacement Therapy among Danish Women Aged 45–65 Years: Prevalence, Determinants, and Compliance. *Obstetrics and Gynecology* 90, no. 2: 269–277.

Oliver, M. F. 1997. Should We Treat Hypercholesterolaemia in Patients Over 65? *Heart* 77, no. 6: 491–492.

Palmlund, I. 1997. The Marketing of Estrogens for Menopausal and Postmenopausal Women. *Journal of Psychosomatic Obstetrics and Gynecology* 18, no. 2: 158–164.

Pickar, J. H., R. A. Wild, B. Walsh, E. Hirvonen, and R. A. Lobo. 1998. Effects of Different Hormone Replacement Regimens on Postmenopausal Women with Abnormal Lipid Levels. Menopause Study Group. *Climacteric* 1, no. 1: 26–32.

Pitkin J. 2002. Compliance with Estrogen Replacement Therapy: Current Issues. *Climacteric* 5: 12–19.

Quill, T., M. Lipkin, and P. Greenland. 1988. The Medicalization of Normal Variants: The Case of Mitral Valve Prolapse. *Journal of General Internal Medicine* 3, no. 3: 267–276.

Rahn, D. W. 2001. Lyme Vaccine: Issues and Controversies. *Infectious Disease Clinics of North America* 15, no. 1: 171–187.

Roberts, C. 2002. 'Successful Aging' with Hormone Replacement Therapy: It May Be Sexist, but What If It Works? *Science as Culture* 11, no. 1: 39–60.

Rossouw, J. E., G. L. Anderson, R. L. Prentice, A. Z LaCroix, C. Kooperberg, M. L. Stefanick, R. D. Jackson, S. A. Beresford, B. V Howard, K. C. Johnson, J. M. Kotchen, and J. Ockene, Writing Group for the Women's Health Initiative Investigators. 2002. Risks and Benefits of Estrogen Plus Progestin in Healthy Postmenopausal Women: Principal Results. From the Women's Health Initiative Randomized Controlled Trial. *JAMA* 288, no. 3: 321–333.

Schwartz, L., S. Woloshin, F. J. Fowler, and H. G. Welch. 2004. Enthusiasm for Cancer Screening in the United States. *Journal of the American Medical Association* 291, no. 1: 71–78.

Strauss, G. M. 1999. Screening for Lung Cancer: An Evidence-based Synthesis. *Surgical Oncology Clinics of North America* 8, no. 4: 747–774.

———. 2000. Randomized Population Trials and Screening for Lung Cancer. Breaking the Cure Barrier. *Cancer* 89, no. 11: 2399–2421.

Stumpf, P. G., and M. P. Trolice. 1994. Compliance Problems with Hormone Replacement Therapy. *Obstetrical and Gynecological Clinics of North America* 21, no. 2: 219–229.

Varas-Lorenzo, C., L. A. Garcia-Rodriguez, C. Cattaruzzi, M.B. Troncon, L. Agostinis and S. Perez-Gutthann. 1998. Hormone Replacement Therapy and the Risk of Hospitalization for Venous Thromboembolism: A Population-based Study in Southern Europe. *American Journal of Epidemiology* 147, no. 4: 387–390.

Varas-Lorenzo, C., L. A. Garcia-Rodriguez, S. Perez-Gutthann and A. Duque-Oliart. 2000. Hormone Replacement Therapy and Incidence of Acute Myocardial Infarction. A Population-based Nested Case-control Study. *Circulation* 101, no. 22: 2572–2578.

Wailoo, K. 1997. *Drawing Blood: Technology and Disease Identity in Twentieth-Century America*. Baltimore: Johns Hopkins University Press.

Watkins, E. S. 2001. Dispensing with Aging Changing Rationales for Long-term Hormone Replacement Therapy, 1960–2000. *Pharmacy in History* 43, no. 1: 23–37.

Wenger, N. K. 2002. Usefulness of Lipid-lowering Therapy in Elderly Patients. *American Journal of Cardiology* 90, no. 8: 870–871.

Wilson, Robert A. 1966. *Feminine Forever.* New York: Evans (with Lipincott).

Wines, M. 1983. Scandals at EPA May Have Done in Reagan's Move to Ease Cancer Controls. *National Journal* 15: 1264–1269.

Worcester, N., and M. H. Whatley. 1992. The Selling of HRT: Playing on the Fear Factor. *Feminist Review* 41: 1–26.

Wynder, E. L. 1997. Tobacco as a Cause of Lung Cancer: Some Reflections. *American Journal of Epidemiology* 146: 687–694.

Young, A. 1995. *The Harmony of Illusions: Inventing Post-traumatic Stress Disorder.* Princeton: Princeton University Press.

# The Jewel in the Federal Crown?

## History, Politics, and the National Institutes of Health

The National Institutes of Health (NIH), the United States' (and the world's) largest single funder of biomedical research, have grown enormously since World War II. Over this period, health research grew faster than other kinds of research, and the growth was greater in the United States than in other countries, in both absolute and relative terms. What are the reasons for this exceptional—and consistent—growth over six decades?

The policy story is one of bipartisan support for the National Institutes of Health through many election cycles, persisting through changes of Republican and Democratic control of Congress and the presidency. We believe this story is best understood through complementary approaches: history, political analysis, and identification of national values embraced by both major political parties. Citizen advocates emerged as credible champions for health research and academic health centers became a potent constituency. NIH stepped forward to support research during a five-year period when general support for a National Research Foundation was debated, and by the time the National Science Foundation took shape in 1950, NIH was already becoming the mainstay for health research. Other mission agencies likewise embraced basic as well as applied research. As a consequence, the United States never formed a central research ministry. The strong separation of legislative and executive branches of the U.S. government made Congress a target for health-research constituencies. All these factors converged to produce consistent, dramatic growth in health research over five decades.

## Post-World War II Growth of Research

The National Institutes of Health grew out of a single institute for federally funded research in bacteriology, which was originally created as part of the United States Public Health Service in 1887—and thus initially designed to understand infectious and contagious diseases. As disease patterns shifted, so did the federal research emphasis. The creation of the National Cancer Institute (NCI) in 1937 made the institutes plural—and also heralded new patterns for future development. NCI was unusual among federal research agencies in the prewar period—except for the Department of Agriculture—in making extramural grants to individuals and organizations outside of government as well as conducting its own in-house (intramural) research. NCI established the precedent for the flowering of research programs based on specific conditions or diseases that was to mark the politics of NIH after World War II. In the 1940s, however, the NIH was small and chiefly occupied with intramural research. It was about to begin its transformation into an extraordinary national biomedical research engine, powered by tax funds and run through sprawling organizations.

The growth of health research after World War II can be, and often is, viewed as just one more example of the rise of postwar science and technology. Government funding increased for many kinds of research, flowing from wartime experience that demonstrated the value of research and development. There is some truth to this. Federal expenditures for R&D increased more than twenty-two percent a year in the 1950s, nearly three times a quickly as overall federal expenditures, and about seven percent a year in the 1960s, in line with the growth of total federal spending in those years (U.S. Bureau of the Census 1975). The NIH budget no doubt benefited from general expansion in government support of R&D, although the absolute increase in R&D expenditures was mostly due to the buildup in the defense and then the space programs. NIH funding grew faster than the overall R&D budget, however, because it started from a much smaller base, but it accounted for less than four percent of net growth in annual R&D from 1950 to 1960 and less than eight percent from 1960 to 1970.

The remarkable attribute of NIH funding has been its steady growth, year in and year out, while funding in other major areas of R&D has fluctuated, largely in response to external events. The strong bipartisan support in Congress for NIH funding reflects the development of strong constituency groups that campaign for annual increases, the general public's concern about disease, and public faith in biomedical research.

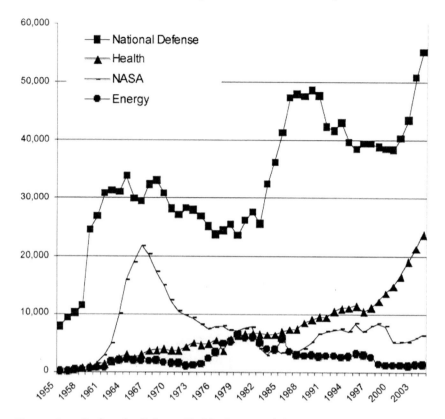

**Figure 8.1** Outlays for Defense, Health, Space, and Energy R&D, FY 1955–FY 2004 (in millions of constant dollars).

Source: OMB, Historical Tables, Budget of the U.S. Government, FY 2004, Table 9.8

In the immediate postwar period science was widely credited with helping win the war. An analysis of newspaper articles and editorials from 1945 concluded:

> Americans expected science to give them great economic, medical, and strategic benefits. Science would facilitate the return to a peacetime economy by promoting new industries that would in turn create new markets and more jobs. It was believed that science should not only ensure the country's prosperity, but would also, through scientific research in medicine, enable Americans to live healthier, longer lives. Finally, Americans expected science to provide the means to protect the healthy, prosperous nation from foreign aggressors.    (Jones 1976, 39)

Vannevar Bush, serving as President Roosevelt's wartime science advisor, captured this widely shared consensus in his report, *Science–The Endless*

*Frontier,* as the war neared its end (Bush 1945). That report is often seen as a touchstone of postwar science policy and a blueprint for government support of science. It was a seminal document, but it was not the path for postwar science.

Bush's central structural recommendation for a single agency to support research, which he called the National Research Foundation, was ultimately rejected by Congress and President Harry Truman (and after him, Dwight Eisenhower). Bush's notion that government should fund science with a light hand and respect the autonomy of the scientific community did, however, become the norm guiding a postwar R&D boom. Those policies include a preference for funding most science through grants rather than contracts, informing governmental R&D policy through elaborate systems of gathering advice from nongovernment scientists, and making scientific and technical merit (usually but not always through peer review) a primary criterion for funding projects. Merit review was not purely technical as "merit" included social need and potential social impact of the research, additional factors that helped guide planning and funding. Mechanisms to seek and heed technical advisors pervaded science policy at all levels and distinguished postwar American science from other models such as formula funding (fixed formulas for allocation) and institutional funding (allocation directly to research institutions rather than individual projects). High regard for scientific autonomy survived as a legacy of Vannevar Bush's proposals.

Vannevar Bush did not foresee, however, that the armed services would fund basic research in academia under arrangements that allowed freedom of inquiry. Bush also underestimated the biomedical research community's resolve for a separate agency, and he did not realize the importance of health-research advocates, who became a major force in championing federal funding for research to combat specific diseases. Bush was a scientific mandarin, and health advocates came largely from outside science. Struggle for control between scientists and lay advocates became a recurrent theme of health-research politics. While the two major health-research constituencies—scientists and disease research advocates—often differed over how and to what degree research should be planned and "targeted," they shared the common goal of increasing research funding.

Vannevar Bush's inattention to the disease advocate constituency that would prove so powerful in postwar health research was understandable for two reasons. First, his vision grew directly from wartime R&D experience. The signal biomedical achievement of the war was production of penicillin.

Penicillin was discovered a decade before the war in England, but its large-scale production was largely an American wartime story directed by the War Production Board and a group of American pharmaceutical companies (Kingston 2000; Swann 1988; Neushul 1993). Penicillin takes pride of place in the opening sentence of *Science–The Endless Frontier*.[1] The story of penicillin had little to do with disease advocates. It was instead a story of technical development of large-scale manufacturing driven by the need to treat soldiers' infections. Other examples of wartime biomedical successes included the development of atabrine and the discovery and development of chloroquine as antimalarials, development of better blood substitutes and methods for preserving and transporting whole blood, and the development of DDT, all conducted under the auspices of the Committee on Medical Research of the wartime Office of Scientific Research and Development (Baxter 1946).

## The Emergence of Health-Research Advocates as a Powerful Constituency

The power of disease advocacy became more apparent after the war. It reached its apogee with the discovery, development, and deployment of the polio vaccine in the early 1950s through what is now the March of Dimes (Smith 1990; Wilson 1963). Fear of polio was pervasive. President Roosevelt was infected by polio mid-career and became a champion for combating it. Grass-roots fund-raising against polio was a staple of American society, and the National Foundation for Infantile Paralysis (which became the March of Dimes) funded medical care for those affected by polio. The foundation also planned and funded a research program that culminated in the Salk and Sabin vaccines. The research, clinical testing, and initial use of the vaccines were predominantly funded through contributions to the March of Dimes, which raised on the order of $630 million between 1938 and 1962 (Wilson 1963, 66). Only about eleven percent of that total went to research, but that sum was quite large compared to other sources of funding. Indeed, it was the March of Dimes that funded James Dewey Watson when he joined Francis H. C. Crick at the University of Cambridge to discover the double helical structure of DNA (Watson and Crick 1953a; 1953b).

Private philanthropy had been the mainstay for funding biomedical research in academe before the war, most notably the Carnegie Corporation, the Rockefeller Foundation, the Guggenheim Foundation, and the March of Dimes (Köhler 1991; Smith 1990; Ginzberg and Dutka 1989). That pattern persisted for several years after the war until government funding displaced private philanthropy as the main funder of academic medical research. From the 1960s until the late 1980s, federal funding for health research also exceeded private research and development expenditures by industry.

The polio effort pushed private philanthropy to the limit. Just as polio vaccines were proving clinically effective, the March of Dimes faced successive financial crises caused by the enormous sums needed to pay for R&D and clinical care. The federal government emerged as a more robust, stable, and readily expandable source of support for biomedical research than individual organizations. Private philanthropy remained important, but these funds began to shift to supporting disease-research advocacy directed at Congress and encouraging the federal government to fund medical research.

One chief architect of the political strategy was Mary Lasker. She was married to Albert Lasker, a major figure in creating the modern advertising and public relations industry in the mid-1900s. During the war, in 1942, Albert and Mary Lasker donated $50,000 to create the Lasker Foundation to fund medical research. The real power of Mary Lasker's disease advocacy, however, took shape when she lobbied for federally funded cancer research. The NCI was not a major force in medical research during the war. Even as Vannevar Bush was writing *Science–The Endless Frontier,* Mary Lasker was creating a potent political force to promote cancer research. She joined the board of the American Association for the Control of Cancer (now the American Cancer Society), who agreed that a fourth of the funds she raised would go to research. In 1945, she and Albert Lasker helped raise four million dollars, a princely sum in its day, and five times more than the association had previously raised (Strickland 1972). Just as important, the Laskers joined forces with Florence Mahoney and her husband Daniel, who owned the Cox newspaper chain. The Lasker-Mahoney collaboration used the emerging techniques of Madison Avenue and the expanding power of public media to promote a candidate for U.S. Senate, Claude Pepper, who agreed with their foremost goal—a substantial role for the federal government in funding medical research. This funding of a political campaign by public-spirited citizens is now considered commonplace, but at the time the Laskers and Mahoneys were inventing a powerful new strategy. It won them, and their cause, long-term allies. Claude Pepper remained committed to biomedical research through his four-decade career in both the House and Senate. Lasker and Mahoney recruited more members of Congress and officials in the Executive Branch and quickly learned that the key positions were in the appropriations subcommittees that made funding decisions for NIH in Congress.[2]

James Shannon was another crucial leader in the advocacy movement. He was NIH director for much of the critical period of its growth spurt

(1955–1968). His main achievement may have been keeping his scientific colleagues from getting in the way of the disease-advocacy juggernaut. Many of his colleagues deeply distrusted lay advocates and feared science would be misdirected. Shannon, understanding the basis for the strong support of NIH funding, supported the disease-oriented categorical structure of NIH and its budget request. He concluded that no simple discipline-based structure existed and that broad groupings of diseases in institutes provided a workable focus for research. Moreover, the categorical approach had "the added advantage of being socially understandable and still amenable to balancing scientific opportunity with perceived social needs" (Shannon 1975).[3]

Lasker and other health research advocates formed alliances with Shannon and those above him in the federal Department of Health, Education, and Welfare. They forged ties to several U.S. Presidents of both parties. They were tireless advocates. Mahoney preferred to use her own network of contacts in the press and in Congress, but Lasker appreciated the skills of hired, professional full-time lobbyists to do direct work with Congress (Robinson 2004; Drew 1967).[4] Both pioneered a political strategy that argued for more funding for NIH as the only long-term solution to combat first mental illness, then heart disease, then cancer. The strategy was picked up by other groups, who formed lobbies for "their" conditions.

The fact that disease-advocacy lobbies were not attempting to pump federal dollars into their own troughs, but rather to fund research at universities, nonprofit research centers, and the government laboratories at NIH enhanced their credibility. To members of Congress, the difference was noteworthy: the mission of disease advocates was to combat disease, not to feather their own nests. While the exercise of such political power was surely a heady reward and produced a modicum of self-interest, there was a stark contrast with most industries and special interests that pleaded for appropriators' largesse. Moreover, members of Congress pushing for increased funding of research on a particular disease could feel they were promoting the general welfare, not just the local interests of their particular constituencies.

Another reason for bipartisan congressional support for medical research relates to periodic attempts to pass a national health insurance program, going back to Harry Truman's efforts in the late 1940s. It was when the national health reform effort failed in 1950 that the Laskers, who had helped fund the lobbying arm of that effort, decided to turn their attention to federal funding of research (Starr 1982, 286). Mary Lasker continued to support national health insurance and was involved in several later unsuccessful efforts to nationalize health-care financing during the administrations of Lyndon Johnson and

Richard Nixon, but she realized that she could have the greatest impact by lobbying for expanded federal research funding.[5] National health insurance
divided Congress, largely along party lines, while medical research was much
safer politically. It produced research results and a public good that could be
distributed widely, and was universally lauded. Moreover, the politics of distribution bred less conflict for legislators because decisions from merit review
panels insulated them from deciding winners and losers. A legislator who
voted for a larger NIH budget campaigned as someone who acted to improve
the nation's health, and a large increase for NIH was a small fraction of the cost
of health-care services.

## The Struggle for Control between Advocates and Scientists

The National Cancer Act of 1971 brought conflict between scientific autonomy
and lay leadership to a head (Rettig 1977). This conflict illuminated the
struggle for control, although the episode was most remarkable as a rare lack of
alignment between Shannon's and Lasker's policy preferences. Mary Lasker
and her allies were frustrated with the pace and direction of leadership for cancer research at NIH. They argued strongly for moving the National Cancer Institute out of NIH, giving it direct presidential authority, and mounting a
well-funded, concerted effort to conquer cancer. Legislation to this effect was
introduced. After a series of hearings convened by Congressman Paul Rogers,
Congress rendered its verdict by passing the National Cancer Act. NCI
remained within NIH, but with some special authorities: a "bypass budget"
that was to go directly to the President and Congress for approval without tran-
siting normal departmental channels; a President's Cancer Panel to monitor
progress and report roadblocks directly to the President; and presidential
appointment of the NCI director.

Shannon and others at NIH and in academic medicine fought hard to preserve NCI within NIH, and in the end, Congress deferred to this scientific elite.
When disease-research advocates and the medical research establishment were
in alignment, they were a powerful force. When the lay advocates came into
direct conflict with the technical experts over the question of scientific autonomy, however, Congress backed the scientists.

James Shannon also presided over the transformation of medical schools
into strong research institutions. Appropriations for extramural awards
increased from sixty-seven percent of NIH's budget of $81.3 million in 1954
(the year before Shannon became director) to seventy-six percent of NIH's
budget of $1.6 billion in 1968 (the year he stepped down). Not only did NIH

build up support of extramural research projects and research training, largely in institutions with academic health centers, it also added programs to fund construction of research facilities (1956), general research support grants (1960), construction of community mental health centers and mental retardation research facilities (1963), grants to medical libraries (1965), education of health professionals (allied health, dental, nursing, and medical, 1968–1973), and construction of educational facilities in medical schools (1968).

The general research support grants were formula grants to health professional schools based on the amount of research performed the previous year. These were intended by Shannon to move NIH beyond "support of medical research in a narrow sense to support of the full structure and range of activities necessary to provide a sound scientific program in medicine and the related sciences for the indefinite future" (Shannon and Kidd 1961, 1400). Such grants reflected Shannon's concern that NIH had been so successful in funding research in academic health centers that they were becoming too dependent on federal funding, which was distorting their educational and health-care-delivery missions.

The programs for health professional education and construction of medical facilities came to NIH through a reorganization of the Public Health Service (PHS) in 1968 that transferred the Bureau of Health Professions to NIH. Shannon campaigned for the transfer, arguing that having one agency administer all programs affecting medical schools would provide a more balanced relationship between the federal government and the medical schools. Now NIH would support the conduct of research, training of future researchers, training of health professionals, and construction of biomedical research and educational facilities. Although the "manpower" bureau only stayed in NIH for five years, and extramural construction funding soon disappeared, NIH helped a major constituency, academic health centers, expand substantially in size and quality in the 1950s and 1960s.

The rise of the academic health center—research universities that included a medical school—was in large part the result of federal policy, and a legacy of James Shannon's guiding philosophy. NIH grew through support of fundamental science, with some attention to clinical application, but moved NIH further and further from its roots in public health—and gave relatively little attention to the system of health care delivery. Over the course of six decades, NIH's growth and its focus on cellular and molecular biology led to a disproportionate growth of life sciences within academic research institutions. A 2004 RAND study noted that two-thirds of the $21.4 billion in federal funds going to colleges and universities went to the study of life sciences, and forty-five percent of funds from the Department of Health and Human Services (mainly NIH) went to medical schools (Fossum et al. 2004).

## The Emergence of Pluralistic Support of U.S. Science through Mission Agencies

One of Vannevar Bush's most cherished goals was a coherent central organization for science. The pluralistic funding structure that emerged after the war thwarted Bush's push for a single designated federal R&D agency. Bush directed the wartime Office of Scientific Research and Development that funded weapons research, medical research, and even the nascent fields of social science and systems research. His proposed National Research Foundation had three major components: research to aid the military services, medical research, and research in the physical and mathematical sciences. Most national governments fund research and development through structures that more closely resemble Bush's template than Bush's own government chose to do. In the United States, support for science, including health research, came to be mainly supported through "mission agencies," that is, departments, bureaus, and agencies with responsibility for domains of government to which science and technology contribute. This was not because Congress and the executive branch considered and then rejected the arguments for a central R&D ministry, but rather because postwar science grew organically out of mission agencies in the United States. The deviation from Bush's template stems from several well-known factors in policy: struggle for control, delay, opportunism, and historical contingency.

The delay in establishing the National Science Foundation (NSF) was linked to a struggle over governance of science. President Truman strongly opposed the system of governance that Bush had proposed, in which the President would appoint "members" of the foundation who, acting as a board, would elect the director (England 1982). In Truman's view, the President should appoint the director, as he would any other agency head in the federal government. Truman's 1947 veto of the NSF bill delayed the establishment of the National Science Foundation until 1950.

Truman's impact on the decentralization of federal research—caused in part by his veto of the first NSF bill—may have been unintended, but his administration very likely would have supported decentralization as a matter of deliberate policy. *Science and Public Policy,* a 1947 report of the President's Scientific Research Board (also known as the Steelman Report after the board's chairman, John Steelman) in effect ratified decentralization by describing in detail the activities of the various R&D agencies in several volumes and only recommending an interagency coordinating committee. The Steelman Report also supported Truman's position that NSF be headed by a presidentially appointed director. But the report strongly supported the rest of Bush's Report in calling for a substantial increase in federal funding of R&D, especially basic research in universities, and for administrative arrangements that would preserve freedom of inquiry by federally funded researchers.

Meanwhile, during the period 1945–1950 opportunistic mission agencies initiated their own extramural research programs. The Navy was first, creating the Office of Naval Research (ONR) to ensure that leading academic scientists would stay involved in defense R&D (Sapolsky 1990). The Army similarly expanded the Army Research Laboratories and funded research at universities as well as government laboratories, and the Air Force Office of Scientific Research was created when the U.S. Air Force was carved out of the Army (White 2002). President Eisenhower, long annoyed by interservice rivalries, was especially frustrated when the Soviet Union shamed U.S. space science by launching *Sputnik* in 1957. Eisenhower attributed the delay in U.S. progress in space to bickering among the military services (especially between the Army and Air Force) for control of outer space for military purposes, and to dithering in Congress and the executive branch about the respective roles of military and civilian uses of space. Eisenhower created a trans-service agency to fund militarily relevant research: the Defense Advanced Research Projects Agency, more familiarly known as DARPA.[6] (*Sputnik* also fueled arguments about the need for a civilian space agency, which led to creating the National Aeronautics and Space Administration.) Across the board, the research units linked to national defense expanded.

Post-*Sputnik* government support for research also grew in health, the other policy domain area where there was broad agreement on a government role in R&D. PHS had established its extramural grant program at the beginning of 1946 with the transfer of research projects from the wartime Office of Scientific Research and Development.[7] By the time NSF was formed in 1950, the budget for health research at NIH (part of the Department of Health, Education, and Welfare) was larger than the $50 million Vannevar Bush expected to ever go toward health research through a National Research Foundation (Bush 1945; Miles 1974). The second appropriation for NSF, in fiscal year (FY) 1952, was $3.5 million, compared with NIH's appropriation of $57.7 million that year.[8] NSF's budget could never catch up, while the science-friendly administration of R&D by mission agencies made the idea of transferring basic research support from the armed services and NIH to NSF essentially moot (England 1982).

The defense R&D agencies not only began to provide substantial support to academic research, including basic research, they also accepted the notion that scientists should initiate research projects and be given substantial leeway in carrying them out. Vannevar Bush's desire to put basic research and applied defense research under an agency controlled by scientists probably stemmed from his experience in World War II, where military direction of research was often unimaginative and controlling (Bush 1970). He did not fully appreciate the degree to which military R&D leaders, as a result of the World War II experience, had become true believers in undirected basic research in the universities. ONR staff visited the campuses to offer leading scientists support of their basic research through flexible contracting arrangements, and ONR's policies and procedures became a model of government-university relations in scientific research (Sapolsky 1990).

NIH adopted this model of external peer review, although the size of its program soon expanded well beyond the project selection systems used by ONR or the wartime Committee on Medical Research. The ONR model was in turn was based on the way that foundations (such as Rockefeller) funded academic research projects before World War II (Mandel 1996). In 1947, the Steelman Report described NIH's approach: "Administration is directed toward giving the greatest amount of freedom to the researcher by reducing necessary controls to an absolute minimum. This is in keeping with the practice of private research foundations" (President's Scientific Research Board 1947).

By the time the National Science Foundation was created, therefore, the two largest domains of R&D, health and defense, were already tightly in the grip of existing research institutions embedded in departments with high-priority government missions. Research on plants and animal husbandry had long been housed in the U.S. Department of Agriculture. Then NASA was created, taking over R&D money needed for space flight and aeronautics. So it was natural that when energy and the environment emerged as policy priorities in the 1970s, the newly created Department of Energy and the Environmental Protection Agency included the funding of science in pursuit of their missions.[9] Pluralistic science was, by then, a uniquely American tradition.

Since its inception, NSF has remained smaller than the research units of the military and NIH. U.S. science has therefore been funded mainly by mission agencies, with NSF serving as a "flywheel" supporting general science and science education, with a role in gathering statistics and analyzing science policy across the board, but never acting as a research ministry. The result is no less fateful than a carefully argued policy choice by Congress and the executive branch.

The decentralized structure of American science means there is no unified "R&D budget" planned as such, as there would be within an R&D ministry. In preparing the President's budget for submission to Congress, there is no federal director of research who would be forced to consider needs for a high-energy physics facility versus research on the molecular biology of cancer, for example. Instead, the units of government that fund science send their budgets up through the administrative channels of their mission agencies. If they are part of a department like NIH, which is part of Health and Human Services, the budget goes through those departments en route to the White House Office of Management and Budget. DARPA, ONR, and the other military R&D units, which are in the Department of Defense (DOD), go through the Pentagon for their funding. The R&D budget request is included with the department's other programs, not with the R&D budget requests of other agencies.

In the congressional appropriations process, R&D budgets are similarly separated, because department and agency budgets, including their R&D funding, are considered by different appropriations subcommittees. For example, NIH is funded from a subcommittee that sets annual appropriations for the Department of Labor and the Department of Education as well as the Department of Health and Human Services. Most funding for DOD is considered by the Defense appropriations subcommittee. The Department of Energy's funding is under the jurisdiction of the Energy and Water appropriations subcommittee. Funding for the VA, NSF, NASA, and EPA is handled in another appropriations subcommittee.

Analysts do look at aggregate science budgets in both Congress and the executive branch, of course. The Science Committee in the House, for example, analyzes science across the board, and NSF gathers funding and activity statistics for R&D throughout the government (and the private sector); government officials in the Office of Management and Budget integrate budgets for the entire government, which often entails cross-department tradeoffs, and the full appropriations committees in both the House and Senate do likewise. Yet the vast bulk of science budgeting is done without tradeoffs between R&D funders; the tradeoffs are much more likely against other "missions" and nonresearch activities than between R&D priorities. This would not have been true in Vannevar Bush's National Research Foundation, where the director of that agency would have been forced to prepare an annual budget spanning a full range of science and technology.

The lack of a central science ministry has likely enabled the R&D components of mission agencies to grow faster than if tradeoffs had been forced between science components. If a boost for molecular biology had, year after year, required lesser increases in chemistry or physics or engineering or the kind of research funded by the Department of Energy or the Department of Defense, the growth rates for NIH might have more closely resembled those for engineering and the physical sciences.

Vannevar Bush's enthusiasm for scientific autonomy also collided with popular democracy. As noted above, President Truman rejected an agency run by and for scientists. Truman's vision and the Steelman Report paid less obeisance to scientific autonomy. Bush and the Steelman Board may have agreed on the instrumental value of science to promote public good and been in favor of federal support for science, but the Steelman Board did not regard pursuit of science as requiring radical departures from democratic governance. This supported Truman's view that science should not be completely autonomous if funded by government. Bush's Boston Brahmanism flew in the face of Truman's populist instincts and strong regard for presidential prerogative.[10]

The separation of powers in U.S. government gave the legislative branch strong control over the popular health research accounts and made Congress the principal ground cultivated by disease research advocates. Both Congress and the executive branch had a high regard for scientific expertise and they ceded considerable autonomy to scientific authority in program design and project selection, responding to assessments of technical merit and scientific opportunity. Macro-allocation and overall governance, however, remained subject to the standard democratic process. The big decisions about the overall NIH budget and the overall structure of NIH were highly political and largely decided by Congress and senior executive branch officials, with strong input from disease advocates and scientists (McGeary and Smith 2002). This compromise is a far cry from Bush's vision of scientific self-governance, but it is also far from a populist democratic ideal.[11]

### The Shift from Public Health to Basic Research

The historical evolution of NIH also helps explain the emphasis on research relative to public-health services at the federal level. At the beginning of 1946, NIH was, with the exception of some extramural grants awarded by NCI, an intramural research organization. It had been founded as the research arm of the PHS and mainly conducted research on infectious diseases and other health problems addressed by the public health system, although by the 1930s PHS leaders wanted NIH to begin to work on chronic diseases.

The main constituency of the PHS was state and local departments of public health, which the agency helped support through intergovernmental grants-in-aid under the Social Security Act of 1935. The leadership of the PHS and

NIH came from the career commissioned officer corps up to the surgeon general. Except for a few program officers at NCI, the Division of Research Grants (DRG) established at the beginning of 1946 *was* the NIH extramural program, with its staff visting universities to solicit applications for funding, organizing the study sections for peer review of grant applications, and administering the grants. (The separation of the peer review function in DRG from the program development and administration functions in the institutes came later.)

The situation changed substantially, even before Shannon became director in 1955. The extramural program quickly became NIH's largest activity and involved NIH with a whole new set of constituents, namely, researchers in universities, medical centers, and other nonprofit research institutions; academic administrators affected by the expanded infrastructure and overhead services that federal research projects required; the scientific and medical societies and associations representing the various scientific disciplines and medical specialties; and of course, the disease advocacy organizations that supported NIH budget increases. Scientists from academia and industry began to work and take leadership positions at NIH instead of becoming career PHS officers. Shannon, for example, came from the Squibb Institute for Medical Research to be associate director for research at the National Heart Institute in 1949 and became associate director of NIH in 1952 before becoming NIH director in 1955.

## The Emergence of Academic Research Centers as a Constituency

Before World War II, the PHS carried out five related functions: public health, health services to special populations (Native Americans and merchant seamen), drug regulation, health resources (facilities and personnel), and medical research. Over time, NIH changed from being the research arm of the federal public health enterprise to being the keystone of the national biomedical research enterprise, and the more it focused on biological research, especially molecular biological research, the more support it enjoyed from its new constituencies (McGeary and Smith 2002).

Shannon helped create a biomedical research enterprise based in academic health centers, which emerged as large, complex organizations with research as their primary mission. Their fate depended on NIH's budget, and NIH's budget depended in part on their technical success and on continued support in Congress and the executive branch. National organizations such as the Association of American Medical Colleges, the Association of American

Universities, the Association of Academic Health Centers, the Federation of American Societies for Experimental Biology, and dozens of others focused on continued political support for biomedical research. They generally joined hands with lay advocacy organizations and disease lobbies, except where control of the scientific agenda conflicted with the agenda for groups focused on particular diseases. Academic health centers took their place on the national stage, their fate tied to the annual NIH budget.

Even as Shannon was building a powerful constituency of academic research institutions to conduct health research, he also curtailed NIH's remaining involvement in public health. In 1956–1957, he transferred the National Heart Institute's heart disease control program and the National Cancer Institute's cancer control program to the Bureau of State Services, the public health arm of the PHS. Citizen advocates were able to reinstate the programs in the War on Cancer Act of 1971 and the National Heart, Blood Vessel, Lung, and Blood Act of 1972, and other successful public health programs, such as the National High Blood Pressure Education Program (also in 1972) have been implemented within NIH. Nonetheless, public health activities have been a relatively low priority at NIH, including research to discover and test improved public-health interventions that the Centers for Disease Control and the Health Resources and Services Administration, as the current public-health arms of the PHS, could implement.

The chasm between health services and health research widened in the 1960s, as the twin federal roles were driven apart by several events. First, in 1965, President Johnson and his advisers decided to create a new agency to administer Medicare rather than put it under PHS, which they viewed as being stodgy and unenthusiastic about Johnson's Great Society programs. Second, Johnson and then Secretary of Health, Education, and Welfare John Gardner and his successor, Wilbur Cohen, decided that a more modern and responsive bureaucracy was needed to administer Great Society health programs (e.g., Health Professions Educational Assistance Act of 1963; Nurse Training Act of 1964; Allied Health Professions Training Act of 1966; and the Health Manpower Act of 1968). In 1968, they stripped the surgeon general of his line authority over the PHS bureaus (including NIH) and his position as head of the commissioned corps of PHS officers and put the bureaus under the assistant secretary for health and scientific affairs, a politically appointed position held by Philip R. Lee, who became the first noncareer head of the PHS (Parascandola 1998). The Office of the Assistant Secretary achieved little coordination, and in 1995, Lee, back for a second tour as the assistant secretary, backed a reorganization in which his office became advisory, and the seven "operating divisions" of the PHS were reorganized to report directly to the secretary. Needless to say, the secretary of an enormous federal department had little time to coordinate the various PHS activities. Power devolved to the agencies, with attempts from time to time to pull it back to the center, such as the "One Department" campaign of former Secretary of Health and Human Services Tommy Thompson to add a layer of oversight for communications, public affairs, legislative affairs, and travel at the departmental level.

### Federal Health Research Linkages
### to Biotechnology and Pharmaceuticals

Pasteur's experimentation on fermentation and baceteriology was driven both by practical interests in brewing and wine-making as well as the desire to develop vaccines for infectious diseases of humans (and animals) (Geison 1995); his research was linked directly to industrial interests. Academic science and commercial products have been connected in obvious ways for more than a century and a half. One root of today's pharmaceutical industry is German industrial chemistry a century ago. When German patents could be disregarded by wartime adversaries in World Wars I and II, firms in France, England, the United States, and other countries built substantial pharmaceutical capacity to support the war effort and strengthened ties to academic scientists (Swann 1988). The pharmaceutical industry's strong dependence on academic science emerged as one of its most distinctive features, as corroborated by economic and bibliometric quantitative studies (Cockburn and Henderson 1996; OTA 1993).[12]

Two trends of the 1980s are particularly important to note. One was the emergence of a "biotechnology industry" comprised of companies dedicated to exploiting commercial opportunities arising from molecular and cellular biology, mainly applied to medicine and agriculture. The other was a remarkable increase in R&D funding among research-intensive pharmaceutical firms.

The term *biotechnology* was used intermittently before the 1980s, but it took its common current meaning from Wall Street analysts who used it to refer to new startup firms capitalized to exploit cell fusion and recombinant DNA technologies. These new companies were premised on technologies that grew directly out of academic and government laboratories, primarily in North America and Europe. The monoclonal antibody methods of Köhler and Milstein (1975) were discovered in the United Kingdom, but their commercial exploitation was mainly by U.S. startup firms. Even more companies stepped forward to use recombinant DNA, and a new "industry" was born. It was not actually an industry so much as a group of companies eager to use the new technologies to develop products and services—new outcroppings of existing pharmaceutical, medical device, and agricultural industries. Recombinant DNA was discovered in 1973 by Stanley Cohen and Herbert Boyer. Cohen joined the Board of Cetus Corporation in 1975, as it incorporated recombinant DNA into its business plan; Boyer helped found Genentech in 1976 (Hughes 2001). Genetech "went public" (offering stock for public sale) in 1980 with a big splash, and Cetus followed suit in 1981.

Biotechnology was well positioned to instantiate the emerging "technology transfer" framework emerging in Congress. The Bayh-Dole Act passed in 1980, which mandated efforts to commercialize inventions arising from federally funded research by encouraging grantees and contractors to secure patent rights. Stanford University filed a patent on recombinant DNA technology in November 1974 on behalf of itself and the University of California. The first of three patents was issued on December 2, 1980, just before the Bayh-Dole Act passed. The invention was a direct result of federal and nonprofit funding, acknowledging NIH, NSF, and the American Cancer Society (see U.S. Patents 4,237,224, 4,468,464, and 4,740,470). Another seminal patent for expression of proteins from eukaryotic (nucleated) cells, issued to Columbia University, was based on the work of Richard Axel and others that had been supported by federal funding. This resulted in three patents between 1983 and 1993 (see U.S. Patents 4,399,216, 4,634,655, and 5,179,017). These patents were licensed similarly by Stanford and Columbia, charging relatively low royalty rates on products that embodied use of the technology to produce valuable protein therapeutics such as insulin, erythropoietin, tissue plasminogen activator, and others. The universities did not charge licensing fees for academic institutions using the methods. Nevertheless, these patents were highly lucrative, generating hundreds of millions of dollars for the institutions over the patent term.

Recombinant DNA technology found its way into commercial use relatively quickly. Recombinant insulin was approved in 1981. Monoclonal antibodies were slower to prove commercially viable, although by the end of the 1990s many were either products themselves or were used in conjunction with instruments and reagents. Many of the patents on monoclonal antibodies were held by academic research centers or first-generation biotechnology startup firms that had grown directly out of university laboratories. When the Office of Technology Assessment analyzed the emergence of commercial biotechnology in the United States in 1984, it judged that government support for basic research was the most important determinant of U.S. dominance in biotechnology (OTA 1984). NIH was far and away the most important single funder of biotechnology-related research (OTA 1988). It is not an overstatement to say that biotechnology was spawned by publicly funded academic science.

Even as dedicated biotechnology companies came to be called an "industry," an investment boom in R&D among established pharmaceutical firms began to gather force. Most such spending remained focused on clinical trials and product development, but the companies also began to move deeper and deeper into molecular and cellular biology, overlapping with academic science, to augment the industry's "absorptive capacity" for new product ideas and new methods of drug discovery (Fabrizio 2005; Cockburn and Henderson 1998). One of the leaders of this movement toward biological science was P. Roy Vagelos, a former academic scientist who rose through the R&D ranks at Merck to become CEO. Vagelos's career embodied the trajectory from academic science to industrial R&D to commercial success, as Merck became the world's largest pharmaceutical firm for most of a decade, largely based on its R&D prowess (Vagelos and Galambos 2003).

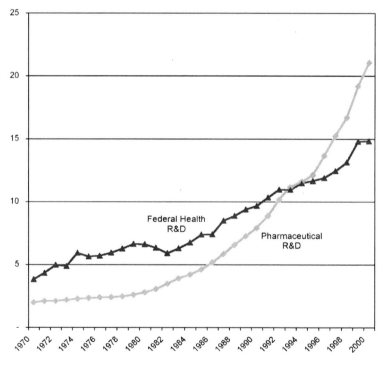

**Figure 8.2**   Federal Health R&D and Pharmaceutical R&D Expenditures 1970–2000 (in billions of 1996 dollars).

Source: National Science Foundation, Survey of Federal Research and Develpment Fundings by Budget Function, various years; Pharmaceutical Research and Manufacurers' Association, Annual Survey of R&D, various years, OMB deflator applied by authors.

Both medical biotechnology and pharmaceuticals changed in the 1990s, as marketing, strategic acquisitions, and attention to distribution networks grew in importance in determining financial success. Industrial R&D continued to draw heavily on academic science, and a highly complex mutualism developed. R&D was also vital in pharmaceuticals and biotechnology, but the grounds of competition broadened to marketing and distribution channels.

In the first years of the new twenty-first century, some fissures in the academic-industrial complex began to widen into public controversies. Longtime science and technology analyst Daniel S. Greenberg wrote about how science had come to be dominated by the self-interests of academic scientists and their institutions, and pointed to "ethical erosion" (Greenberg 2001). Bioethicist Daniel Callahan called for priorities beyond profit and life extension to guide biomedical research (Callahan 2003). Academic scholars began to reevaluate the success attributed to the Bayh-Dole Act, giving it credit for increasing academic patent activity, but also pointing to many other factors contributing to the process of converting academic science into socially valuable goods and services, most notably a very long history of academic-industrial relations in American universities and the very practical value of "open science" research results as inputs to industrial R&D (Cohen et al. 2002; Mowery et al. 2004).

A remarkable shift with portent for policy change came from scandal. A series of congressional hearings, in part a reaction to press accounts led by David Willman of the *Los Angeles Times* (Willman 2003; 2004), focused on senior administrators at NIH who received substantial payments from industry partners. A spate of books argued that the relationships between industry, academic medicine, and government had become too cozy. Two former editors of *The New England Journal of Medicine* and several academics wrote muckraking books about how the pharmaceutical industry systematically biased science in its favor (Abramson 2004; Angell 2004; Kassirer 2004; Avorn 2004; Goozner 2004). The debate was framed as "conflict of interest" and invoked powerful moral language of exploitation, greed, deceit, and corruption. The controversies had policy consequences. In September 2004, NIH seriously constrained intramural scientists' partnerships with industry, and new rules were codified in February 2005 (DHHS 2005a), as extramural academic research institutions braced for a similar storm.

The doubling of NIH's budget gave way to several years of relatively low growth, mingled with renewed concerns about scandal and conflict of interest, even as NIH's appropriation hearings became more cursory. NIH's vaunted "most favored agency" status and bipartisan congressional support seemed newly fragile, with unpredictable consequences for its continued growth.

## Conclusion

The result of NIH's focus on basic research has been a steadily expanding science budget relative to the other functions of the PHS. In FY 2004, NIH's appropriation of $27.7 billion constituted sixty percent of the total amount appropriated to the seven PHS agencies, four times the appropriation for the Health Resources and Services Administration, the next largest PHS agency, and six times the appropriation for the Centers for Disease Control and Prevention, the third largest (DHHS 2005b). In FY 1955, the NIH appropriation of $81.3 million was twenty-six percent of the overall PHS appropriation (DHEW 1955).[13]

NIH's concentration on science has immensely expanded knowledge about the biology of disease, with particular strength in molecular and cellular biology. NIH has been spectacularly successful at funding high-quality science over the long haul. That science base has greatly strengthened the biotechnology and pharmaceutical industries, which have drawn on a science commons produced through public expenditure. The relative de-emphasis of public-health and health-services research, however, has meant a weaker evidence base for general health. Lack of systematic research into health goods and services has led to a relative paucity of evidence on which to base decisions about the goods and services the federal government purchases through Medicare, Medicaid, Veterans Affairs, the Indian Health Service, and the military health services. The Agency for Healthcare Research and Quality (and its predecessors) is small, and the health-services research base has been funded through various streams, none of them remotely comparable in size to NIH's. This relative dearth of public-health research and health-services research has major implications for private sector health-care delivery as well, because no private party can take responsibility for public health, and no one payer, purchaser, or insurer can mount the research effort needed to build evidence for coverage and reimbursement decisions.

NIH's relationship to industrial R&D has grown in intensity. Before World War II, NIH was a bit player in biomedical research. By the dawn of the recombinant DNA era, it was the dominant partner. The 1980s saw a resurgence of pharmaceutical R&D and the birth of a new medical biotechnology sector; and by the end of that decade, privately funded R&D once again surpassed the NIH budget. A powerful academic-government-industrial mutualism produced a welter of goods and services, but also a complex web of relationships that called attention to conflicts of interest and allegations of corruption and avarice contaminating academic health research.

The postwar history of the NIH is thus first a story of stunning success—creating an enormously powerful engine to fund science that has fueled the development of innumerable drugs, devices, procedures, and other technical improvements in health care. It is also, however, a cautionary tale of relative inattention to public health and the delivery systems for health care, and to the powerful inducements of money—as opposed to burden of illness—on research priorities. Both the strengths and weaknesses trace their roots to fateful decisions made in the 1950s and 1960s about constituency, focus, and mission.

## Notes

Paper prepared for the Robert Wood Johnson Health Policy Investigators Program History and Health Policy Cluster Working Group.

1. "We all know how much the new drug, penicillin, has meant to our grievously wounded men on the grim battlefronts of this war—the countless lives it has saved—the incalculable suffering which its use has prevented. Science and the great practical genius of this Nation made this achievement possible" (Bush 1945, 10).

2. Lasker and Mahoney learned this the hard way. Their initial success was the drive to create the National Institute of Mental Health (NIMH) in 1947. They learned to their chagrin that authorizing legislation was one thing, while appropriations were another matter, handled by a different committee. NIMH was not funded until 1949 (Strickland 1972).

3. Shannon did not support continuing proliferation of institutes, however, opposing the establishment of the National Eye Institute in 1968, elevation of the National Institute of Environmental Health Sciences to institute status in 1969, and establishment of the National Institute on Aging in 1974.

4. Unfortunately, there is no biography of Lasker, but Elizabeth Drew's contemporaneous article captured the essence of her strategies for promoting biomedical-research funding (Drew 1967).

5. Lasker was instrumental in Johnson's establishment of the Commission on Heart Disease, Cancer, and Stroke in 1964, whose report called for a national network of heart disease, cancer, and stroke centers for research, training, and patient care. She was also a member of Walter Reuther's new committee for national health insurance in 1969.

6. DARPA is perhaps best known for its support of interactive computing and the Internet (see Norberg and O'Neill 1996). For its first year, however, it was the nation's main space agency, and it has been involved in a broad range of military research programs.

7. The authority to award extramural grants was contained in the Cancer Act of 1937 and became available to the rest of NIH when NCI and NIH were merged in the Public Health Service Act of 1944, but NCI had funded few grants and so NIH's extramural research program effectively started at the beginning of 1946. For a more detailed account of the early history of NIH grants, see Fox 1987 and Strickland 1989.

8. NSF's first appropriation in FY 1951 was for $225,000, to be used to organize the new agency, not fund programs.

9.  At the beginning of the Eisenhower Administration, the Bureau of the Budget tried again to centralize support of basic academic research in NSF but lost the battle once and for all when Eisenhower issued an executive order in 1954 that assigned "general-purpose basic research" to NSF but sanctioned continued support of basic research by other agencies "in areas which are closely related to their missions" (E.O. 10521, "Administration of research by agencies of the federal government," quoted in Penick and Pursell 1972, 34).

10. Reingold 1987. For a full biography of Bush, see Zachary 1997.

11. Columbia University philosopher Philip Kitcher (2003) describes the ideal of "well ordered science" guided by scientific opportunity, but also taking into account social need through deliberative democracy. Kitcher points to how health research deviates from this ideal, although arguably the involvement of health advocacy organizations brings it closer to that ideal in the United States than most other countries, and compared to other fields of science. Cary Gross and others have noted the correlation between NIH funding by disease and burden of illness measures (Gross, Anderson, and Powe 1999). This is grist for the mill of both NIH critics, who urge stronger weight for social need guiding scientific priorities, and NIH supporters, who note the generally positive correlations above chance suggest NIH spending does respond to the biggest health needs.

12. See also Gambardella 1995; Mansfield 1991, 1995; Narin and Olivastro 1992; Narin and Rozek 1988.

13. The Food and Drug Administration was not part of the PHS in 1955 and has been excluded, for comparative purposes, from the PHS appropriation for FY 2004 (including it would have reduced NIH's share to 51 percent).

## References

Abramson, John. 2004. *Overdo$ed America: The Broken Promise of American Medicine.* New York: HarperCollins.

Angell, Marcia. 2004. *The Truth About Drug Companies: How They Deceive Us and What to Do About It.* New York: Random House.

Avorn, Jerry. 2004. *Powerful Medicines: Benefits, Risks, and Costs of Prescription Drugs.* New York: Alfred Knopf.

Baxter, James Phinney. 1946. *Scientists against Time.* Boston: Little, Brown.

Bush, Vannevar. 1945. *Science–the Endless Frontier.* Washington, DC: Office of Scientific Research and Development.

———. 1970. *Pieces of the Action.* New York: William Morrow.

Callahan, Daniel. 2003. *What Price Better Health? Hazards of the Research Imperative.* Berkeley: University of California Press.

Cockburn, Iain, and Rebecca M. Henderson. 1998. Absorptive Capacity, Coauthoring Behavior, and the Organization of Research in Drug Discovery. *Journal of Industrial Economics* 46, no. 2: 157–182.

———. 1996. Public-Private Interaction in Pharmaceutical Research. *Proceedings of the National Academy of Sciences* 93: 12725–12730.

Cohen, Wesley M., and John P. Walsh. 2002. Public Research, Patents and Implications for Industrial R&D in the Drug, Biotechnology, Semiconductor and Computer Industries. In *Capitalizing on New Needs and New Opportunities: Government–Industry Partnerships in Biotechnology and Information Technologies,* ed. C. W. Wessner, 223–243. Washington, DC: National Academy Press.

Department of Health, Education, and Welfare (DHEW). 1955. *Annual Report of the U.S. Department of Health, Education, and Welfare.* Washington, DC: U.S. Government Printing Office.

Department of Health and Human Services (DHHS). 2005a. Interim Final Rule, Supplemental Standards of Ethical Conduct and Financial Disclosure Requirements for Employees of the Department of Health and Human Services. *Federal Register* 70: 5543–5565.

———. 2005b. *FY 2006 Budget in Brief.* www.dhhs.gov/budget/06budget/FY2006Budget inBrief.pdf (accessed 27 June 2005).

Drew, Elizabeth. 1967. The Health Syndicate: Washington's Noble Conspirators. *Atlantic Monthly,* December, 75–82.

England, J. Merton. 1982. *A Patron for Pure Science: The National Science Foundation's Formative Years, 1945–57.* Washington, DC: National Science Foundation.

Fabrizio, Kira R. 2005. Absorptive Capacity and Innovation: Evidence from Pharmaceutical and Biotechnology Firms. Unpublished working paper, Haas School of Business, University of California, Berkeley.

Fossum, Donna, L. S. Painter, E. Eiseman, E. Ettedgui, and D. M. Adamson. 2004. *Vital Assets: Federal Investment in Research and Development at the Nation's Universities and Colleges.* Arlington, VA: RAND.

Fox, Daniel M. 1987. The Politics of the NIH Extramural Program, 1937–1950. *Journal of the History of Medicine and Allied Sciences* 42: 447–466.

Gambardella, Alfonso 1995. *Science and Innovation: The U.S. Pharmaceutical Industry during the 1980s.* New York: Cambridge University Press.

Geison, Gerald L. 1995. *The Private Science of Louis Pasteur.* Princeton: Princeton University Press.

Ginzberg, Eli, and Anna B. Dutka. 1989. *The Financing of Biomedical Research.* Baltimore: Johns Hopkins University Press.

Goozner, Merrill. 2004. *The $800 Million Pill: The Truth behind the Cost of New Drugs.* Berkeley: University of California Press.

Greenberg, Daniel S. 2001. *Science, Money, and Politics: Political Triumph and Ethical Erosion.* Chicago: University of Chicago Press.

Gross, Cary P., G. F. Anderson, and N. R. Powe. 1999. The Relation between Funding by the National Institutes of Health and the Burden of Disease. *New England Journal of Medicine* 340, no. 24: 1881–1887.

Hughes, Sally Smith. 2001. Making Dollars Out of DNA: The First Major Patent in Biotechnology and the Commercialization of Molecular Biology, 1974–1980. *Isis* 92: 541–575.

Jones, Kenneth Macdonald. 1976. The Endless Frontier. *Prologue* 8, no. 1: 35–46.

Kassirer, Jerome. 2004. *On the Take: How Big Business Is Corrupting American Medicine.* New York: Oxford University Press.

Kingston, William. 2000. Antibiotics, Invention, and Innovation. *Research Policy* 29: 679–710.

Kitcher, Philip. 2003. *Science, Truth, and Democracy.* New York: Oxford University Press.

Köhler, Georges J. F., and César Milstein. 1975. Continuous Cultures of Fused Cells Secreting Antibody of Predefined Specificity. *Nature* 256, no. 5517: 495–497.

Kohler, Robert E. 1991. *Partners in Science: Foundations and Natural Scientists, 1900–1945.* Chicago: University of Chicago Press.

Mandel, Richard. 1996. *Half a Century of Peer Review: History of the Division of Research Grants 1946–1996*. Bethesda, MD: National Institutes of Health, Division of Research Grants.

Mansfield, Edwin. 1991. Academic Research and Industrial Innovation. *Research Policy* 20 February: 1–12.

———. 1995. Academic Research Underlying Industrial Innovations: Sources, Characteristics, and Financing. *Review of Economics and Statistics* 77: 55–65.

McGeary, Michael, and Philip M. Smith. 2002. Organizational Structure of the National Institutes of Health. Background paper for the National Academies' Committee on the Organizational Structure of the National Institutes of Health. Washington, DC: National Academy of Sciences.

Miles, Rufus, Jr. 1974. *The Department of Health, Education, and Welfare*. New York: Praeger.

Mowery, David C., Richard R. Nelson, Bhaven N. Sampat, and Arvids A. Ziedonis. 2004. *Ivory Tower and Industrial Innovation: University–Industry Technology Transfer Before and After the Bayh-Dole Act*. Stanford, CA: Stanford Business Books.

Narin, Francis, and D. Olivastro. 1992. Status Report: Linkage between Technology and Science. *Research Policy* 21: 237–249.

Narin, Francis, and R. P. Rozek. 1988. Bibliometric Analysis of U.S. Pharmaceutical Industry Research Performance. *Research Policy* 17, no. 3: 139–154.

Neushul, Peter. 1993. Science, Government, and the Mass-Production of Penicillin. *Journal of the History of Medicine and Allied Sciences* 484: 371–395.

Norberg, Arthur L., and Judy E. O'Neill. 1996. *Transforming Computer Technology: Information Processing for the Pentagon, 1962–1986*. Baltimore: Johns Hopkins University Press.

Office of Technology Assessment (OTA). 1984. *Commercial Biotechnology: An International Analysis*. OTA-BA-218, NTIS order #PB84-173608. Washington, DC: Government Printing Office. Also available at www.wws.princeton.edu/~ota/.

———. 1988. *New Developments in Biotechnology. U.S. Investment in Biotechnology*. OTA-BA-360, NTIS order #PB88-246939. Washington, DC: Government Printing Office. Also available at www.wws.princeton.edu/~ota/.

———. 1993. *Pharmaceutical R&D: Costs, Risks, and Rewards*. OTA-H-522. GPO stock #052-003-01315-1. NTIS order #PB93-163376. Washington, DC: Government Printing Office. Also available at www.wws.princeton.edu/~ota/.

Parascandola, John L. 1998. Public Health Service. In *A Historical Guide to the U.S. Government*, ed. G. T. Kurian, 487–493. New York: Oxford University Press. Also available at lhncbc.nlm.nih.gov/apdb/phsHistory/resources/phs_hist/pub_phs01.html.

Penick, James L., and Carroll W. Pursell, eds. 1972. *Politics of American Science, 1939 to the Present*. Revised ed. Cambridge, MA: MIT Press.

President's Scientific Research Board. 1947. *Science and Public Policy*. 4 Vols. Washington, DC: U.S. Government Printing Office.

Reingold, Nathan. 1987. Vannevar Bush's New Deal for Research; or, the Triumph of the Old Order. *Historical Studies in the Physical and Biological Sciences* 17, no. 2: 299–344.

Rettig, Richard. 1977. *Cancer Crusade: The Story of the National Cancer Act of 1971*. Princeton: Princeton University Press.

Robinson, Judith. 2001. *Noble Conspirator: Florence S. Mahoney and the Rise of the National Institutes of Health*. Washington, DC: Francis Press.

Sapolsky, Harvey. 1990. *Science and the Navy: The History of the Office of Naval Research*. Princeton: Princeton University Press.

Shannon, James A. 1975. The Background of Some Contemporary Problems. Presented at Conference No. 3 on the Biomedical Sciences, Macy Foundation. Available at Office of NIH History, Building 31, Room 5B38, MSC 2092. Bethesda, MD: National Institutes of Health.

Shannon, James A., and Charles V. Kidd. 1961. Federal Support of Research Careers. *Science*. 134, no. 3488: 1399–1402.

Smith, Jane S. 1990. *Patenting the Sun: Polio and the Salk Vaccine*. New York: William Morrow.

Starr, Paul. 1982. *The Social Transformation of American Medicine*. New York: Basic Books.

Strickland, Stephen P. 1972. *Politics, Science, and Dread Disease: A Short History of United States Medical Research Policy*. Cambridge, MA: Harvard University Press.

———. 1989. *The Story of the NIH Grants Programs*. Lanham, MD: University Press of America.

Swann, John P. 1988. *Academic Scientists and the Pharmaceutical Industry: Cooperative Research in Twentieth Century America*. Baltimore: Johns Hopkins University Press.

U.S. Bureau of the Census. 1975. *Historical Statistics of the United States, Colonial Times to 1970*. Washington, DC: U.S. Government Printing Office. Also available at www2.census.gov/prod2/statcomp/.

Vagelos, P. Roy, and Louis Galambos. 2003. *Medicine, Science, and Merck*. New York: Cambridge University Press.

Watson, James D., and F. H. C. Crick. 1953a. A Structure for Deoxyribonucleic Acid. *Nature* 171, no. 4356: 737–738.

———. 1953b. Genetical Implications of the Structure of Deoxyribonucleic Acid *Nature* 171, no. 4361: 964–967.

White, Robert P. 2002. *History of the Air Force Office of Scientific Research*. OSR Brief 0108. Arlington, VA: Air Force Office of Scientific Research. www.afrlhorizons.com/Briefs/Mar02/OSR0108.html (accessed 27 June 2005).

Willman, David. 2003. Stealth Merger: Drug Companies and Government Medical Research. *Los Angeles Times*, 7 December.

———. 2004. National Institutes of Health: Public Servant or Private Marketeer? *Los Angeles Times*, 22 December.

Wilson, John Rowan. 1963. *Margin of Safety*. Garden City, NJ: Doubleday.

Zachary, G. Pascal. 1997. *Endless Frontier: Vannevar Bush, Engineer of the American Century*. New York: Free Press.

# A Marriage of Convenience

## The Persistent and Changing Relationship between Long-Term Care and Medicaid

It is impossible to discuss the nation's need for affordable long-term care services without concurrently discussing America's Medicaid program. Since it was established in 1965, Medicaid has often, in passing, been called our health-care program for "the poor." In truth, the program has always been at once more and less than that. Medicaid is less than that meager description because it has always systematically excluded certain categories of poor people.[1] However, Medicaid is also much more than a program for "the poor" because it provides long-term care services to elderly who resided, and whose families reside, firmly in the middle class. Today, nearly seventy percent of nursing home residents are dependent on Medicaid to finance at least some of their care. While about forty percent of nursing home residents are "poor enough" to be eligible for Medicaid upon admission, another forty-five percent begin as private paying residents, spend down their resources, and eventually become Medicaid eligible (Weiner 1999; Cohen et al. 1993). Many senior citizens who receive Medicaid do not have a history of poverty, yet they have long consumed a substantial proportion of Medicaid's resources.[2] While the elderly and disabled constitute about thirty percent of program recipients, they consume about seventy percent of program expenditures (CMS website).

Policies that purport to provide a safety net for the poor yet leave millions of people uninsured and with little or no access to medical coverage, while extending "welfare medicine" to America's middle class for the provision of long-term care services, may seem unfair. Not surprisingly, policy makers have questioned the appropriateness of using Medicaid for America's long-term-care program (Grogan 2005; Grogan and Patashnik 2003a). Indeed, some policy makers, health-policy advocates, and analysts have suggested that Medicaid was a mere afterthought and never intended to be America's long-term-care program (Kane et al. 1998; Weiner, 1999).

The purpose of this chapter is to debunk that myth. I will show that the inclusion of nursing home coverage under Medicaid in 1965 was not only intentional, but front and center. The courtship between medical aid for the poor and long-term care for the elderly began unintentionally in 1935 with the establishment of Old-Age Assistance (OAA), but two important subsequent events served to intensify and solidify the relationship: the creation of medical vendor payments in 1950 and the enactment of Medical Assistance to the Aged (MAA) under the Kerr-Mills Act in 1960. From 1935 to 1965 there was a dramatic increase in the number of nursing homes. This was not an accident; it was clearly encouraged by the aforementioned public policies. These homes, supported largely with public dollars, became the primary American response to problems of chronic disease in an aging population. They were, of course, only a partial response, since individuals who must live in nursing homes because of debilitating, persistent, and sometimes multiple chronic conditions represent a small, if important, minority (only about four percent) of Americans sixty-five and over (Jones 2002). However, while the number of elderly living in institutions is relatively small, the proportion at risk for ending up in a nursing home is quite high: over half of women and almost one-third of men sixty-five years of age can expect to use a nursing home sometime before they die (Murtaugh et al. 1990).

I devote the first part of this chapter to explaining the Medicaid/long-term care (LTC) courtship by detailing the rise of nursing homes and the policies that encouraged the increase. I then turn briefly to Medicaid's enactment in 1965 to illustrate that LTC was not an afterthought; indeed, the inclusion of nursing home care was inevitable. In part three, I highlight the main tensions in this Medicaid/LTC marriage since 1965, tensions arising primarily from changes in public perceptions about both the Medicaid program and the deservingness of the elderly.

## The Courtship from 1935 to 1965

The history of the modern American nursing home industry began with a concerted effort by the federal government to close almshouses (also known as poorhouses or poor farms) and thereby abandon institutionalization as a legitimate method for addressing the concerns of poverty. Institutionalization of the poor began with fervor in the 1820s when a demographic explosion and economic changes bolstered the view that the causes of poverty could be located

squarely within the individual. With this view in mind, almshouse administrators undertook to change individual behavior through work and punishment
(Holstein and Cole 1996).

While these institutions, which housed the poor of all ages, including the
sick and mentally ill, grew quite rapidly during the nineteenth century, social
reformers at the turn of the twentieth century began designing institutions for
specific groups with an effort to reform, rehabilitate, and educate. For example,
children were sent to orphanages, the insane to mental institutions, and the
physically disabled to special schools. Not surprisingly, the chronic, incurable
condition of most elderly almshouse inmates did not fit nicely with the reform
and rehabilitation rhetoric of that time (Holstein and Cole 1996). Because there
was no "reform movement" for the elderly, they were simply left in the
almshouses. As a result, the vast majority of inmates were sick, elderly persons
with chronic conditions (Stewart 1925; Katz 1986).

While this shift happened unintentionally, many physicians and social
reformers began touting almshouses as the appropriate place not only for
poor elderly, but for the non-poor elderly who needed long-term-care services
as well. Physicians and hospital administrators liked almshouses as a solution to "caring" for elderly individuals with chronic care needs. They defined
old age as the deterioration of health and therefore favored a medical institutional model with some type of skilled care to deal with the problems of
old age (Stewart 1925; Katz 1986; Haber 1983). Hospitals, however, were
developing a new improved image as places where sicknesses could be
cured. The elderly with chronic conditions that could not be cured had no
place in these new institutions (Stevens 1971; Rosenberg 1987; Vladeck
1980). Despite this "professional" support, the general condition of almshouses continued to deteriorate, and the elderly and their families continued
to fear the poorhouse.

In the early twentieth century this fear turned into activism, coalescing
around the idea of publicly funded old-age pensions for two reasons. First, the
Depression shifted public opinion about the causes of poverty from question-
able individual behavior to forces over which the individual had no control.
As widespread unemployment, sickness, old age, and death of a spouse thrust
hard-working Americans into poverty through no fault of their own, the American public looked to the federal government to help solve the problem of basic
economic need (Katz 1986; Stevens and Stevens 1974).

Second, the horrendous, inhumane conditions of the almshouses became
more widely recognized. New Deal activists argued that old-age pensions would
allow elderly persons to live with dignity outside of such institutions (Vladeck

1980; Stevens and Stevens 1974). When the federal government passed Old-Age Survivors Insurance (OASI, what we commonly call Social Security today) and a federal-state, means-tested program (OAA) for poor elderly persons, politicians and Social Security administrators made it quite clear in the statutes that no assistance would be given to almshouse inmates (Vladeck 1980; Holstein and Cole 1996). This clause was inserted in the landmark Social Security Act of 1935 with the clear intent of closing the poorhouses.

The poorhouse did die out. However, institutional care for the elderly did not. Indeed, on the contrary, it grew (Senate Committee on Finance, January 23, 1950, 186).[3] Because many elderly people still needed services for chronic conditions and families either could not or would not care for their elderly relatives, many of the elderly used their OAA funds to pay for *private* institutional care. Historians Martha Holstein and Thomas R. Cole (1996) sum up this irony nicely: "Hatred for the almshouse created a resistance to any public provision of nursing home care; thus, the almshouse . . . led to the now-dominant proprietary nursing home industry" (29).

### Medical Vendor Payments: 1950

In 1950, states could include the cost of medical care in their determinations of need for public assistance payments (that is, payments for OAA, Aid to Dependent Families, Aid to the Blind), but they were pragmatically constrained by federally defined maximums on payment amounts. Many states argued that the federal maximums were so low that states could not include the "true" costs of medical care, and yet they argued further that it was often sickness and medical-care expenditures that then caused poverty (Senate Committee on Finance 1950; Vladeck 1980; Stevens and Stevens 1974). Moreover, several public welfare administrators realized that OAA recipients were using a large proportion of their checks to pay for nursing home care in private institutions.

In an effort to address these concerns, medical vendor payments were created under the Social Security Amendments in 1950. This program allowed states, under a separate federal financial matching formula, to pay medical providers directly for services rendered to public assistance recipients (Stevens and Stevens 1974). The bill also lifted the prohibition against federally financed cash payments to elderly persons living in public institutions. Moreover, because federal policy makers feared that medical vendor payments would be used, yet again, to finance poorhouses, a regulatory clause was included in the Social Security Amendments requiring states to establish and maintain standards so that these public institutions "met the definition of a medical institution, not just the old-fashioned poorhouse" (Senate Committee on Finance 1950, 60).

Thus, for the first time, states—with federal financial assistance—could set the level and terms of payments to medical providers including physicians, hospitals, and, most importantly, nursing homes for public assistance recipients. Moreover, a regulatory apparatus was established to begin thinking about the appropriate quality of care provided to public assistance recipients in nursing homes.

Despite these important expansionary seeds, the significance of medical vendor payments was largely overlooked at the time of the bill's passage for two main reasons. The first reason is simply that other questions seemed more pressing. The Social Security Amendments bill expanded the original bill in four other ways:

1. It called for substantial increases in benefits and expanded eligibility under OASI.
2. It created a major new category of federal–state aid to the totally and permanently disabled.
3. It included a change in the federal matching rate formula to use state per capita income.
4. It considered extending ADC (Aid to Dependent Children) eligibility to include children with needy parents (not just single or widowed mothers).

Among the state representatives coming to testify before Congress, the vast majority focused foremost on the OASI expansions. To the small extent that other issues were discussed, medical vendor payments competed for attention with these two other pressing issues. For example, among public welfare administrators from twenty different states who came to testify in favor of the 1950 Social Security Amendments, only a few even mentioned the medical vendor payment provision. When they did, no discussion ensued.

The second, and more important, reason for the lack of attention to medical vendor payments is that proponents of national health insurance then (and throughout most of Medicaid's history) viewed public assistance as a residual program that could be done away with when national health insurance was enacted. Those in favor of national health insurance did not perceive medical vendor payments as a win for their opponents (as one might presume since conservatives tended to favor relatively small means-tested approaches); rather, they viewed this provision as a small public assistance expansion that would not harm and might help some vulnerable people a little. For example, when the lone questioner, Senator Millikin from Colorado, wondered about the potential significance of this seemingly small provision, Commissioner Altmeyer—a key proponent of national health insurance from the Truman Administration—quickly assured him that any such significance could not adhere to such meager provisions for public assistance recipients:

> *Senator Millikin.* What control do they [states] have over the doctor or the theory of medicine?
>
> *Mr. Altmeyer.* I do not think they would have any control by reason of this amendment. Many states and localities now of course have made arrangements with the local doctors of one kind or another, and they would make similar arrangements under this amendment, except that they could make payments directly to the doctors instead of including an amount in the cash assistance which is then paid to the doctors.
>
> *Senator Millikin.* But at the state level the states can make any sort of regulations that they want to make so far as the payments are concerned, can they not? . . . Would some sort of restriction on the extent of that control be desirable in connection with a bill of this kind?
>
> *Mr. Altmeyer.* I do not know what restriction or control would be envisaged. I do not think it is necessary. I do not recall that it has ever been a burning question in the states. The whole problem that has vexed the welfare departments and the doctors is some way by which they can get payment as directly as possible, without a lot of red tape.
>
> *Senator Millikin.* What I am getting at is, one of the objections to the proposed social medicine plan is that in the natural tendency of governmental affairs the first thing you know the Government will be telling the doctors what medicines to prescribe and be setting up all sorts of qualifications for the doctors who receive the money, various kinds of controls, hospital rules and regulations, and so forth and so on. I am just wondering whether the same sort of objection, without discussing its merits at all, would be open to this.
>
> *Mr. Altmeyer.* . . . I do not think the same question that concerns the medical profession in the case of health insurance is involved in making the necessary arrangements to pay the medical profession or the hospitals for services given to these recipients of public assistance.
>
> (Senate Committee on Finance 1950, 57–58)

Part of the reason public assistance programs were discussed as residual is because they were usually viewed in relation to increasing social insurance. Indeed, every state-level public welfare administrator emphasized in their testimony that federally funded social insurance should be increased and federal-state public assistance would then be allowed to decrease. The following statement from Loula Dunn, director of the American Public Welfare Association, illustrates this common theme:

> I think the first and most important thing to do, Senator, is to extend and broaden your social insurances . . . the lack of balance which we find today in the number of people receiving public assistance and getting insurances is, one might say, almost the opposite of what we had hoped for at the time the Social Security Act was passed. Public assistance is larger than the insurances; and in my judgment it should be exactly the reverse. And I think if you extended your coverage and your benefits and stepped up your rate of payments, you would find that you would have a decline, then, of the pressures on your public-assistance programs. (Senate Committee on Finance 1950, 166–170)

While many policy makers agreed with the concept of increasing social insurance, there was general skepticism (even among many supporters) that a substitution effect would occur. This skepticism is illustrated by Senator Millikin's response to Ms. Dunn:

> May I suggest that your logic is impeccable; but, if I may put out a thought of my own, I doubt very much, despite the good quality of your logic, that it will decrease public assistance $1. Because public assistance is intimately related with politics in the states and at the federal level. (Senate Committee on Finance 1950, 166–170)

This concern about uncontrollably increasing government expenditures is exactly the reason why even supporters of the means-tested public assistance approach to health care were not avid supporters of medical vendor payments. For example, conservative Senator Taft, who was a strong opponent of national health insurance, said in relation to the federal government assuming the cost of medical care: "It seems to me we are getting to a point where there is just so much free cash going to so many millions of people that you are getting into a very dangerous over-all situation" (Senate Committee on Finance 1950, 72).[4]

Indeed, the creation of medical vendor payments did foster the type of supply-side political pressure that worried Senators Millikin and Taft. Health providers had a windfall to gain. While health-care providers were relatively silent about the medical vendor payment provision in the 1950 Social Security Amendments, they nonetheless understood its significance. The Inter-Association of Health, composed of top-ranking officials from the major provider groups,[5] submitted a statement in support of the need for earmarked funds (through medical vendor payments) to finance medical care for public assistance recipients. Like Senator Millikin, they understood that various financing schemes *would* influence their practice and therefore included in their statement "the further view that any provision to finance medical care for assistance recipients . . . should have the support of those six organizations" (Senate Committee on Finance 1950, 171). In a separate statement the American Hospital Association also prophetically recommended that medical assistance include long-term care for chronic diseases "because of the constantly expanding span of life of the aging population" (Senate Committee on Finance 1950, 1073). There was, however, not (yet) an established nursing home "industry." Though a variety of homes existed for a variety of purposes, they were of widely different standards and were almost entirely unregulated.

As fiscal conservatives feared, public assistance programs continued to increase in the 1950s—despite increases in OASI—in large part due to expansions in medical vendor payments. Although this particular provision did not have much financial significance in the few years following its passage, the provision allowed for a series of revisions and expansions in 1953, 1956, 1958, and 1960, culminating in the passage of Medicaid in 1965 (Poen 1982; Stevens and Stevens 1974). In 1953 a separate federal-state matching rate for medical vendor payments (apart from cash payments) was established, and the individual medical maximums and federal matching rate for vendor payments subsequently expanded in each of the years listed above. The 1946 Hill-Burton Act also provided funds for nursing home (as well as hospital) construction.[6] Taken cumulatively, these incremental expansions continued and strengthened the tie between nursing homes and public assistance that began with the public almshouse. The Kerr-Mills Act, included under the 1960 Social Security Amendments, added more fire to this courtship.[7]

### The Kerr-Mills Act of 1960

After Truman's failure to enact national health insurance and in the wake of medical vendor payments, the two camps of experts and politicians—those supporting social insurance and those supporting public assistance—shifted their positions a bit. Proponents of national health insurance decided to restrict their goals to expanding hospital benefits only for OASI beneficiaries—in other words, elderly persons over sixty-five. A series of events solidified this compromise strategy (Gordon 2003; Marmor 1973). Oscar Ewing, from the Social Security Administration (SSA), publicly proposed this limit in June of 1951,[8] and SSA's Annual Report released in April of 1952 also recommended such a limit. In addition, in April 1952, Senators Murray and Humphrey and Representatives Dingell and Celler introduced bills in Congress with this limit, and, by the end of that year, President Truman publicly endorsed such a limit (Gordon 2003; Marmor 1973). Based on this consensus, Senator Forand introduced the original "Medicare" bill in 1957, proposing universal coverage for the elderly with a restricted hospital-based benefit package administered and financed on a contributory basis by the federal government (Marmor 1973).

In response to the Forand bill and mounting public pressure to do something for the aged, Representative Wilbur Mills and Senator Kerr proposed (similar to Senator Taft before them in the 1940s) a means-tested alternative to forestall Forand's "social insurance" scheme. In general, conservative southern Democrats and Republicans favored the Kerr-Mills approach, while liberal Democrats from the North favored the Forand bill.[9] This alternative passed in 1960 and came to be called the Kerr-Mills Act. Two crucial provisions were embedded in Kerr-Mills that would profoundly influence Medicaid's subsequent policy evolution: the concept of medical indigency and comprehensive benefits. Kerr-Mills was designed to be distinct from welfare and its continuing stigma of public assistance. The "medically indigent" were older persons who needed assistance when they became sick (but not otherwise), because they had large medical expenses relative to their current income. Proponents emphasized that the "medically indigent should not be equated with the totally indigent"; that is, those who receive cash assistance (Fein 1998). The concept of medical indigency was put in place with the idea that sickness should not cause impoverishment.

While it is unclear how much the elderly were helped under Kerr-Mills, the program had a huge impact on the growth and use of nursing homes. From 1960 to 1965, vendor payments for nursing homes increased almost tenfold, consuming about a third of total program expenditures (Vladeck 1980). Even at this time, it was increasingly difficult to view these programs as simply residual ones that would wither away under increases in social insurance. They had achieved a life and a purpose of their own. Indeed, by 1960 there was general recognition of the need for nursing homes, as well as other chronic long-term care services. President Eisenhower's proposal, presented in a last-ditch effort to counter Kerr-Mills in 1960, not only emphasized the need for chronic long-term care services for the elderly and relied on state administration, but called for establishing national eligibility and benefits standards—something advocates have long sought to attain under Medicaid (Senate Committee on Finance 1960).

## The Arranged Marriage: Medicaid in 1965

The Social Security Amendments of 1965 (the Medicare and Medicaid legislation) combined three approaches to financing medical care into a single package. By all accounts, the creation of this massive "three-layer" cake took nearly everyone by surprise (Stevens and Stevens 1974; Marmor 1973). The first layer was Medicare Part A, a hospital insurance program based on the Social Security contributory model. The second layer was Medicare Part B, a voluntary supplemental medical insurance program funded through beneficiary premiums and federal general revenues. The third and final layer was the Medicaid program (originally called Part C), which broadened the protections offered to the poor and medically indigent under Kerr-Mills. The Kerr-Mills means test was liberalized in order to cover additional elderly citizens, and eligibility among the indigent was broadened to include the blind, permanently disabled, and adults in (largely) single-headed families and their dependent children.

The adoption of Medicaid in combination with Medicare in 1965 was in keeping with a thirty-year historical pattern; that is, adopting a limited social insurance program and "supplementing" it with public assistance. I put "supplement" in quotation marks because, starting with OAA in 1935, these public assistance programs were hardly supplemental. America's social insurance programs (OASI and Medicare) have been so sufficiently limited that the inevitable public assistance programs (OAA and Medicaid) were vital—and grew substantially. Despite this history, once again legislators perceived Medicaid as a relatively minor piece of the 1965 Social Security legislation, of much less significance than Medicare. Government estimates of Medicaid's future budgetary costs assumed the program would not lead to a dramatic expansion of health-care coverage (Stevens and Stevens 1974). Even assuming that all fifty states would implement the new program, the federal government projected Medicaid expenditures to be no more than $238 million per year above what was currently being spent on medical-welfare programs. As it turned out, this expenditure level was reached after only six states had implemented their Medicaid programs. By 1967, thirty-seven states were implementing Medicaid programs, and spending was rising by fifty-seven percent per annum (CRS 1993, 30).

The hope for a small increase in Medicaid given the enactment of Medicare was in keeping with how policy makers, administrators, and advocates had long discussed the relationship between public assistance and social insurance. That this substitution did not occur, however, should not have come as a surprise to anyone looking closely at medical vendor payments and the Kerr-Mills MAA program. The fastest growing and most expensive component of these two public assistance programs was the cost of nursing homes for chronically ill elderly persons. By 1965, every state had medical vendor payments for public assistance recipients, and forty states had implemented a Kerr-Mills MAA program for the medically indigent (Stevens and Stevens 1974). Because these forty state programs provided nursing home coverage, and while long-term-care coverage was essentially ruled out under Medicare, it would have been political suicide to withdraw such benefits from existing Kerr-Mills recipients. Kerr-Mills and medical vendor payments were consolidated under the new program called Medicaid, and nursing home expenditures continued to increase.

While the increase in nursing home expenditures was perhaps unplanned, three summary points are important to note:

1. This increase in nursing home expenditures is part of a larger trajectory that started fifteen years before Medicaid.
2. Medicaid's enactment in 1965 was not an afterthought, but business as usual.
3. The inclusion of nursing home care coverage under Medicaid was clearly inevitable.

## A Difficult Marriage: 1965 to 1995

The same tension that existed between OASI (Social Security insurance) and OAA (public assistance programs) throughout the 1940s and 1950s emerged between Medicaid and Medicare in the 1970s. Federal policy makers were surprised by the level of state responsiveness under what they had thought would be another meager public assistance program. In response, in 1967—only two years post-enactment—the federal government clamped down on these state liberalization efforts (Grogan and Patashnik 2003b; Stevens and Stevens 1974). Although this retrenchment was aimed in part at preventing states from using Medicaid as a stepping stone to universal health coverage, the action solidified an image of Medicaid as a stingy welfare program not worthy of the elderly. Among the four witnesses who discussed concerns about nursing home coverage in a 1970 Senate hearing on the "Sources of Community Support for Federal Programs Serving Older Americans," only one witness mentioned Medicaid and then only in passing. After describing the details of Medicare nursing home coverage (or lack thereof), he said "these shortcomings apply equally to Medicaid situations" (Senate Committee on Aging 1970).

General concern about long-term care was growing. In a 1981 congressional hearing on "The Impact of Alzheimer's Disease on the Nation's Elderly" several witnesses discussed the problem of nursing homes rejecting patients with dementia due to a lack of mental-health coverage. Although this was clearly a limitation in Medicaid policy, almost all the policy recommendations made at this hearing focused on amending Medicare policy.

Medicaid's restrictiveness was also a problem, as nicely illustrated in a congressional hearing that dealt with the "Impact of Federal Budget Cuts on the Elderly" in 1981. Long-time advocate for the elderly and chairman of the committee Representative Claude Pepper described the "less fortunate" elderly: "In spite of Social Security, one-sixth, over sixteen percent, of the elderly live below the poverty line. . . . They lack decent housing. Medicare only pays thirty-eight percent of their medical costs. They live under fear of serious disease when they would not have the aid of Medicare. They wouldn't be eligible for Medicaid because if you have anything at all to speak of, you are not eligible for Medicaid" (House Hrg: 82-H141–22).

Although there were valid concerns about the elderly having to impoverish themselves to become eligible for Medicaid/LTC services and there were no spousal protections in place at this time, by 1982 Medicaid nursing home expenditures greatly exceeded out-of-pocket payments for nursing home care. Nonetheless, the Medicaid program was generally dismissed out-of-hand as too stingy and stigmatizing to be an acceptable reform strategy for the elderly. There was very little discussion about Medicaid reform because (like OAA) it was viewed as a residual program, while Medicare (like OASI) was viewed as the appropriate program for advocacy efforts.

### Medicaid As a Needed Safety Net

Despite the persistence of this framing as a residual program, the Medicaid program experienced significant changes during the 1980s that were difficult to ignore. In contrast to Medicaid's policy-retrenchment era during the 1970s, the program expanded during the 1980s, through two main policies: first, an intentional expansion for children and pregnant women, and second, a somewhat unintentional expansion for low-income elderly financed by Medicaid (Grogan and Patashnik 2003b). The cumulative force of these expansionary policies in the 1980s created a new framing of the Medicaid program by the early 1990s, allowing policy makers to view both the program and the elderly's relationship to it in a different light. By 1990 very few described the program as residual. Instead, twenty-plus years post-enactment, the program was recognized as a crucial safety net for many diverse needy groups.

A rhetoric of the elderly emerged that they are politically privileged to the detriment of younger generations. Under this new understanding of the program, elderly middle-class inclusion in Medicaid was often discussed as problematic. The middle-class elderly were portrayed as too deserving for "welfare," but also as unfairly consuming the limited resources provided for the poor under means-tested Medicaid.

By the mid-1980s, low-income seniors not covered under Medicaid spent on average one-quarter of their annual income on medical bills (Rosenbaum 1993). Because Medicare did not (and still does not) cover most long-term care needs, the out-of-pocket costs associated with Medicare's co-payments and deductibles reached catastrophic proportions for many elderly people with serious medical conditions.

In keeping with the historical tendency to advocate for expanded social insurance to replace public assistance, advocates for long-term care coverage primarily lobbied for Medicare expansions. The Medicare Catastrophic Care Act (MCCA) of 1988 was the federal government's response to this advocacy. The act expanded coverage to include outpatient prescription drug benefits and long-term hospital care and was the largest expansion to the Medicare program since its inception in 1965. To finance MCCA, however, the legislation made a sharp break from Medicare's social insurance tradition and required Medicare beneficiaries, rather than current workers, to shoulder the financial burden of the new provisions. In particular, Medicare beneficiaries were asked to pay special premiums according to family income to cover the cost of expanded benefits. Controversy over this new financing scheme (and several other reasons) ultimately led to MCCA's repeal just one year later.[10] Medicare prescription drug benefits were then shelved until 2003.

Set against MCCA's repeal in 1989, however, were two major expansionary policies that remained intact within the Medicaid program. The first provided protections against spousal impoverishment by increasing the amount of money that seniors in the community could retain when their institutionalized spouses received Medicaid benefits. The second expansion was the creation of the Qualified Medicare Beneficiary (QMB) program. This program required the Medicaid program to buy into the Medicare program for low-income seniors and persons with disabilities. Specifically, since 1989, Medicaid has been required to pay Medicare Part B premiums and cover any deductibles or cost-sharing expenses for elderly persons under 100 percent of the poverty level (in 1990 premium support was expanded to elderly with incomes up to 120 percent of poverty).

While budget constraints and a relatively large federal deficit were significant motivating factors behind MCCA's passage and its financing scheme, a new rhetoric of intergenerational equity also contributed to its support in Congress. This new rhetoric emphasized that relatively few resources were devoted to needy children because of large public costs imposed by the elderly and, second, that families were financially burdened due to contributory transfers from young to old to support large expensive federal programs, such as Social Security and Medicare (Cook 1994). Several scholars have documented the emergence of the intergenerational equity theme during the 1980s around discussions about the elderly more generally and the passage and repeal of MCCA (Pierson and Smith 1994; Quadagno 1989; Cook et al. 1994). Not surprisingly, given the significant expansions that remained for the elderly within the Medicaid program after the MCCA repeal, this intergenerational equity discourse became infused into Medicaid's political discourse as well.

## Intergenerational Equity

Intergenerational equity concerns probably emerged first among state actors. It had been the case since the emergence of medical vendor payments in 1950 that while the elderly comprised less than fifteen percent of Medicaid recipients, they accounted for more than thirty percent of the program's costs, in large part because of their nursing home care (Rosenbaum 1993). In light of these statistics, some advocates for poor children began in the 1980s to argue that it was inappropriate for a disproportionate share of Medicaid dollars to support the elderly while younger people were struggling to pay for their health care (Benjamin, Newacheck, and Wolfe 1991). With federal mandates in the 1980s that expanded benefits to both "cost-effective" pregnant women and children and to the "expensive" elderly, representatives from the states started to voice concerns that they could not legitimately finance expansions to both groups. Difficult choices, they said, needed to be made or expanding long-term care costs would result in fewer services for poor families. A representative from the State Medicaid Directors' Association put the issue starkly:

> Obviously, for the private payer, the spousal protections . . . are very desirable and very needed. As you reduce their share of the cost, you are again passing those increases onto the Medicaid program. I'm not suggesting that you not do it, only to keep in mind that those Medicaid budgets are being consumed by long-term care expenditures. Because state revenues and local revenues are not limitless, again choices have to be made. What we are seeing in effect is Medicaid by default becoming a long-term care budget and not being able to cover more of the primary health-care needs of women, children, and families.
>
> (House Subcommittee on Health
> and the Environment 1988, 433)

This intergenerational concern within Medicaid became even more heated as the expansions in coverage for the elderly were implemented at the state level in the early 1990s. Illustrative testimony from a Michigan state congressman not only emphasized the disproportionate share of the Medicaid budget consumed by the elderly, but also suggested that such expenses were used inappropriately for expensive care during the last year of life.

> Congressman, two-thirds of our health care dollars are spent in the last year of life, and two-thirds of those are spent in the last 90 days. This is the fastest-growing part of our population. We have a dramatically aging society spending more and more on health care. The health care share of our budget in Michigan has gone from 20 percent of the budget in 1980, to 26.8 percent in 1990. Medicaid is one of the major problems and you will hear across the country, Medicaid is eating up state budgets.
>
> (House Subcommittee on Health and
> the Environment 1991, 272–273)

In a series of hearings discussing Medicaid during the early 1990s and continuing throughout the decade, representatives from the states stressed the explosive costs of long-term care and how these costs forced them to choose between needy population groups. Many mentioned the "truly" needy groups that Medicaid should cover but could not because of expensive long-term care costs, such as working families without insurance. The North Carolina Medicaid director vividly encapsulated the rhetoric of the times:

> The Medicaid program is up a creek. . . . In the creek are two islands. They are filled with people who need help with their medical bills.
>
> One island contains infants, children, teenagers, their parents. This island threatens to sink just by the sheer weight of the numbers of the people on the island, twice as many as occupy the second island.
>
> The second island has fewer people, but they are all severely disabled or elderly. The weight of their problems is twice as great as those on the first island. This island, too, is sinking fast, but, ironically, there is a boat docked here at the second island named Medicare, the good ship Medicare. It should be carrying the elderly and disabled to shore, but it is so filled with holes it is of little use to the would-be patients. It does not go where the patients want to go.
>
> The Medicaid program is the only available boat in the river, and its course is not clearly charted. Should it head toward the island and save the children and their parents or should it head in the opposite direc-

tion, tow Medicare's boat and bring those patients aboard? The answer is it must do both. Its seating capacity is unlimited by law.

(House Subcommittee on Health<br>and the Environment 1991, 303)

Note that in addition to emphasizing an either-or choice facing the states (taking care of the children versus the elderly), this image designates Medicare as the culprit in creating this tension within Medicaid, and concludes that Medicaid has no choice—it must take care (somehow) of both populations. How Medicaid could possibly do both, and whether Medicaid could and should remain a means-tested program and make hard choices between needy groups, was largely swept under the rug.

Perhaps, alternatively, Medicaid could become something else in order to accommodate the diverse needs of program recipients as well as other groups that need help. But what? This question infused the third framing of the Medicaid program that began to emerge in the early 1990s and became most pronounced during the 1995 debate about the Republican proposal that was viewed by most Democrats as an attempt to retrench the Medicaid program.[11] This view emphasized Medicaid as a core social entitlement that appropriately included middle-class elderly who need long-term care. In contrast, the intergenerational equity view implicitly painted Medicaid as a means-tested program that had to choose between needy groups.

### Medicaid as a Social Welfare Program

The third view of the Medicaid program recognized it as a major social welfare program that reached into the middle class—far from its rhetorical beginnings, which defined it as a residual "poverty" program. In a 1990 congressional hearing titled "Medicaid Budget Initiatives," Chairman Henry Waxman highlighted the middle-class aspect of Medicaid in his opening statement:

Most people who need nursing home care eventually find themselves dependent on Medicaid. . . . It is absurd, and it is unacceptable that an individual could work hard for their entire life, set aside a fund for his or her retirement, then become—then have to be impoverished and go on welfare in order to take advantage of facilities and services and aids that flow from the Medicaid system. With the passage of Representative Kennelly's bill, my state and nine others are proposing to offer an alternative.

(House Subcommittee on Health<br>and the Environment 1991, 2)

The Kennelly bill referred to by Chairman Waxman called for demonstration projects to develop private-public partnerships to encourage middle-class elderly to purchase long-term care insurance. Under this bill,

> if and when an individual exhausts his or her insurance and applies for Medicaid, each dollar that the insurance policy has paid out in accord with state guidelines will be subtracted from the assets Medicaid considers in determining eligibility. In other words, coverage of long-term care expenses by private insurance would count as asset spend-down for the purpose of Medicaid eligibility.
>
> (House Subcommittee on Health
> and the Environment 1991, 23)

Although Representative Waxman as chairman of the Subcommittee on Health and the Environment expressed general support for Kennelly's bill in his opening remarks, he raised concerns about whether this bill would create a new category of Medicaid eligibility—one that expanded eligibility to middle-class (or even upper-income) elderly by allowing Medicaid to be used to protect assets and to finance the transfer of wealth.[12] Kennelly's response to Waxman's concerns put to the forefront the question of whether Medicaid was still a truly means-tested program or had expanded to something beyond that.

> First let me say that I think part of the reason you and I have different perspectives on this issue [whether her bill creates a new category of Medicaid eligibility] is that we start from very different points. You seem to see Medicaid solely as a means-tested entitlement for the poor. While I agree, I also see Medicaid as a program where, at least based on Connecticut figures, over forty percent of those who receive Medicaid long-term care services did not start out poor.
>
> I hear of financial planners teaching seniors how to transfer their assets and access Medicaid benefits and I feel there ought to be a better way. . . . Our society has changed markedly in the twenty-five years since the enactment of the Medicaid program to the point where many of those receiving Medicaid are not included in our traditional definition of 'poor.'
>
> The current Medicaid long-term care program is a means-tested program in name only. The major asset most seniors possess is a house which is typically protected by Medicaid. . . . Given the political pressures associated with the aging of the population, we are likely to see even more proposals to further increase the amount of assets exempted from Medicaid.

In that context, my proposal . . . may be the ONLY proposal that has the potential of actually protecting Medicaid against further erosion of its means-tested origin.

(House Subcommittee on Health<br>and the Environment 1991, 23)

This quote is important for two reasons: first, as mentioned above, it reiterates a long-term fear about the growth of public assistance programs. Like Ms. Dunn who earlier worried about OAA taking over state budgets unless OASI was expanded, Representative Kennelly worried about Medicaid expansions unless a private solution was created.[13] Most noteworthy is the loss of the substitution theme by the mid-1990s. Policy makers and advocates no longer talked about the necessity of expanding Medicare—our social insurance program—so that we could dismiss Medicaid—our residual public assistance program. Waxman's description of Medicaid as a core social entitlement was stated quite clearly in a 1991 hearing investigating the Medicaid program:

Medicaid is an enormously important and enormously complex program. It is the major source of health care reform for the poor in this country, covering more than twenty-eight million poor people, roughly half of whom are children. It is the single largest payer for maternity care. . . . It is the single largest payer for nursing home care. . . . It is the single largest payer for residential services for individuals with mental retardation. . . . [The] program has been asked to solve almost every major problem facing this society, from infant mortality to substance abuse to AIDS to the need for long-term care. . . . Despite all of the current interest in health care reform, nothing will be enacted tomorrow . . . [and] the poor in this country, mothers and children, the disabled, the elderly will continue to rely on Medicaid for access to basic health care.

(House Subcommittee on Health<br>and the Environment 1991, 3-4)

Indeed, even during hearings about transforming the Medicaid program in 1995, Republican legislators in favor of block granting Medicaid went to great pains to stress that their goal was to strengthen and not to dismantle the program. For example, in Chairman Bilirakis's opening statement he said: "We all have very personal and compelling views about Medicaid. No one involved in this reform effort sees our objective as dismantling a program that is essential to millions of low-income Americans. In fact, we are motivated in this effort by the conviction that what we are doing will strengthen and preserve the

Medicaid program for years to come, and that's our goal" (House Subcommittee on Health and the Environment 1996, 164).

Liberal Democrats might discard the sincerity of such statements as pure rhetoric, but it is important to note that the program had changed significantly enough that conservative Republicans felt compelled to frame their argument in this way.

Even President Clinton recast Medicaid as a middle-class entitlement during the 1995 debates. It was not surprising that he sought to rally public opinion against the GOP budget package by arguing that it would entail huge cuts in spending for Medicare, education, and environmental protection— three federal programs with obvious appeal for middle-class voters. However, quite startling was Clinton's explicit support for *Medicaid* on par with these other universal (that is, middle-class) programs (Grogan and Patashnik 2003a). In explaining why protecting Medicaid was so vital, Clinton emphasized that it was a key support for senior citizens residing in nursing homes, that many of these seniors were middle class before they depleted their resources, and that they had middle-class children and grandchildren. Stated Clinton in one address:

> Now, think about this—what about the Medicaid program? You hardly hear anything about Medicaid. People say, oh, that's that welfare program. One-third of Medicaid does go to help poor women and their poor children on Medicaid. Over two-thirds of it goes to the elderly and the disabled. All of you know that as well [commenting on Republican proposals]. You think about how many middle-class working people are not going to be able to save to send their kids to college because now they'll have to be taking care of their parents who would have been eligible for public assistance.
>
> (President Clinton speech to Senior Citizen Group,
> reported by U.S. Newswire 15 September 1995)

Note the huge political significance of this framing of the issue: by 1995, Medicaid's long-term care role and financial protection policies were so sufficiently recognized that it was acceptable for the President in a major public address to explain Medicare and Medicaid as comprising a health-care *package* for the mainstream elderly (Grogan and Patashnik 2003a). In sum, Clinton sought to cast Medicaid as broad social entitlement that incorporated the middle class.

Emphasizing the incorporation of the elderly middle-class into Medicaid is an important aspect of the core social entitlement framework. All advocates for the elderly mentioned this incorporation of the middle class during the 1995 hearings. For example, a representative from the American Association of Retired Persons began her testimony by saying "[I] testify today on behalf of the almost five million older Americans who rely on Medicaid." She then went on to say, "Many who need long-term care start off as taxpaying middle-class Americans. They worked hard and saved" (House Subcommittee on Health and the Environment 1996, 288–289). Note the change in discussion about the elderly middle class in Medicaid. In 1990, Representative Kennelly recognized the importance of Medicaid for the elderly middle class and offered a bill to keep them out of the program and preserve Medicaid's means-tested origins. In 1995, advocates, members of Congress, and the President mentioned the elderly middle class in Medicaid as a central reason why the program should be viewed as a core social entitlement.

### Conclusion: A Marriage of Acceptance?

While some might look back at the Medicaid/LTC marriage and dislike the results, it is important to recognize its logic. Very early on, indeed even before the New Deal, health-care providers recognized the importance of long-term care services for the elderly. Their answer, and policy makers subsequent answer—institutional care—is often viewed by LTC advocates as a huge mistake. But it is false to then say that Medicaid (or our public assistance programs prior to Medicaid) was never intended to be our answer to long-term care.

Medicaid's predecessors—medical vendor payments in 1950 and Medical Assistance to the Aged (MAA) under the Kerr-Mills Act in 1960—provided public funding, which encouraged a dramatic increase in the number of nursing homes. As a result, the inclusion of nursing home coverage under Medicaid in 1965 was not only inevitable and intentional, but front and center. Medicaid continued to be the primary funder for elderly institutional care, and this became the primary American response to problems of chronic disease in an aging population.

Critics have argued for a long time that this response is inappropriate and inadequate, not only because of the persistent concerns about the quality of care provided in many of the nation's nursing homes (Mendelson 1974; Vladek 1980; Senate Committee on Aging 1996), but, more importantly, because most elderly individuals would rather not live in even high-quality nursing homes but rather reside in a more independent, "home-like" setting (Kane and Kane 1985; Kane et al. 1998). Quality concerns and concerns about Medicaid's institutional focus, however, do not explain why advocates for long-term care reform shunned Medicaid throughout the 1970s and 1980s and often fought instead for a Medicare expansion. That attitude is explained by a larger historical pattern in American social policy of limiting social insurance and using public assistance as a supplement to fill in the inevitable gaps. Indeed, when Medicaid was enacted alongside Medicare it was viewed as a residual program that could be dismantled when the social insurance Medicare program expanded.

However, as Medicaid nursing home costs (as well as other parts of the program) continued to grow and Medicaid-funded, community-based LTC services began to emerge, Medicare stayed largely in place, and it became more and more difficult to refer to Medicaid as simply a residual program (or a supplement to Medicare) (Oberlander 2003). Today, Medicare is rarely invoked as a privileged program ready to expand and replace Medicaid. Instead, Medicaid is often described as a core safety net that needs protection. Key to describing that core is the provision of long-term care services for the elderly and their middle-class families. While the Medicaid/LTC marriage has been problematic, we seem to have reached a point of acceptance, and divorce no longer appears imminent. Indeed, while the burden of the marriage on Medicaid's purse strings is still clearly in view, the political advantages that the marriage affords—namely, to reframe Medicaid as a core social entitlement for America's middle class—has been used strategically and is gaining recognition. While advocates for improved LTC quality and universal LTC coverage have traditionally favored a Medicare expansion, this history suggests that their focus may be misplaced. The key to policy improvements probably lies where LTC began—with the Medicaid program.

### Notes

1. Poor as defined by the federal poverty level.
2. For more information on "Middle-class Medicaid," see Grogan and Patashnik 2003a and a GAO study titled Medicaid Estate Planning, 1993. For more information on the "excluded poor," see McLaughlin 2004 and Brown 1991.
3. Table on Persons 65 Years of Age and Over Living in Institutions was inserted into the record by Wilbur Cohen. Source: Special report on institutional population 1940, table 12, Bureau of the Census.
4. See Patashnik and Zelizer (2001) for a discussion about the important influence of financial concerns during this period.
5. The six organizations: American Medicaid Association, American Hospital Association, American Nurses Association, American Dental Association, American Public Health Association, and the American Public Welfare Association.
6. See Holstein and Cole (1996) for a discussion of how SBA and FHA construction loans encouraged the building of private for-profit nursing homes.
7. Named after its Democratic congressional sponsors, Senator Robert Kerr and Representative Wilbur Mills.

8. At Press Conference, 25 June 1951, 2:30 P.M., Room 5246, Federal Security Agency, 330 Independence Avenue, SW, Washington, DC.
9. Interestingly, President Eisenhower offered what could be defined as a slightly more generous proposal, but it did not gain much attention.
10. For a book-length discussion that explains Medicare Catastrophic Coverage Act's passage and repeal see Himelfarb 1995.
11. There is some debate about this, but most policy makers and analysts at the time were concerned that the Republicans' proposal to block-grant the Medicaid program would have reduced federal funding and eliminated recipients' entitlement rights to the program.
12. This is taken from Kennelly's testimony and prepared statement for the record where she responds to Chairman Waxman's questions and concerns about her bill.
13. Obviously, there is a larger story, which I don't have the room to discuss herein, about the emergence of a private approach as the new legitimate substitute for Medicaid—our public assistance approach (see Hacker 2002 and Klein 2003 for more on historical origins of private approach).

### References

Benjamin, A. E., P. W. Newacheck, and H. Wolfe. 1991. Intergenerational Equity and Public Spending. *Pediatrics.* 88, no. 1: 75–83.

Brown, Lawrence D. 1991. *Health Policy and the Disadvantaged.* Durham, NC: Duke University Press.

Centers for Medicare and Medicaid Services (CMS). Department of Health and Human Services. http://www.cms.hhs.gov.

Cohen, Marc A., Nanda Kumar, and Stanley S. Wallack. 1993. Simulating the Fiscal and Distributional Impacts of Medicaid Eligibility Reforms. *Health Care Financing Review* 14, no. 4: 133–150.

Congressional Research Service (CRS). 1993. *Medicaid Source Book: Background Data and Analysis (A 1993 Update).* Washington, DC: U.S. Government Printing Office.

Cook, Fay Lomax. 1994. The Salience of Intergenerational Equity in Canada and the United States. In *Economic Security and Intergenerational Justice,* eds. Theodore R. Marmor, Timothy M. Smeeding, and Vernon L. Greene, 91–129. Washington, DC: The Urban Institute Press.

Fine, Sidney. 1998. The Kerr-Mills Act: Medical Care for the Indigent in Michigan, 1960–1965. *Journal of the History of Medicine* 53: 285–316.

Gordon, Colin. 2003. *Dead on Arrival: The Politics of Health Care in Twentieth-Century America.* Princeton: Princeton University Press.

Grogan, Colleen M. 2005. The Politics of Aging within Medicaid. In *Age-Based Politics in the 21st Century,* ed. Robert B. Hudson. Baltimore: Johns Hopkins University Press.

Grogan, Colleen M., and Eric M. Patashnik. 2003a. Universalism within Targeting: Nursing Home Care, the Middle Class, and the Politics of the Medicaid Program. *Social Service Review* 77, no. 1: 51–71.

———. 2003b. Between Welfare Medicine and Mainstream Entitlement: Medicaid at the Political Crossroads. *Journal of Health Politics, Policy and Law* 28, no. 5: 821–858.

Haber, Carole. 1983. *Beyond Sixty-five: The Dilemma of Old Age in America's Past.* New York: Cambridge University Press.

Himelfarb, Richard. 1995. *Catastrophic Politics: The Rise and Fall of the Medicare Catastrophic Coverage Act of 1988.* University Park: Pennsylvania State University Press.

Holstein, Martha, and Thomas R. Cole. 1996. The Evolution of Long-Term Care in America. In *The Future of Long-Term Care: Social and Policy Issues*, eds. Robert H. Binstock, Leighton E. Cluff and Otto Von Mering, 19–48. Baltimore: Johns Hopkins University Press.

House Committee on Aging. 1982. *Impact of Federal Budget Cuts on the Elderly: Seattle, Washington*. Hearing 14 November.

House Subcommittee on Health and the Environment of the Committee on Energy and Commerce. 1988. *Medicare and Medicaid Catastrophic Protection*. Hearing, Serial No. 100–74. 21, 27, and 28 May, 2 June 1987.

———. 1991. *Medicaid Budget Initiatives*. Hearing, Serial No. 101–206. 10 and 14 September 1990.

House Subcommittee on Health and the Environment of the Committee on Commerce. 1996. *Transformation of the Medicaid Program—Part 3*. Hearing, 26 July and 1 August 1995.

Jones, A. 2002. The National Nursing Home Survey: 1999 Summary. National Center for Health Statistics. *Vital Health Statistics* 13, no. 152: 12, Table 7.

Kane, Robert, and Rosalie Kane. 1985. *A Will and a Way: What the United States Can Learn from Canada about Caring for the Elderly*. New York: Columbia University Press.

Kane, Robert, Rosalie Kane, and R. C. Ladd. 1998. *The Heart of Long-Term Care*. New York: Oxford University Press.

Katz, Michael B. 1986. *In the Shadow of the Poorhouse: A Social History of Welfare in America*. New York: Basic Books.

Marmor, Theodore R. 1973. *The Politics of Medicare*. New York: Aldine.

McLaughlin, Catherine G. 2004. *Health Policy and Uninsured*. Washington, DC: Urban Institute Press.

Mendelson, Mary Adelaide. 1974. *Tender Loving Greed: How the Incredibly Lucrative Nursing Home Industry Is Exploiting America's Old People and Defrauding Us All*. New York: Knopf.

Murtaugh C. M., P. Kemper, B. C. Spillman. 1990. The Risk of Nursing Home Use in Later Life. *Medical Care* 28, no. 10: 952–962.

Oberlander, Jonathan. 2003. The *Political Life of Medicare*. Chicago: University of Chicago Press.

Patashnik, Eric M., and Julian E. Zelizer. 2001. Paying for Medicare: Benefits, Budgets and Wilbur Mills's Policy Legacy. *Journal of Health Politics, Policy and Law* 26, no. 1: 7–36.

Pierson, Paul, and Miriam Smith. 1994. Shifting Fortunes of the Elderly: The Comparative Politics of Retrenchment. In *Economic Security and Intergenerational Justice: A Look at North America*, eds. Theodore R. Marmor, Timothy M. Smeeding, and Vernon L. Greene, 21–59. Washington, DC: The Urban Institute Press.

Poen, Monte M. 1982. The Truman Legacy: Retreat to Medicare. In *Compulsory Health Insurance*, ed. Ronald L. Numbers, 97–114. Westport, CT: Greenwood Press.

Quadagno, Jill. 1989. Generational Equity and the Politics of the Welfare State. *Politics and Society* 17, no. 3: 353–376.

Rosenbaum, Sara. 1993. Medicaid Expansions and Access to Health Care. In *Medicaid Financing Crisis: Balancing Responsibilities, Priorities, and Dollars*, eds. Diane Rowland, Judith Feder, and Alina Salganicoff, 4582. Washington, DC: AAAS Press.

Rosenberg, Charles E. 1987. *The Care of Strangers: The Rise of America's Hospital System*. New York: Basic Books.

Rosenberry, Sara A. 1982. Social Insurance, Distributive Criteria and the Welfare Backlash: A Comparative Analysis. *British Journal of Political Science* 12, no. 4: 421447.

Senate Committee on Aging. 1970. *Sources of Community Support for Federal Programs Serving Older Americans.* Hearing 18 April.

Senate Committee on Aging. 1996. *Medicaid Reform: Quality of Care in Nursing Homes at Risk.* Hearing, 26 October 1995.

Senate Committee on Finance 1950. *Social Security Revision: Hearing on R. R. 6000.* 81st Congress, 2d session. 23–31 January, 1–3 and 6–10 February.

Senate Committee on Finance. 1960. *Social Security Amendments of 1960: Hearing on H.R. 12580.* 86th Congress, 2d session. 29–30 June.

Stevens, Robert B., and Rosemary Stevens. 1974. *Welfare Medicine in America: A Case Study of Medicaid.* New York: Free Press.

Stevens, Rosemary. 1971. *American Medicine and the Public Interest.* New Haven, CT: Yale University Press.

Stewart, Estelle M. 1925. The Cost of American Almshouses. *U.S. Bureau of Labor Statistics, Bulletin No. 386.* Washington DC: U.S. Government Printing Office.

Taft, Robert A. 1950. *Social Security Revision.* Committee on Finance Hearing. Senate, 81st Congress, 2d session on H.R. 6000, 23–31 January, 1–3 and 6–10, February. Washington DC: U.S. Government Printing Office.

Thompson, F. J., and J. J. DiIulio eds. 1999. *Medicaid and Devolution: A View from the States.* Washington, DC: Brookings Institution Press.

Vladeck, Bruce C. 1980. *Unloving Care: The Nursing Home Tragedy.* New York: Basic Books.

Wiener, Joshua. 1999. Long Term Care. In *Medicaid and Devolution: A View from the States,* eds. F. J. Thompson and J. J. DiIulio, chapter 6. Washington, DC: Brooking Institution Press.

# Part IV

# Policy Management and Results

# Rhetoric, Realities, and the Plight of the Mentally Ill in America

Deinstitutionalization of persons with mental illnesses is now a fact of life. Many have criticized its consequences and insisted that the policy has been disastrous (Isaac and Armat 1990). Few, however, have demanded that we return to institutional solutions for care of persons with mental illnesses. Public mental hospitals in the United States have largely been emptied, with only approximately 54,000 patients in long-term state mental hospitals at the beginning of the twenty-first century. In today's context, however, the meaning of *deinstitutionalization* has changed; it now refers to barriers to long-term inpatient residence. Patterns of care have changed radically as well. Hospital care is now largely limited to short-term admissions during florid episodes of disorders or when patients are believed to pose significant risks to themselves or others.

The debates about deinstitutionalization continue with wide appreciation that realities have deviated greatly from the intentions and expectations of its proponents. Few look back on its history as one of policy triumph, and retrospective examination suggests that many of the same factors that diverted earlier aspirations still distort policy today, although in different ways. Most important among these are the effects of financing programs and incentives on locations, types, and patterns of treatment, the expansion of concepts of mental illness that obfuscate the differences between serious mental illness and other forms of psychological distress, the confusion between wishful thinking about prevention and evidence of its efficacy, and the role of advocacy and ideology in shaping medical policy. Understanding public mental-health policy also requires attention to the cross-cutting issue of the tensions between federal and state authorities, their respective historical responsibilities, and the fundamental role of federal health and welfare programs, constructed mostly with other client populations in mind, in the evolution of mental-health policies.

Most observers looking back on mental-health policy note the failure to develop the promised integrated and coordinated community systems of mental-health care that were seen as an alternative to the hospital. Even major special demonstration programs funded with generous private funds have had difficulty improving care and patient outcomes through integrating community services (Lehman et al. 1994; Rosenheck et al. 2002). These failures are not separate from the more general problem in American health policy of building coordinated health-care organizations that successfully integrate care at the clinical level (Shortell et al. 1996). In considering future possibilities, therefore, it is necessary to think deeply about whether the traditional visions of community mental health are compatible with our general health and welfare policies or whether it might be more realistic to encourage disease-oriented specialized systems of care that predominate in other parts of the general health sector.

On superficial appraisal, one might be tempted to view the abandonment of long-term hospital care as simply an economic result of government's and private payers' attempts to reduce expenditures and budgets. That this is too facile an explanation is made clear by the large concomitant growth of incarceration in the criminal justice system supported by both policy makers and the public. Estimates of the extent of "criminalization" of the mentally ill are controversial, but one important consequence of the dispersion of persons with mental illnesses into a broad array of institutional settings, from nursing homes to jails and from residential care to scattered housing, is that it fundamentally changed the visibility of mental illnesses as a societal problem requiring earmarked support. New forms of mental-health advocacy have emerged, including the National Alliance for the Mentally Ill, a strong family-based organization with national and state lobbying offices. Nevertheless, the challenge of advocacy is more difficult with the dispersion of care responsibility among many different programs and bureaucracies.

The deinstitutionalization narrative is usually told in global terms as a national and even international phenomenon, and one extending as well to other populations, including persons with physical and developmental disabilities (Scull 1977). While some features of deinstitutionalization have been shared here and abroad, a closer look reveals large variations among states and nations, which must be understood in the context of their history, values, and socio-political, economic, and health and welfare traditions (Mechanic and

Rochefort 1992). Some countries such as Japan built up their private mental hospital sector in the 1970s, substantially increasing the number of long-term patients and substituting inpatient hospital care for informal care. Although the United Kingdom did much early work on alternatives to hospitalization and rehabilitation approaches, it reduced its mental hospital populations only slowly. In contrast, following the radical ideology of Franco Basaglia, a Venetian psychiatrist, Trieste and other areas in Italy closed their mental hospitals rapidly (Mechanic 1999).

In the United States, an appropriate understanding of the history of reductions in public mental hospital residents and the range of alternatives requires appreciation of variations among states, the character of their mental-health systems, and the opportunities seen by sophisticated state administrators to take advantage of federal programs and thus to shift costs (Mechanic and Rochefort 1992). Central to this story, still substantially untold, is how state administrators used programs such as Medicaid, Supplemental Security Income (SSI), and Disproportionate Shares funding not only to empty their public hospitals but also to design alternative systems of care.

Many states closed mental hospitals at an early date; California reduced its state hospital population by three-quarters between 1955 and 1973. Others reduced populations on a more gradual basis; in Nevada the decrease over the same period was only fifteen percent. Some states (for example, New Hampshire) actually built new mental hospitals or replaced older ones, while Vermont closed down its mental hospital entirely. Different states developed or used different alternatives to replace older patterns of care, in part reflecting their preexisting institutional and treatment resources. In short, the processes we call deinstitutionalization varied by place and time and were dependent on the configuration of preexisting mental-health facilities, the structure of state governments, the strength of related advocacy and special interest groups, the knowledge and sophistication of state policy makers, and dominant community values and ideologies (Mechanic and Rochefort 1992).

## The Causes of Deinstitutionalization

Deinstitutionalization is commonly attributed to the "pharmaceutical revolution" and the introduction of thorazine in large state institutions in the mid-1950s. New medications were important in reducing the symptoms of psychosis, such as delusions and hallucinations, and gave hope and confidence to therapeutic staff, administrators, and families that patients could be managed with fewer restraints. However, the introduction of new pharmaceuticals was not sufficient to explain changes in patterns of care. Individual studies have shown that in some localities, both in the United States and abroad, deinstitutionalization preceded the introduction of new drugs. Individual hospitals in the UK, for example, introduced administrative changes prior to the introduction of new drugs that significantly reduced resident inpatients without the new medications (Brown et al. 1966; Scull 1977). Much the same occurred in the United States. At Worcester State Hospital in Massachusetts, a change in outlook and administrative practices in the early 1950s hastened rates of release back into the community. These changes, which also occurred elsewhere at such institutions as Boston Psychopathic Hospital and the Butler Health Center in Providence, antedated the introduction of drugs. Moreover, the average length of stay declined as well (Bockoven 1972). The introduction of drugs simply facilitated a trend that was already transforming institutional practices.

The main thrust of deinstitutionalization was a function of both federal policy and circumstances in the various states. In most states the highest rates of deinstitutionalization occurred between 1966 and 1980, and followed the introduction of new federal policies and entitlements. For example, mental hospital resident populations between 1955 and 1965 declined from 558,922 to 475,202, a reduction of only fifteen percent. Between 1965 and 1975, by contrast, the number of residents declined to 193,664, a reduction of sixty percent. These figures, however, conceal much variability. Between 1955 and 1973 the rate of reduction varied from less than twenty percent in Delaware to more than seventy percent in Illinois, Utah, and Hawaii (Mechanic and Rochefort 1992).

There were influences which hastened the pace of deinstitutionalization that were national in scope, even international among Western European nations: the ideologies of equality and community associated with the war against totalitarianism; the growth of the social sciences with their bias toward environmental causes; the emergence of a social-science literature documenting the deleterious impact of mental hospitals; and the pressures for improved standards of hospital care that inevitably increased costs (Mechanic 1999).

In the United States some unique circumstances contributed to the policy of deinstitutionalization. The military's success during World War II in treating psychiatric symptoms and returning soldiers to their units led to a faith that outpatient treatment in the community was more effective than confinement in remote institutions that broke established social ties. The war also hastened the emergence of psychodynamic and psychoanalytic psychiatry with its emphasis on the importance of life experiences and socioenvironmental factors (Appel and Beebe 1946). Taken together, these changes contributed to the belief that early intervention in the community would be effective in preventing hospitalization and thus avoid chronicity. Finally, the introduction of psychological and somatic therapies (including, but not limited to, psychotropic drugs) held out the promise of a more normal existence for persons with mental illnesses outside of institutions (Grob 1991).

Perhaps the most significant element in preparing the groundwork for the emergence of deinstitutionalization, however, was the growing role of the federal government in social welfare and health policies. For much of American history major responsibility for health and welfare rested with state and local governments. By the early twentieth century, change, albeit slow, was evident. A program to assist disabled Civil War veterans, for example, had become a universal disability and old-age pension program for veterans and their dependents; by 1907 perhaps twenty-five percent of all those aged sixty-five and over were enrolled, and payments accounted for nearly thirty percent of all federal expenditures. The passage of the Social Security Act of 1935 proved another milestone. After World War II federal welfare and health activities expanded exponentially and, equally important, diminished the authority of state governments.

The passage of the National Mental Health Act of 1946 and the subsequent creation of the National Institute of Mental Health (NIMH) thrust the federal government into mental-health policy, an arena historically reserved for state governments. Under the leadership of Robert H. Felix, the NIMH dedicated itself to bringing about the demise of public mental hospitals and substitute a community-based policy (Felix and Bowers 1948). The passage of the Community Mental Health Centers Act in 1963 culminated two decades of agitation. The legislation provided federal subsidies for the construction of community mental-health centers (CMHCs), but left their financing to local communities. These centers were intended to be the cornerstone of a radical new policy. Free-standing institutions with no links to mental hospitals (which still had an inpatient population of about half a million), the centers were supposed to facilitate early identification of symptoms and offer preventive treatments that would both diminish the incidence of mental disorders and render long-term hospitalization superfluous. Ultimately the hope was that traditional mental hospitals would become obsolete. These centers, moreover, would be created and operated by the community in which they were located (Grob 1991).

The Community Mental Health Centers Act, however, ignored key facts about the context in which hospitalized persons with severe and chronic mental illnesses received care. In 1960, forty-eight percent of patients in mental hospitals were unmarried, twelve percent were widowed, and thirteen percent were divorced or separated. The overwhelming majority, in other words, may have had no families to care for them. Hence the assumption that persons with mental illnesses could reside in the community with their families while undergoing psychosocial and biological rehabilitation was unrealistic (Kramer 1967). The goal of creating two thousand CMHCs by 1980 was equally problematic. If this goal had been met, there would have been a severe shortage of qualified psychiatrists or a dramatic change in the manner in which medical graduates selected their specialty. Indeed, training a sufficient number of psychiatrists to staff centers would have decimated other medical specialties without a large expansion of medical education. To be sure, there could have been an increase in the training of other mental-health professionals, but the law as passed included no provision to facilitate training. The subsequent absence of psychiatrists at CMHCs proved significant, given the importance of drugs in any treatment program. The legislation of 1963, in other words, reflected a victory of ideology over reality.

The ideological debates in the Kennedy Administration could have led to a significant transformation; the improvement of mental hospitals and construction of a more integrated system of mental-health care was a viable option in the early 1960s. The concept that the mental hospital could act as a therapeutic community took shape during the preceding decade. Given concrete form by Maxwell Jones, a British psychiatrist who had worked with psychologically impaired servicemen and repatriated prisoners of war, the therapeutic innovations of the 1950s were popularized in the United States by such figures as Alfred Stanton, Morris Schwartz, Milton Greenblatt, and Robert N. Rapoport (Jones 1953; Stanton and Schwartz 1954; Greenblatt et al. 1955; Rapoport 1960). The Council of State Governments (representing the nation's governors) and the Milbank Memorial Fund sponsored studies that emphasized the potential importance of community institutions (Council of State Governments 1950; Milbank Memorial Fund 1956; 1957). Indeed, the concept seemed to presage a policy capable of realizing the dream of providing quality care and effective treatment for persons with mental illnesses. The simultaneous development of milieu and drug therapy indicated a quite specific direction: drug therapy would make patients amenable to milieu therapy; a more humane institutional environment would facilitate the release of large numbers of patients into the community; and an extensive network of local services would, in turn, assist the reintegration of patients into society and oversee, if necessary, their varied medical, economic, occupational, and social needs (Grob 1991).

Those in policy-making positions in the NIMH, however, had a public-health view of mental illnesses and prevention, a strong belief in social etiology, and a pervasive suspicion and distrust of the mental hospital system and state mental-health authorities. They believed that state governments were a barrier to fundamental change and that enlightened federal officials should take the lead. That many states opposed passage of civil rights and voting legislation only confirmed this negative perception.

The provisions of the Community Mental Health Centers Act were vague, although the goal—as President Kennedy remarked when he signed the bill into law—was to replace custodial hospitals with local therapeutic centers. The act left the responsibility of defining the essential services of CMHCs to the U.S. Department of Health, Education, and Welfare (HEW). The regulations as promulgated in effect bypassed state authorities and gave more power to local communities. The most curious aspect of the regulations was the omission of state hospitals. In one sense this was understandable, given the belief that centers would replace mental hospitals. Nevertheless, the absence of linkages between centers and hospitals was striking. If centers were designed to provide the comprehensive services and continuity of care specified in the regulations, how could they function in isolation from a state system that still retained responsibility for nearly half a million patients with severe mental illnesses? Not surprisingly, there were deep and bitter divisions over mental-health issues between state and federal officials in the early 1960s (Grob 1991; Foley and Sharfstein 1983). These resentments even continue to the present and are reflected in some of the federal-state debates over the administration of Medicaid. Such acrimonious relations hardly offer the best organizational framework for cooperation in improving mental-health services systems.

In theory the Community Mental Health Centers were to receive patients discharged from mental hospitals and take responsibility for their aftercare and rehabilitation; in fact, this did not occur. Indeed, previous studies had already raised serious questions about the ability of community clinics (as they were known in the 1950s) to deal with persons with serious mental disorders. Three California researchers found evidence that there were "marked discontinuities in functions" between hospitals and clinics. Those patients who required an extensive social support network were not candidates for clinics that provided no assistance in finding living quarters or employment (Sampson et al. 1958, 76).

Such findings were largely ignored by those caught up in the rhetoric of community care and treatment. Using an expanded definition of mental illness and the mental-health continuum, CMHCs served largely a new set of

clients who better fit the orientations of mental-health managers and professionals trained in psychodynamic and preventive perspectives. The treatment
of choice at most centers was individual psychotherapy, an intervention especially congenial to the professional staff and adapted to a middle-class, educated clientele who did not have severe disorders. Moreover, many CMHCs
were caught up in the vortex of community activism characteristic of the
1960s and 1970s and devoted part of their energies to social reform. The most
famous example of political activism occurred at the Lincoln Hospital Mental
Health Services in the southeast Bronx. Hospital officials sought to stimulate
community social action programs in order to deal with the chronic problems
of urban ghettos. The result, however, was not anticipated. In early 1969 non-
professional staff workers went on strike and demanded that power be transferred from professionals associated with a predominantly white power
structure to the poor, African Americans, and disfranchised persons. However
laudable the intention, such activities removed centers still further from a
population whose mental illnesses often created dependency (Peck 1969;
Shaw and Eagle 1971). The result was exacerbated discordance between the
work of CMHCs and the system of mental-health services administered by the
states. The former's agendas were primarily focused on stress, psychological
problems, and preventive activities in community settings, while the latter
maintained their traditional responsibility for persons with severe and persistent mental illness. It was in this context that deinstitutionalization policies
proceeded (Grob 1991).

In many respects the key turning point in mental-health policy was the
decision in 1964 by the federal government to bypass states and work directly
with communities to develop CMHCs and establish priorities. In addition to
shifting the focus of services from those with more serious illness to clients
with less disabling disorders, these policies and the way they were implemented left many state administrators embittered. During the years of Jimmy
Carter's Presidential Commission on Mental Health and the developments
leading to the passage of the Mental Health Systems Act in 1980, the divisions
about the role of states made achieving a consensus difficult and weakened the
final legislation. Moreover, the fiscal impact of the Vietnam War diminished
federal support for CMHCs, and the Nixon Administration manifested hostility to expanded mental-health initiatives. When Ronald Reagan came into
office in 1981, the Mental Health Systems Act—the result of years of hard effort
during the Carter Administration—was repealed and responsibility for persons
with mental disorders again devolved predominantly to the states. The NIMH
retreated from providing services to focus almost exclusively on its research

mission. The federal role in mental health now came largely through programs such as Medicaid, Social Security Disability Income (SSDI), Supplemental Security Income (SSI), and Section 8 Housing, all of which were designed with other client populations in mind. Since the 1980s, CMHCs have depended on Medicaid for their survival and states have reasserted their authority in establishing guidelines and priorities.

### Deinstitutionalization and Federal Health Policy

Much attention was focused on preventive and community-based mental health in the early 1960s but, oddly enough, the Community Mental Health Centers Act and the hubbub that surrounded it played a relatively minor role in deinstitutionalization. Lyndon Johnson's Great Society initiative proved far more important. In particular, the passage of Medicare and Medicaid in 1965 had the largest influence. These two programs, with the addition of SSI in 1972, housing programs, and a variety of other safety-net supports, established the conditions that made implementation of community-based care possible.

In some respects the term *deinstitutionalization* is a misnomer. The first stage of deinstitutionalization actually involved a lateral transfer of patients from state mental hospitals to long-term nursing facilities. Medicare and Medicaid encouraged the construction of nursing home beds and the Medicaid program provided a payment source for patients transferred from state mental hospitals to nursing homes and general hospitals. Although states were responsible for the full costs of patients in state hospitals, they could now transfer patients and have the federal government assume from half to three-quarters of the cost, depending on the state's economic status. This incentive encouraged a massive transinstitutionalization of long-term patients, primarily elderly patients with dementia who had been housed in public mental hospitals for lack of other institutional alternatives. Although it is difficult to provide precise estimates, careful analysis suggests that between 1964 and 1977, 102,000 patients were transferred from public mental hospitals to nursing homes (Kiesler and Simpkins 1993; Goldman, Adams, and Taube 1983). In 1963, nursing homes cared for nearly 222,000 individuals with mental disorders, of whom 188,000 were sixty-five or older. Six years later the comparable figures were 427,000 and 368,000. Similarly, the availability of federal cost-sharing made it possible to provide inpatient care for persons with serious mental illnesses in general hospitals and contributed to the growth of specialized psychiatric units.

It is noteworthy how the availability of federal funding substantially transformed institutional infrastructures and made it possible to modify patterns of care for good and bad. In 1963 there were 16,370 nursing homes with 568,546 beds; by 1977, 18,900 nursing homes had more than 1.4 million beds and admissions increased over the period by more than 200 percent (Kiesler and Simpkins 1993). Although a large number of patients in nursing homes had dementia, depression, and other psychiatric illnesses, the vast majority came from general hospitals and the community. Nevertheless, the direct transfer from mental hospitals to nursing homes involved a significant proportion of the elderly mental hospital residents.

One might reasonably ask why public mental hospitals had such large numbers of old people with dementia in the first place, persons who could have been cared for more humanely and appropriately in smaller old-age homes commonly found in other countries. Hospitalization had little to offer in the way of treatment or even kind care. This pattern was shaped by presumably innovative public policies, adopted in large states such as New York and Massachusetts, and put in place to improve care and focus responsibility and accountability. At the end of the nineteenth and early in the twentieth centuries these and other states enacted care acts mandating that localities send insane persons to state hospitals where care was supported by state taxes. The goal of these laws was to provide individuals with a higher level of care. Local officials, however, saw an opportunity to shift costs to the state by closing locally funded almshouses (which in the nineteenth century served in part as old-age homes) and redefined dementia as insanity (Grob 1983).

A similar buildup occurred in general hospitals in response to federal funding. In 1963, there were 622 short-term nonfederal hospitals with areas for inpatient psychiatric services; only a few had specialized psychiatric units. By 1977 there were 1,056 such hospitals and 843 of them had specialized inpatient psychiatric units (Kiesler and Sibulkin 1987, 60). Discharges of patients with a first-listed diagnosis of mental illness grew from 678,000 in 1965 to 1.7 million by 1977. The number of private mental hospitals also more than tripled between 1970 and 1992, with inpatient admissions quadrupling, although these institutions accounted for only a small proportion of total hospital days. Average length of stay in general hospitals for patients with psychiatric illness in the period 1965–1988 was approximately twelve to thirteen days in contrast to inpatients stays of months and even years in state mental hospitals in prior years (Mechanic, McAlpine, and Olfson 1998).

One must not assume, however, that the clients with mental illness in general hospitals were necessarily those who would have been patients in state and county long-term mental hospitals. Between 1963 and 1977 a series of developments facilitated the growth of services to new populations: the growth of private and public insurance coverage for inpatient psychiatric care; an expanded definition of mental illness and the need for treatment; a substantial increase in mental health personnel; and greater public acceptance of psychiatric care. In 1955, for example, there were only 1.7 million episodes of mental illness treated in organized mental-health facilities; by 1983 the numbers of treated episodes had risen to 7 million (Mechanic 1999).

In 1947 there were 4,700 American psychiatrists and 23,000 mental health professionals in the core areas of psychiatry, clinical psychology, psychiatric social work, and psychiatric nursing. Assisted by federal training programs beginning in the 1950s, the number of mental health personnel expanded dramatically. Definitions of professional work are often unclear and numbers are difficult to collect accurately, but by the early 1990s there were between 33,000 and 38,000 active psychiatrists, approximately 30,000 practicing clinical psychologists, about 85,000 social workers with master's degrees doing mental health work, and something in excess of 10,000 nurses with master's degrees in psychiatric nursing. Several hundred thousand more workers provided mental-health services in a variety of nursing, social work, and paraprofessional roles. By 1992 there were almost 600,000 scheduled full-time equivalent positions in mental-health organizations (Mechanic 1999).

Rather than leading to improved organization, state policy decisions to reduce public mental hospital populations and to make admission to these hospitals more difficult—in association with other changes in public attitudes, treatment ideologies, and social and economic factors—supported the development of a confusing array of settings for the treatment of persons with mental illnesses. The mental-health system since the 1970s has included a bewildering variety of institutions: short-term mental hospitals, state and federal long-term institutions, private psychiatric hospitals, nursing homes, residential care facilities, community mental-health centers, outpatient departments of hospitals, community care programs, community residential institutions with different designations in different states, client-run and self-help services, among others. This disarray and the lack of any unified structure of insurance coverage or service integration has forced many patients with serious mental illnesses to survive in homeless shelters, on the streets, and even in jails and prisons.

## Some Consequences of Mental Health Policies

The first wave of deinstitutionalization and transinstitutionalization occurred largely in the 1960s and early 1970s, and involved two distinct populations. The first included long-term patients already in mental hospitals. They were transferred to other institutions, returned to their families (when such families existed and were willing to accept the patient), or relocated in a variety of community programs and facilities. The second included new cohorts of persons with mental illnesses coming to public notice for the first time, who encountered a much-modified system of services. These new patients were typically treated during short inpatient stays in general hospitals, in outpatient settings, and by community programs run by hospitals and community mental-health centers. Most received only outpatient care. Patients with serious mental illnesses who faced chronic difficulties could no longer easily reenter the public mental hospital and often had to make do with whatever services they could garner in the community (Pepper and Ryglewicz 1982; Lamb 1984).

Two important consequences for appropriate care followed from deinstitutionalization patterns. First, treatment in the community for clients with complex needs became a more difficult challenge. In the mental hospital all of the functions of care were brought together under one roof and coordinated. That such institutions did not meet all of their obligations was obvious, yet, at a time when alternatives were not available, mental hospitals served an indispensable function. In communities (and particularly in large cities), by contrast, clients were widely dispersed and their successful management depended on bringing together needed services administered by a variety of bureaucracies, each with its own culture, priorities, and preferred client populations. Although a number of efforts were made to integrate these services (psychiatric care, social services, housing, social support) in a meaningful way, the results in most localities were, and remain, dismal. Second, it proved extraordinarily difficult to supervise clients with serious disorders in the community, and many became part of the street culture where the abuse of alcohol and drugs was common. Substance abuse in particular increased the complexities of providing care, and most providers were unprepared for and even resistant to working with patients with dual disorders. Many psychiatric clinics excluded patients who were abusing drugs despite their growing population; this problem persists today in many treatment settings. Moreover, during and after the 1960s the antipsychiatry movement promoted the idea that mental illness was a myth and that psychiatrists and psychologists were controlling people with unconventional behavior (Szasz 1960, 1963). Many young street persons with mental illnesses were influenced by these views and contended that they were not mentally ill and were victimized because of their nonconformist behavior.

The second wave of deinstitutionalization was a phenomenon of the 1970s. An increasing number of lawyers who came to maturity during the civil right struggles of the 1960s transferred their allegiances and labored to protect the rights and liberties of persons with mental illnesses. Many of these lawyers were appalled by the visible abuses and insufficient care in mental hospitals, but they also shared a hostility toward psychiatry and were committed to a libertarian perspective. As Bruce Ennis, who led the Civil Liberties and Mental Illness Litigation Project in New York, wrote, in 1972, speaking of patients in mental hospitals,

> Many of them will be physically abused, a few will be raped or killed, but most of them will simply be ignored, left to fend for themselves in the cheerless corridors and barren back wards of the massive steel and concrete warehouses we—but not they—call hospitals. . . . So vast an enterprise will occasionally harbor a sadistic psychiatrist or a brutal attendant, condemned even by his colleagues when discovered. But that is not the central problem. The problem, rather, is the enterprise itself. . . . They are put away not because they are, in fact, dangerous, but because they are useless, unproductive, "odd," or "different."
>
> (Ennis 1972, vii–viii)

The 1970s was a decade of litigation on behalf of persons with mental illnesses. Lawyers contested involuntary civil commitment, insisted on a right to treatment, argued that patients had the right to refuse medication, and supported the concept of treatment in the least restrictive community alternative (Appelbaum 1994; Stone 1975). The attack, particularly on the practices of mental hospitals, motivated hospital administrators and states to reduce their resident populations further in order to meet court-mandated standards of care for those remaining in the hospital. The reduction in the number of patients and the maintenance of level funding increased per capita expenditures and satisfied court-ordered standards of hospital care, but it did little for the quality of care for most patients now in the community (Mechanic 1976).

The passage of SSI in 1972 facilitated deinstitutionalization by providing income that allowed patients to live in a variety of housing arrangements including sheltered-care facilities and group homes. Typically, the SSI allowance went to the proprietor, who in turn gave patients a small allowance and kept the rest as a payment for their care. It was never clear that these community arrangements, or those in nursing homes, provided a standard of care comparable to that available in any decent hospital, and there was much documentation of neglect, abuse, and fraud in these facilities. Nevertheless, studies of clients indicate that the vast majority preferred community residence, with all its difficulties, to hospital living.

In the heady days of deinstitutionalization advocacy few anticipated the extent of transinstitutionalization; the failure to develop even minimum community-care alternatives; the abdication of responsibility by CMHCs; the difficulties of integrating services across sectors; the complications of mental disorders by substance abuse, victimization, and homelessness; and the "criminalization" of serious mental illnesses. Lawyers and judges, many of whom had noble motives in struggling to protect the rights and liberties of mental patients and to establish a minimum decent standard of care, did not anticipate that state mental-health authorities would simply empty their hospitals without providing reasonable community alternatives. In setting specific treatment requirements for hospitals, judges often unwittingly limited institutional flexibility and innovation in providing care for persons with serious mental illnesses. In designing legislation and entitlements for people who were disabled and poor, policy makers manifested little awareness of the ways that various community actors, from state administrators to proprietors of private hospitals and hospital chains, would manipulate and subvert the payment mechanisms embodied in these programs.

One result of the failure of community-care alternatives for patients released from state mental hospitals has been the "criminalization" of persons with mental illness. Dependence on community treatment and the gross inadequacies of most programs of community care, particularly in high-density populations, ensures that many of these individuals will be in public places where their behavior is disturbing to others who may complain to the police. Although persons with mental illnesses are not at particularly high risk of engaging in serious criminal behavior, persons during florid psychotic states and those who abuse alcohol and drugs have a higher prevalence of violence than others in the population and are more likely to engage in disruptive behaviors leading to arrest (Steadman et al. 1998; Link and Stueve 1998).

A significant number of persons in prison for serious offenses have a mental illness. A study by the Justice Department in 1998 estimated that there were 280,000 people with mental illnesses in jails and prisons and more than a half million on probation (Ditton 1999). These numbers are difficult to interpret because there have always been many people with psychiatric disorders in jails and prisons who attracted little attention. Moreover, as concepts of mental illness have expanded and have come to include substance abuse, the number of incarcerated persons who are mentally ill—by definition—has increased. If, as epidemiological studies tell us, approximately a third of the population has had a mental illness in the prior year, there obviously will be many people in jails and prisons who fit these expansive mental-illness definitions. Estimates of serious mental illness in the prior twelve months that take functional impairment into account are much smaller, in the vicinity of five percent (approximately ten million people in the early 1990s) (Kessler et al. 1996).

Ultimately, the "criminalization" debate is really about whether individuals who commit offenses should be treated within the criminal justice or in the mental health system. Police are known to make "compassionate arrests" to get persons with disturbing behavior off the streets. Whether police bring such persons to mental-health facilities or jails depends on the behavior involved, police policy and programs, the availability of mental health treatment facilities, and the cooperation between treatment facilities and the police.

Those who oppose the criminal justice system point to the stigma associated with arrest and incarceration and the risks of victimization by other offenders. Others argue that persons with mental illnesses must be responsible for their behavior just like any other citizen, that such policy deters irresponsible behavior, and that some patients commit serious crimes that require prosecution. If treatment is required, they argue, it should be provided within the correctional system. Collaboration is possible between the two systems, but often cooperation is difficult to achieve because of the different perspectives, values, and cultures of the two sectors.

### Conclusion

History, of course, never quite repeats itself, but we clearly live with the results of the earlier complicated history of mental-health treatment and policy. While much has changed, we continue to hear the same dissatisfaction and laments. The President's New Freedom Commission on Mental Health, launched in April 2002, reported in its first communication to President George W. Bush in October that

> America's mental health services delivery system is in a shambles. We have found that the system needs dramatic reform because it is incapable of efficiently delivering and financing effective treatments. . . . Responsibility for these services is scattered among agencies, programs, and levels of government. There are so many programs operating under such different rules that it is often impossible for families and consumers to find the care that they urgently need. . . . Too many Americans suffer needless disability, and millions of dollars are spent unproductively in a dysfunctional service system.          (Hogan 2002)

In the aftermath of 9/11, the war on terrorism, and the growth of federal and state deficits, publicly financed services are again being cut back, and mental health coverage is typically among the first to be reduced. States that responded to the opportunities presented by federal programs some forty years ago have now built much of their service systems for persons with mental illnesses as part of the Medicaid program. The role of the state has shifted over time from direct provider, through its support of state hospitals and hospital aftercare programs, to purchaser, payer, and regulator of services largely provided through the private sector. In the process, there has been less direct public accountability. As budgets tighten, the pressures intensify to reduce eligibility and breadth of services and to push more persons with disabilities into managed-care arrangements as an acceptable means of cutting costs (Mechanic 2003). The average length of stay for psychiatric inpatients in general hospitals continues to be pushed down, averaging about 7.3 days in general nonprofit hospitals and 6.7 days in public general hospitals in the year 2000.

It is difficult to talk about mental-health policy as such because the future of mental-health services, particularly for persons with the most severe and persistent disorders, depends more than in earlier decades on the politics of health care generally, on insurance coverage, and on the quality of the safety net. The earlier system of state and county mental hospitals with their interested constituencies—including communities and hospital employees—were a significant political force for funding, but with the reduction of this sector such political power has eroded. Within Medicaid and other programs, advocates for persons with mental illnesses are but one constituency and, as these programs are amended to deal with fiscal pressures, not the first group policy makers have in mind. In recent years mental-health expenditures have fallen as a proportion of all medical expenditures, and the evidence suggests that these services are managed more stringently than other medical or surgical services (Mechanic and McAlpine 1999).

Some of the debates of earlier eras have emerged in new forms. In the 1950s, with the expansion of concepts of mental functioning, serious effort was given to define not only mental disorders but also positive mental health (Jahoda 1958). The community-mental-health movement, with its strong public health and preventive orientation, had a much-expanded view of its responsibilities and saw psychiatrists intervening in a wide range of community settings, working with teachers, judges, parents, and others to promote mental health (Caplan 1964). Although contemporary psychiatry has moved closer to medicine, a coalition of mental-health professionals, pharmaceutical companies, mental-health advocates, and even the federal government now promote a much-expanded concept of mental illness and define the need for treatment to involve a significant proportion of the population. Many problems of living—including substance disorders, eating disorders, inattention in school, and distressed responses to stressful events—are now included among disorders requiring treatment. The significant policy issue is whether such an expansion of concepts will take away from the more profound needs of the smaller population suffering from severe and persistent mental disorders.

History suggests some broad themes that are useful to keep in mind when developing policy decisions. At the very least, it teaches us that there is a price for implementing ideology ungrounded in empirical reality and for making exaggerated rhetorical claims. The ideology of community mental health and the facile assumption that residence in the community itself promotes adjustment and integration did not take into account the extent of social isolation, the exposure to victimization, substance abuse, homelessness, and the "criminalization" of persons with mental illnesses. The idea that CMHCs would take responsibilities for aftercare and rehabilitation of persons discharged from mental hospitals without mechanisms of accountability and control invited the centers to focus on the more amenable patients with less severe problems. There is risk that this problem is repeating itself as states turn to managed care for persons with serious mental illnesses. The evidence is limited, but it indicates that managed care leads to a "democratization" of service provision, reducing the intensity of services for patients with more profound disabilities and needs (Mechanic and McAlpine 1999). Moreover, as we expand definitions of psychiatric disorders and psychiatric need, advocate untested views about prevention, and market new pharmaceuticals aggressively to the general public, we again establish the conditions that can lead to even greater neglect of those who are truly disabled and most in need. At every level of mental-health-policy decision making, from development of financing and reimbursement arrangements to litigation and court decisions on patients' rights, historical review reveals extraordinary effects that were neither anticipated nor desired and consequences that had dire effects on the lives of those who were most vulnerable.

The basic premise that it was possible and useful to provide most treatment in community settings was not unsound if reasonable systems of community care had been developed. But few communities had the foresight or commitment to finance and provide such services and simply dumped patients to make their way among the uncoordinated array of programs, providers, and services that happened to be in the community. In many cases patients who remained sick and disabled had to fend on their own, often with unfortunate consequences. The challenges are even more difficult than most policy makers imagine, as large-scale efforts to integrate have demonstrated. Not only must a coordinated system be in place but specific attention must be given to the quality of services and implementation of each specific service such as housing, psychiatric treatment, and supported employment.

The history of mental mental-health until the end of World War II was largely the history of public mental hospital systems that cared for a relatively small proportion of persons compared to those now diagnosed with mental disorders. As awareness has grown of the prevalence of mental disorders, as new therapies have been developed for depression and other disorders, and as mental health treatment has gained greater acceptability, the population that could benefit from mental-health services has expanded. Many persons who have these disorders, however, lack insurance coverage or have insurance that excludes many mental-health services (Mechanic 2002).

In recent years, advocates at both the federal and state levels have fought for insurance coverage for mental illness comparable to that available for other disorders. Although many states have passed so-called parity legislation, mental illnesses still face stigma and discrimination by policy makers and employers who provide insurance coverage for their workers. Resistance to parity in part reflects an antipsychiatry ideology in the general culture but also relates to concerns that the definitions of mental illness are unbounded and that extensions would cause a flood of demand that would increase medical-care costs and add to the loss of insurance coverage. A key question is what differentiates mental illnesses from the distress and problems of normal life. One solution is to restrict parity to a limited set of serious diagnoses; another is to extend parity to all but only within managed-care arrangements. The evidence indicates that increased costs for this latter solution would be modest (Sturm 1997).

The parity issue, which occupies the attention of policy makers and advocacy groups, is not as central as the public debate seems to suggest, particularly as it applies to vulnerable populations with the most serious illnesses. Parity relates only to the insured population, and many persons with serious mental illness remain uninsured. Of those who have insurance, many are covered by Medicare and Medicaid, which have their own elaborate policy configurations. More importantly, the medical, social, and rehabilitation services needed by persons with severe illness are not typically covered by private insurance benefits. Thus, parity does not really solve the issue of meeting the needs for assertive case management, rehabilitation, housing, social services, supported employment, and other services that such clients require.

A broad solution to mental-health deficiencies requires above all an understanding that the problems of persons with serious and persistent disabilities are different from those of people with mild and moderate disorders. This is a lesson we once understood but has been lost as problems of living become medicalized and the needs of very different populations are intermixed. It may seem trite, since it is an old understanding, but effective community care for those who were once kept in hospitals must make up for the range of functions that hospitalization was intended to provide, from housing and supervision to treatment and rehabilitation. Failure to understand this lesson will contribute to the continuation of the sorry state of the deinstitutionalization saga.

## References

Appel, J. W., and G. Beebe. 1946. Preventive Psychiatry: An Epidemiologic Approach. *Journal of the American Medical Association* 131: 1469–1475.

Appelbaum, P. S. 1994. *Almost a Revolution: Mental Health Law and the Limits of Change.* New York: Oxford University Press.

Bockoven, J. S. 1972. *Moral Treatment in Community Mental Health.* New York: Springer Publishing Co.

Brown, G. W., M. Bone, B. Dalison, and J. K. King. 1966. *Schizophrenia and Social Care.* London: Oxford University Press.

Caplan, G. 1964. *Principles of Preventive Psychiatry.* New York: Basic Books.

Council of State Governments. 1950. *The Mental Health Programs of the Forty-eight States: A Report to the Governors' Conference.* Chicago: Council of State Governments.

Ditton, P. M. 1999. Mental Health and Treatment of Inmates and Probationers. U.S. Department of Justice Statistics (NCJ-174463). Washington, DC: U.S. Government Printing Office.

Ennis, B. 1972. *Prisoners of Psychiatry: Mental Patients, Psychiatrists, and the Law.* New York: Harcourt Brace Jovanovich.

Felix, R. H., and R. V. Bowers. 1948. Mental Hygiene and Socio-Environmental Factors. *Milbank Memorial Fund Quarterly* 26: 125–147.

Foley, H. A., and S. S. Sharfstein. 1983. *Madness and Government: Who Cares for the Mentally Ill?* Washington, DC: American Psychiatric Press.

Goldman, H. H., N. H. Adams, and C. A. Taube. 1983. Deinstitutionalization: The Data Demythologized. *Hospital & Community Psychiatry* 34: 129–134.

Greenblatt, M., R. H. York, E. L. Brown, and R. W. Hyde. 1955. *From Custodial to Therapeutic Patient Care in Mental Hospitals.* New York: Russell Sage Foundation.

Grob, G. N. 1983. *Mental Illness and American Society 1875–1940.* Princeton: Princeton University Press.

———. 1991. *From Asylum to Community: Mental Health Policy in Modern America.* Princeton: Princeton University Press.

Hogan, M. F. 2002. Interim Report of the President's New Freedom Commission on Mental Health. *Achieving the Promise: Transforming Mental Health Care in America. Final Report.* DHHS Pub. No. (SMA) 03–3832, Rockville, MD. Available online at http://www.mentalhealthcommission.gov/reports/Interim_Report.htm.

Isaac, R. J., and V. C. Armat. 1990. *Madness in the Streets: How Psychiatry and the Law Abandoned the Mentally Ill.* New York: Free Press.

Jahoda, M. 1958. *Current Concepts of Positive Mental Health.* New York: Basic Books.

Jones, M. 1953. *The Therapeutic Community: A New Treatment Method in Psychiatry.* New York: Basic Books.

Kessler, R. C., P. A. Berglund, S. Zhao, P. J. Leaf, A. C. Kouzis, M. L. Bruce, R. M. Fridman, et al. 1996. The Twelve-Month Prevalence and Correlates of Serious Mental Illness (SMI).1996. In *Mental Health, United States, 1996,* eds. R. W. Manderscheid and M. A. Sonnenschein. DHHS Pub. No. (SMA) 96–3098, Washington, DC: U.S. Government Printing Office.

Kessler, R. C., K. A. McGonagle, S. Zhao, C. B. Nelson, M. Hughes, S. Eshleman, H. U. Wittchen, et al. 1994. Lifetime and 12-Month Prevalence of DSM-III-R Psychiatric Disorders in the United States: Results from the National Comorbidity Survey. *Archives of General Psychiatry* 51: 8–19.

Kiesler, C. A., and A. E. Sibulkin. 1987. *Mental Hospitalization: Myths and Facts about a National Crisis.* Newbury Park, CA: Sage Publications.

Kiesler, C. A., and C. G. Simpkins. 1993. *The Unnoticed Majority in Psychiatric Inpatient Care.* New York: Plenum.

Kramer, M. 1967. Epidemiology, Biostatistics, and Mental Health Planning. *American Psychiatric Association Psychiatric Research Report* 22.

Lamb, H. R., ed. 1984. *The Homeless Mentally Ill: A Task Force Report of the American Psychiatric Association.* Washington, DC: American Psychiatric Association.

Lehman, A. F., L. T. Postrado, D. Roth, S. W. McNary, and H. H. Goldman. 1994. Continuity of Care and Client Outcomes in the Robert Wood Johnson Foundation Program on Chronic Mental Illness. *Milbank Quarterly* 72: 105–122.

Link, B. G., and A. Stueve. 1998. New Evidence on the Violence Risk Posed by People with Mental Illness. *Archives of General Psychiatry* 55: 403–404.

Mechanic, D. 2003. Managing Behavioral Health in Medicaid. *The New England Journal of Medicine* 348: 1914–1916.

———. 1976. Judicial Action and Social Change. In *The Right to Treatment for Mental Patients,* eds. S. Golann and W. J. Fremouw, 47–72. New York: Irvington Publishers.

———. 1999. *Mental Health and Social Policy: The Emergence of Managed Care.* Fourth ed. Boston: Allyn & Bacon.

———. 2002. Removing Barriers to Care Among Persons with Psychiatric Symptoms. *Health Affairs* 21: 137–147.

Mechanic, D., and D. D. McAlpine. 1999. Mission Unfulfilled: Potholes on the Road to Mental Health Parity. *Health Affairs* 18: 7–21.

Mechanic, D., D. D. McAlpine, and M. Olfson. 1998. Changing Patterns of Psychiatric Inpatient Care in the United States, 1988–1994. *Archives of General Psychiatry* 55: 785–791.

Mechanic, D., and D. Rochefort. 1992. A Policy of Inclusion for the Mentally Ill. *Health Affairs* 11: 128–150.

Milbank Memorial Fund. 1956. *The Elements of a Community Mental Health Program.* New York: Milbank Memorial Fund.

———. 1957. *Programs for Community Mental Health.* New York: Milbank Memorial Fund.

Peck, H. B. 1969. A Candid Appraisal of the Community Mental Health Center as a Public Health Agency. *American Journal of Public Health* 59: 459–469.

Pepper, B., and H. Ryglewicz, eds. 1982. *The Young Adult Chronic Patient.* San Francisco: Jossey-Bass.

Rapoport, R. N. 1960. *Community as Doctor.* Springfield, IL: C. C. Thomas.

Rosenheck, R. A., J. Lam, J. P. Morrissey, M. O. Calloway, M. Stolar, F. Randolph, and the ACCESS National Evaluation Team. 2002. Service Systems Integration and Outcomes for Mentally Ill Homeless Persons in the ACCESS Program. *Psychiatric Services* 53: 958–966.

Sampson, H., D. Ross, B. Engle, and F. Livson. 1958. Feasibility of Community Clinic Treatment for State Mental Hospital Patients. *Archives of Neurology and Psychiatry* 80: 71–77.

Scull, A. T. 1977. *Decarceration: Community Treatment and the Deviant.* Englewood Cliffs, NJ: Prentice Hall.

Shaw, R., and C. J. Eagle. 1971. Programmed Failure: The Lincoln Hospital Story. *Community Mental Health Journal* 7: 255–263.

Shortell, S. M., R. R. Gillies, D. A. Anderson, K. M. Erickson, and J. B. Mitchell. 1996. *Remaking Health Care in America: Building Organized Delivery Systems.* San Francisco: Jossey-Bass.

Stanton, A. H., and M. S. Schwartz. 1954. *The Mental Hospital: A Study of Institutional Participation in Psychiatric Illness and Treatment.* New York: Basic Books.

Steadman, H. J., E. P. Mulvey, J. Monahan, P. C. Robbins, P. S. Appelbaum, T. Grisso, L. H. Roth, et al. 1998. Violence by People Discharged from Acute Psychiatric Inpatient Facilities and by Others in the Same Neighborhoods. *Archives of General Psychiatry* 55: 393–401.

Stone, A. A. 1975. *Mental Health and the Law: A System in Transition.* Rockville, MD: National Institute of Mental Health, Center for Statistics of Crime and Delinquency (USDHEW publication no. ADM), 75–176.

Sturm, R. 1997. How Expensive is Unlimited Mental Health Care Coverage under Managed Care? *Journal of the American Medical Association* 278: 1533–1537.

Szasz, T. S. 1963. *Law, Liberty, and Psychiatry: An Inquiry into the Social Uses of Mental Health Practices.* New York: Macmillan.

———. 1960. The Myth of Mental Illness. *American Psychologist* 15: 113–118.

U.S. Congress. 1963. *Mental Health: Hearings before a Subcommittee on Interstate and Foreign Commerce House of Representatives.* Washington, DC: Government Printing Office.

# Emergency Rooms

## The Reluctant Safety Net

So what you're saying is, you're sick,
you're broke, you're unemployed and uninsured—yeah, sure, come on over.

Frank, desk clerk on NBC's *ER*
(aired February 6, 2003)

In the face of its unwillingness to guarantee health care to all, the United States
has increasingly depended on the emergency room as a de facto safety net for
people with nowhere else to go. Since the public knows that ERs are a place
where "they can't turn you away," hospital emergency departments have
become crowded, not only with true emergencies, but with people seeking routine medical attention. Hospital advocates insist that they are in the midst of
an emergency-care "crisis": overworked doctors and nurses toiling in overcrowded ERs with little or no hope of being reimbursed for much of the high
volume of care they provide.

This chapter will examine how emergency rooms developed into an unintended response to the inadequacies and limitations of the U.S. health-care
system. The ER's status as a doctor's office for all types of patients, from the
poor and uninsured to the middle class, emerged in piecemeal and mostly
unanticipated ways, long before the issue was addressed by law or policy.
Many argue that using the ER as a health-care safety net is irrational both medically and economically, since it encourages the most expensive type of serv-

ice and forces hospitals and doctors to provide uncompensated care, especially since the passage of federal emergency care requirements in 1986. However, patients' insistence on access to emergency rooms for all types of medical care emerged as a relatively rational response to the difficulties of access elsewhere in the health-care system. Emergency rooms are heavily used by both low-income, uninsured patients and middle-income patients with insurance. Both types of patients seek something they cannot find elsewhere: the right to be seen by a practitioner at any time of day or night.

Most literature on the subject assumes that the emergency-room crisis is a recent phenomenon, born of the dramatic upsurge in the uninsured population since the 1980s (Richardson, Asplin, and Lowe 2002). But the crisis began much earlier, in the 1950s, when the use of hospital emergency departments for both urgent and nonurgent care grew at an exponential rate. While ER utilization has continued to rise fairly steadily since 1970, the most dramatic jump came in the twenty-five years after World War II (American Hospital Association 1963–2001). By the late 1950s, the "overcrowding" of emergency rooms—which hospitals blamed on too many patients with seemingly non-emergency conditions—had become the norm. Understanding this earlier "crisis," as well as today's, requires examining the historical transformation of the emergency room from a minor hospital function to a centerpiece of U.S. health care.

## The Rise of the Emergency Room

The expectation that every hospital should have an emergency room was a phenomenon of the mid-twentieth century. Earlier definitions of emergencies were quite narrow, referring solely to accidents and trauma rather than disease or other conditions. Most accident victims in the 1800s were rushed to their homes, not the hospital, to await attendance by a physician. Large urban hospitals may have had an "accident room" or "first-aid room" for urgent cases, but these areas, like the rest of the facility, lacked round-the-clock physician coverage, and patients could wait hours to be seen. In order to handle a growing number of factory and railroad accidents, some smaller industrial cities built emergency clinics that later grew into general hospitals (Rosenberg 1987). Most patients taken to first-aid rooms and emergency clinics were travelers or transients, too far from home to call their own doctor, or people who lacked private physicians, such as industrial workers and the unemployed.

In the 1920s and 1930s, an increase in accident and trauma cases (mostly due to the automobile) combined with surgical advances and the growing prestige of hospitals led to an expansion of hospitals' emergency-care facilities. As more middle- and upper-class patients chose hospital-based surgery, larger hospitals began to offer after-hours operations for accidents and traumas, and some attending physicians took on the role of "night surgeons." New facilities adopted new technologies especially suited to emergencies, such as portable operating tables, quick sterilizers, and faster x-ray machines. As municipalities developed modern police, fire, and ambulance services, some hospitals opened special entrances to receive vehicles carrying incoming emergency patients (Raffensberger 1997; Hart 1933; Brown 1976).

Despite these developments, by the 1930s only a small minority of hospitals—mostly large, urban teaching institutions in the Northeast—had an officially designated "emergency ward." Just a few decades later, in 1960, 93.1 percent of them had one (USDHEW 1963). This astonishing growth paralleled the vast postwar expansion of U.S. hospital capacity purchased by the federal Hill-Burton Hospital Survey and Construction Act of 1946. Hill-Burton dollars allowed many hospitals to create new emergency wards with their own entrances. Hospitals that already had emergency facilities used Hill-Burton funds to add new emergency rooms or to expand their emergency services. In 1940 the average floor space given to emergency care in a sampling of Midwestern and Eastern hospitals was 63,000 square feet; by 1955 it had more than doubled, to 159,280 square feet (Shortliffe, Hamilton, and Noroian 1958, 22). Brand-new "modern" hospitals built with federal subsidies, particularly in nonurban areas, were now expected (but not required) to include an emergency room.

Hospitals added or expanded emergency care not just because funds were available to do so, but also because of the rise of a distinct science of emergency medicine that demanded its own technology and facilities. Battlefront medical advances during World War II gave physicians new abilities to revive the unconscious, prevent shock, and transfuse blood. Antibiotics made dramatic, immediate surgery safer; the discovery of heart defibrillation in the early 1940s made the hospital and its emergency ward the scene of "miraculous" new lifesaving techniques. By 1940 the hospital residency had become the approved training path for the medical specialties, giving more teaching hospitals around-the-clock physician coverage for their emergency rooms (Stevens 1989; Eisenberg 1997; Ludmerer 1999).

Emergency rooms became increasingly important to hospital incomes—a significant number of inpatient admissions originated in the ER—and to their attempts to build their status as community institutions. To maximize this potential, hospitals aggressively advertised their emergency capabilities. National Hospital Week, the American Hospital Association's (AHA) annual public relations event, featured the hospital's emergency role and emphasized the continuous availability of care. "Night and day . . . 'round the clock . . . the hospitals in [your area] stand ready to serve your every health need," touted a 1949 AHA radio spot. Ten years later, an AHA press release made the same point but this time referred to the ER's literal visibility as the nation's night light: "When the windows of homes and stores are dark and the whole city seems to be sleeping, a light can be seen behind a door marked 'Emergency Entrance' in your hospital" (Suggestions and Promotional Material . . . 1949).

The nation's growing emergency-care system had to make room for rapidly growing numbers of patients. Studies of the postwar decades show a spectacular increase in visits to hospital emergency departments. The AHA and American College of Surgeons determined in 1962 that "emergency room visits have increased fourfold since 1945," and a major study in *The New England Journal of Medicine* also found that emergency-room visits had increased 400 percent from 1940 to 1955. Hospital journals featured similarly high figures: the emergency department of Methodist Hospital in Indianapolis reported an increase in patient load of 380 percent from 1949 to 1959; emergency visits at Good Samaritan Hospital in Phoenix grew from 3,000 in 1950 to 26,000 in 1960 (Horgan 1962; Shortliffe, Hamilton, and Noroian 1958; Duncan 1961; Fahey 1964). Until at least the 1970s demands were more pronounced for the ERs of community general hospitals than those of university teaching hospitals serving large urban populations, and while today we often associate heavy use of emergency rooms with poverty, some studies found that "the greatest increase in utilization of hospital emergency departments occurred in middle-income groups" (*Hospital Topics* 1970; Webb and Lawrence 1972).

Observers puzzled over the reasons for this stunning growth in demand. In some ways it seemed a natural result of a swelling population, new facilities, and rising public expectations of medical care. ER volume was also increasing in Europe and Canada, although not as rapidly as in the United States (Blalock 1966; Seifert and Johnstone 1966). The popularity of emergency care could certainly be traced to the growing acceptance after World War II of the hospital as the center of the American health-care system. "The role of the general hospital has changed from that of a last resort," noted the authors of one emergency-care study, "to a community resource for a broad spectrum of general medical care." Rates of accidents and trauma rose after the war, mostly due to automobile crashes and industrial injuries, but these could account for only part of the increase. In several ERs studied in the early sixties "accidental injuries constituted only about one-third of the total emergency service cases." The huge jump in automobile ownership, however, played another role in ER use, since patients with cars—including women at home with children—simply found it easier and quicker to get to the hospital than those who depended on walking or public transport (Weinerman and Edwards 1964, 56; Seifert and Johnstone 1966, 58).

One explanation that hospitals repeatedly mentioned for the rise in ER visits was "the orientation of the public to the hospital as a place where one can receive aid at all times" (Shortliffe, Hamilton, and Noroian 1958, 23). The public's willingness to use the emergency room could not have come without wide awareness of the ER's role as an around-the-clock resource for care—an awareness that had been promoted by hospitals and providers via National Hospital Week and other forums. "The light over the emergency room door is the most trusted and comforting light known to the American public. It spells security," gushed the journal *Medical Economics* (Fahey 1964, 66). Hospitals wanted the patients to come, but their public relations campaign was, perhaps, too successful. By the late 1950s it was becoming evident that many, and in some cases most, of the patients arriving at the ER doors did not have an emergency condition at all.

### The "Crisis" of Nonemergency Care

In 1960 a study in *The Modern Hospital* commented that the emergency room "has now become a sort of a community health center to which many patients come for care of non-emergent illnesses." "Is the 'Accident Room' Evolving into the Community Medical Center?" echoed the *Bulletin of the American College of Surgeons* in 1961, a question that would be reiterated with growing urgency over the next decade (Duncan 1961; *Bulletin of the American College of Surgeons* 1961).

By 1965, professional journals and popular news media were featuring "sensational" headlines "referring to the 'emergency room crisis' or the 'great emergency room emergency'" (Michigan Blue Cross 1965). Patients were using the ER for purposes other than emergencies in such large numbers that the nation's shiny new emergency wards were transformed into overcrowded purgatories, staffed by gruff administrators and harried nurses and physicians, where patients waited for hours and people with the common cold drew resources away from those with chest pains and broken bones. In addition, the crowded waiting rooms and rushed staff left all patients feeling ill-treated and damaged the hospital's reputation.

The percentage of ER visits classified as "nonurgent" or "nonemergency" in the 1950s and 1960s was substantial, in some cases much greater than it is today. Hospitals reported rates of nonemergency visits ranging from forty-two percent to as high as seventy percent of their total caseloads. At one Indianapolis ER, 84.5 percent of visits were of a "less than urgent" or "non-emergency" nature (McCarroll and Skudder 1960; Fahey 1964; Duncan 1961).[1] The wide variation probably reflected the lack of consensus on the definition of "emergency" (aside from traumatic injuries). Emergency medicine did not become a professional specialty until the late 1970s, and in the absence of official standards, nurses, administrators, physicians, and researchers came up with their own classifications. Patients labeled nonurgent included those with stomach pains or upset; headache; cold or flu symptoms; ear, nose, and throat problems; allergies; minor injuries; scrapes and bruises; and those asking for diagnostic tests, prenatal or newborn care, prescription drugs, or follow-up care (Michigan Blue Cross 1965). In the 1950s and 1960s complaints that today would be considered urgent—such as a cut needing stitches, a minor fracture, or a child's ingestion of a suspect household chemical—might also be classed as nonemergency since it was expected that they would be taken care of in a doctor's office.

Hospital journals in the fifties and sixties began to study the problem in earnest, determined to understand what was drawing patients to emergency rooms for their routine care. No one was able to find a single, overarching reason, but several explanations stood out.

### Lack of a Private Physician

Some patients came to the ER because they had no doctor of their own. An increasing emphasis on specialization meant that fewer MDs were becoming primary-care doctors. Between 1950 and 1965, the number of general practitioners in the United States dropped from 95,000 to 68,000, and many only treated patients part-time (Blalock 1966; Somers and Somers 1961). Some commentators hypothesized that population mobility after World War II meant people were less likely to have a regular personal physician. For example, in Harvey, Illinois, a suburb of Chicago whose population had nearly doubled between 1952 and 1962, ER visits were rising at the rate of twenty-six percent a year. Hospital officials surmised that "most of the newcomers [to the town] hadn't bothered to get a family doctor" and that the ER had simply replaced the personal physician in the minds of these patients (Fahey 1964, 99; Seifert and Johnstone 1966).

### Reduced Access to Private Physicians

Students of ER overcrowding were, however, bewildered to find that patients who *did* have their own personal physicians also came to the hospital with both emergency and nonemergency conditions. A 1965 survey of twenty-two Michigan hospitals, for example, found that only eight percent of ER patients reported that they did not have a family doctor (Michigan Blue Cross 1965). On second glance, the phenomenon of patients turning to the ER rather than their doctor's office is less surprising; it was clearly related to structural changes in medical practice after World War II. The era of the house call was coming to an end, and private physicians were increasingly unwilling or unable to see patients outside of limited office hours (Somers and Somers 1961).

The authors of a 1958 study asked hospitals, "To what do you attribute the change in the use of the Emergency Room?" The most frequent reason, cited by 46.1 percent of respondents, was that patients could not find a physician at night or on weekends (Shortliffe, Hamilton, and Noroian 1958). Doctors were famously unavailable on Wednesdays, but not just on Wednesdays: "Sundays!" moaned one emergency physician, "That's when MDs send us their patients because the MDs don't want to make house calls—but they don't want to lose the patients, either!" (Horgan 1962, 54). The Michigan hospital survey found that "the patient load was greater on Sunday than on any other day of the week. . . . Only forty percent of all visits occurred during the daytime hours of 8 am to 4 pm" and "daytime visits increased on Wednesdays and Sundays" (Michigan Blue Cross 1965, 34–35).

Some blamed the problem on the public's impatience: "If people can't get their own doctors within a half hour, they head straight for our emergency room," complained the attending physician at Parma Community General Hospital in Ohio. But others thought the responsibility lay with practitioners. A writer for *Medical Economics* warned that private doctors could expect patients to visit their offices before the emergency room only "by becoming as accessible as the ER. Short of that, it would seem, physicians have forfeited the privilege of first consideration by a patient when he thinks he needs medical help fast, whether it's an emergency or not" (Fahey 1966, 85, 103). Physicians "have been partially responsible for fostering care of non-emergent problems in emergency rooms," argued an AMA handbook, and doctors needed to be reminded that "they have a 24-hour responsibility to their patients" (American Medical Association 1966, 6).

### Physician Attitudes toward Emergency Rooms

Physicians were not only less available, but also more willing to use the emergency room as a backup, advising patients to head to the ER for even routine care. The AHA journal *Hospitals* in 1964 reported a "growing tendency among private physicians to refer patients with unscheduled or off-hours requests for care to the hospital emergency department." Some doctors even "instruct their telephone answering service to suggest that callers go to the hospital emergency room if they need care when the doctor cannot be reached." Even during office hours, doctors would sometimes meet patients at the ER and use the facilities for a private consultation (Weinerman and Edwards 1964, 55; Michigan Blue Cross 1965).

Doctors increasingly relied on hospital emergency rooms as sources of newer and better technologies and equipment than they themselves could provide patients. In 1966 an Ohio GP reminisced, "Thirty years ago my office was much better equipped to handle accidents than our hospital emergency room was. I had a nurse, lab technician, x-ray, fluoroscope, EKG, closet full of plaster and splints, Kirschner drills and wire, all kinds of operating sets, facilities for anesthesia, etc. Today, I have no x-ray, no EKG, no lab technician and my office is not cluttered up with splints. . . . Were I to do the procedures I formerly did in my office I would be held for malpractice simply because we now have adequate and better facilities in the hospital emergency room." By the mid-1960s, not only doctors, but also employers, school administrators, police, and fire departments looked to the emergency room as the place of first resort to send the sick or injured (American Medical Association 1966, 6). Many patients arrived on their own, but many others were referred by someone in authority.

## Insurance Coverage

Increasing numbers of Americans in the 1950s and 1960s had hospital insurance, which paid for visits to the hospital—including the ER—but not doctor's offices. "[Insurance] coverage for care in, but not out of, the hospital contribute[s] to the popularity of the emergency service," commented the journal *Hospitals* in 1964 (Weinerman and Edwards 1964, 56). Blue Cross of Michigan was so disturbed by allegations that its coverage policies exacerbated emergency-room overcrowding (or, put less delicately, that they encouraged "Blue Cross abuse") that it surveyed patients in 1965 to determine why they used the ER for nonurgent conditions. Less than one percent mentioned financial reasons, but the study noted, "It can be argued that this figure understates the importance of financial motives because some patients may have been reluctant to admit them." The study's authors suspected that, especially among "repeat visitors" to the ER with nonurgent conditions, "there were some patients who used their hospital coverage to avoid paying physicians' fees." Private doctors may also have been influenced by insurance coverage when they referred patients to the ER. Some MDs admitted they were more likely to send patients to the hospital knowing that they were covered for such care but not for doctor's fees (Michigan Blue Cross 1965, 42, 44; Freidson and Feldman 1958, 7–8).

The expansion of insurance coverage with the creation of Medicare and Medicaid in 1965 also contributed to increasing ER use. Patients who had formerly been classed as "indigent" and were now covered by public insurance found themselves no longer eligible for free outpatient care. These patients moved "from the long, hard benches of the outpatient clinic . . . to the somewhat softer chairs—but equally long wait—in the emergency room" (Gee 1970, 73–75, 182). Indigent patients without any health coverage may also have preferred the ER as a way to avoid means-testing at charity clinics.

**Hospitals Respond to the "Crisis"**

Throughout the 1960s, hospitals became increasingly alarmed by emergency-room overcrowding. They depended on ERs for good public relations and for a significant percentage of profitable patient admissions, and overcrowding with nonemergency cases made it more difficult to deliver "real" emergency care and stole resources from the most urgent cases. When visits to the ER turned into a nightmare for both emergency and nonurgent patients, "A good hospital image that has taken years to acquire can be completely destroyed in a single visit to the emergency room." Hospitals responded with a new kind of public relations campaign. In 1964 the overwhelmed community hospital in Harvey, Illinois, launched publicity designed to reduce ER visits. Twenty thousand leaflets beseeched the public, "Attempt to contact your family physician before coming to the hospital. . . . The primary purpose of the emergency room is to treat only emergency cases." The campaign was found to have some effect in reducing the rate of increase of non-emergency visits, but not in stopping the increase (Fahey 1964, 99–103). By 1972 the AHA was no longer urging Americans to view the emergency room as a welcoming beacon; instead, National Hospital Week staff pleaded with hospitals to educate the public in the "proper use of the emergency room and [the] impact of [the] use of [the] ER as a 'doctor's office' on emergency room services" (For Urban Hospitals 1972).

The "triage" system, in which patients are briefly seen by a doctor or nurse and classified by urgency of condition, had been developed for battlefront medicine but was adapted to address the emergency-room crisis. Some hospitals reported great success with the method, arguing that it allowed patients with true emergencies to be seen almost immediately, while lesser cases were separated for longer waiting times or simply given referrals to a physician (Weinerman and Edwards 1964; Slater 1970). Triage was less successful on the public-relations level, since waiting times for nonurgent cases now stretched to many hours and left patients disgruntled. Some physicians and administrators were opposed to the concept of triage, thinking it appropriate for military medicine but not for "civilian emergency practice, where it is important to treat all patients without delay" (Webb and Lawrence 1972, 76).

Rather than keeping patients away or classifying them by triage, some physicians and administrators thought that emergency departments should adapt to their changing role in the medical system, and that the trend of increasing ER use "represent[ed] an emerging concept of health care that must be recognized and accepted" (Michigan Blue Cross 1965, 5). They argued that instead of restricting care, emergency-room facilities should be expanded to accommodate the growing demand. While for some the nonurgent patient in the emergency room represented a threat, others saw an opportunity to make the hospital into a truly comprehensive center for medical care.

### Crisis in the City

By the mid-1960s the ER "crisis" was also intertwined with the social crisis of America's inner cities. "Perhaps most important of all," wrote two physicians from Connecticut's Grace–New Haven Hospital in 1964 in explaining the increase in ER use, "is the steady trend toward concentration in the urban center, around the large hospitals, of . . . minority population groups, who are often recent arrivals to these old communities and have only remote connections to the 'usual' pattern of private medical care" (Weinerman and Edwards 1964, 56). Although middle-class use of emergency rooms also continued to increase, the media and professional journals turned their focus away from the broader public and toward the "ghetto poor" who were transforming urban ERs into centers for primary care for minorities, migrants, and immigrants.

While middle-class nonurgent patients usually did not lack a personal doctor, for inner city residents there was a growing and severe shortage of physician access as members of the overwhelmingly white medical profession joined the droves of other whites fleeing the city for the suburbs. In Baltimore, the Johns Hopkins's ER received over 100,000 visits in 1968; the neighborhood surrounding the hospital was served by only eight doctors, most of them semi-retired. After another Baltimore neighborhood, Lower Park Heights, shifted rapidly from a mostly Jewish to a mostly African American population, only five physicians remained. In contrast, a nearby white area boasted 114 MDs. In 1960 eighty-four percent of visitors to the emergency room at Sinai Hospital, which served Lower Park Heights, were white; by the end of the decade sixty-nine percent were black (Hoyt 1970; Berman and Luck 1971).

In the Chicago area in 1969, four percent of all physician visits were made in emergency rooms, but "for some of the inner-city poverty areas, between two-thirds and three-quarters of physician visits [took] place in emergency depart-ments, which clearly function[ed] as the major source of primary medical care." Only half of Chicago inner-city ER patients had a private physician (Gibson 1971, 51).

The problem for inner-city hospitals facing growing crowds in the emer-gency room was predominantly financial. Hospital personnel saw middle-class overutilization, while still significant, as a problem of overcrowding more than of reimbursement, since many of these patients had insurance coverage. Inner-city patients usually did not. In the 1960s and 1970s budgets for charity care shrank dramatically and hospitals looked to Medicaid to take up the slack. But government reimbursements for Medicaid proved disappointing, and budget cuts reduced them further while tightening eligibility requirements. As a result, Medicaid patients by the late 1970s were lumped with the uninsured; to hospitals, both represented financial loss. Private hospitals in the inner city, previously expected to take at least some share of low-income patients, began to shift the burdens of overcrowding and uncompensated care onto public institutions (Goldfrank 2003; Opdycke 1999). This led to a new crisis: "patient dumping."[2] The problem was no longer just that of patients using the ER for primary care, but of true emergencies being refused any care.

In the summer of 1981 the *Chicago Tribune* described a harrowing scene at Cook County Hospital, Chicago's gigantic public hospital, where "seriously ill patients could be seen lying on the floor at County's battle-scarred emergency room." Cook County normally took care of 90 to 125 indigent patients trans-ferred from private hospitals each month, but after new Medicaid cuts the number jumped to 365 in July and 560 in August. "Officials at County don't call this 'transferring,'" reported the *Tribune.* "They call it 'dumping,' a delib-erate attempt to get rid of Medicaid patients." Patients who were "dumped" at County included a sixty-year-old woman with severe pain, vomiting, and bowel obstruction who had to be operated on immediately for advanced can-cer and a woman with obvious symptoms of meningitis who was transferred for a CAT scan—even though the transferring hospital was well aware that County had no CAT-scan equipment (Schumer and Longworth 1982).

This was only the beginning of Cook County's crisis, which became the center of national attention in 1986 when the *New England Journal of Medicine* published a study of patients transferred to the hospital's emergency room. Transfers to Cook County had increased from 1,295 in 1980 to 6,769 in 1983. In their study of 467 patients transferred from private emergency rooms over a

six-week period, the authors found that eighty-nine percent were black or His-
panic; twenty-four percent were transferred in unstable condition; death rates
among transferred patients were more than twice that of patients not transferred; and in eighty-seven percent of the cases, the patient was transferred
because he or she had no insurance (Schiff et al. 1986). This and other exposés
led to a public outcry and demands that transferring hospitals be punished, but
there seemed to be little or no legal recourse for preventing such practices.
Patient dumping may have been an affront to ethical standards, but neither federal and state law nor hospital and health-care regulations prevented private
hospitals from refusing emergency cases. Law and policy had lagged far behind
public and medical understandings of the importance of emergency rooms in
the health-care system.

### Emergency Rooms in Law and Policy

"Patient dumping" or emergency refusal had a long history. In the late nineteenth century, for example, New York was scandalized when some patients
died while being transferred from private hospitals to Bellevue (Rosenberg
2004). Most physicians likely felt an ethical obligation to aid patients in emergencies, but the law recognized no such requirement. The common-law principle of "no obligation of rescue" applied to physicians and hospitals as well
as to the general public (Curran 1997). Malpractice law offered no redress for
patients denied emergency care. Although such cases seemed to invite charges
of physician negligence or abandonment, by law these concepts only applied
when treatment had already begun. Neither did hospitals, protected from lawsuits by government and charitable immunity, face any consequences for deny-
ing treatment. *McDonald v. Massachusetts General Hospital,* the famous 1876
case that established hospitals' charitable immunity, held that "no person has
individually a right to demand admission." The first state supreme court case
to address emergency refusal, *Birmingham v. Crews* in 1934, affirmed that
*McDonald* applied even in case of emergency; although a two-year-old girl died
of diphtheria after being turned out of a Birmingham, Alabama, emergency
ward, the court ruled that the hospital was in its rights to "refuse any patient
for any reason." The *Birmingham* ruling made it virtually impossible for
patients or their survivors to win suits for emergency refusal for the next several decades.[3]

State and local statutes, administrative regulations, and voluntary standards on emergency care were slow to develop. Illinois was in the vanguard:
the state had a statute forbidding emergency refusal in 1927 (oddly enough, a
criminal statute), but it seems never to have been enforced. By 1961 Illinois

was still the only state with such a law (Horty 1961a). The Chicago Hospital Council passed what was apparently the first voluntary antidumping guideline in 1947: "Hospitals must accept all patients coming for emergency treatment regardless of their finances, race, creed or color" (Hayt and Hayt 1947, 92). Since "dumping" continued in Chicago into the 1980s, the voluntary guideline was obviously ineffective.

Standards promoted by the nation's professional societies were entirely voluntary and lacked mechanisms for enforcement. The American Medical Association's 1957 revised Code of Ethics stated that physicians be "free to choose whom to serve . . . except in emergencies," but the AMA was silent on such crucial questions as emergency room staffing requirements and specialists' on-call obligations for emergency cases. The American College of Surgeon's emergency-room code suggested that the public's expectation of immediate care in an emergency room "must be accepted as a community obligation" of hospitals (Michigan Blue Cross 1965, 5), but hospitals faced no specific sanctions for failing to adopt the code. Other professional standards and guidelines failed to distinguish emergency from nonemergency care and in some cases even seemed to encourage or turn a blind eye to emergency refusal. In the early 1950s, the American Hospital Association's Manual on Admitting Practices and Procedures stated that admissions departments should be authorized to transfer patients, whether "for *financial reasons* or because they are warranted by the patient's medical condition" (*Trustee* 1951, 10; emphasis added). In its Standards for 1965, the Joint Commission for the Accreditation of Hospitals (JCAH) advised that "adequate appraisal, advice and/or initial treatment shall be rendered to any ill or injured person who presents himself at the hospital," but then carefully added, "based upon community need and the capability of the hospital." Hospitals with limited facilities could transfer particular patients, and the JCAH Standards concluded, "other hospitals may elect to transfer all emergency patients" (JCAH 1965). Voluntary regulations carefully weighed the growing role of emergency rooms in the health-care system against providers' right to refuse care.

In some areas, local authorities attempted to change hospital behavior by using licensing codes and tax regulations. Hospitals who turned away emergency patients might be threatened with loss of their licenses; Kentucky, for example, added a requirement forbidding discrimination in emergencies to its hospital licensing statute in 1961 (Horty 1961b). Since the great majority of hospitals were classed as charities or nonprofits and not required to pay taxes, a threat of revoking tax exemption could be particularly potent. In 1954 a severely burned five-month-old infant died after being turned away from

Chicago's Woodlawn Hospital, a private, tax-exempt institution, allegedly because her mother could not pay the $100 deposit. The baby's parents went to the press, and their story received nationwide coverage. After sensational headlines and raucous public meetings, the Cook County tax authorities, at the request of the state's attorney and Chicago's activist public-health commissioner, removed Woodlawn from the tax-exempt list, and sent the hospital a tax bill of $12,002.88.[4]

"When a climate of public indignation exists," noted one analyst, "the very governmental exemptions and subsidies that hospitals enjoy can become weapons against them" (Horty 1961a, 106). What about the hospitals' most massive government subsidy, the Hill-Burton hospital construction program? As Rosemary Stevens has shown, Hill-Burton legislation had been designed to minimize federal regulation of hospitals, even as federal dollars poured into their construction and expansion (Stevens 1989). Officially, hospitals accepting Hill-Burton funding were required to provide a "reasonable volume" of uncompensated care, but these requirements were ignored until the 1970s. And the law's "separate but equal" provision gave sanction to racially segregated hospitals in the South and served to encourage racial dumping (Smith 1999).[5] In 1963 federal Hill-Burton administrators drew up guidelines specifically for hospital emergency services, but like the professional-society standards they were extraordinarily weak and entirely voluntary, listing only staffing and technical criteria "which might be considered" and making no mention of community-service or nondiscrimination requirements (USDHEW 1963). The legislation establishing Medicare was more specific about ER requirements for participating hospitals, insisting that hospitals provide around-the-clock staffing for emergencies, but it was silent on the question of access (Webb and Lawrence 1972, 69).

Voluntary, unenforceable standards, weak or nonexistent regulations, and the persistence of "dumping" combined with the public's growing reliance on the emergency room to create a climate ripe for legal change. In 1961, the AHA journal *Modern Hospital* reported that in the past five years "there have been more appellate cases involving hospital emergency care situations than in all the previous years in which cases have been nationally reported." For the first time, a legal requirement to provide emergency care was becoming a serious possibility. "Adequate emergency facilities are generally assumed by the public," and hospitals that disappointed public expectations should prepare for litigation, warned the journal (Horty 1961b, 106, 159). In *Wilmington v. Manlove* (1961) the Delaware Supreme Court insisted on hospitals' obligation to provide emergency care, arguing that the very existence of an emergency room meant the hospital was "holding out to the public" a promise to provide care. After two severely burned Mexican children were turned away by a private hospital, the Arizona Supreme Court ruled in *Guerrero v. Copper Queen* (1975) that hospitals "may not deny emergency care to any patient [including non-citizens] without cause."[6] Courts outside Delaware and Arizona, however, generally did not find these rulings sufficient to overturn *Birmingham v. Crews*.

In 1979, after decades of struggling for professional acceptance, emergency physicians established their own specialist certifying board, the American College of Emergency Physicians (Goldfrank 2003). This new professional body was concerned with the training and knowledge emergency specialists should exhibit and was initially silent about hospitals' or physicians' obligations to provide emergency care. There was more action at the state level; by 1984, twenty-two states had some type of emergency-care laws on the books, but again, these were rarely enforced. Patients denied emergency treatment might look to a bewildering variety of legal precedents, local and state laws, regulations, and standards to claim a right to care, but there was still no concerted or coordinated effort, either in law or in the health-care system, to prevent emergency refusals (Dowell 1984).

## EMTALA: The Right to Emergency Care

Chicago's crisis quickly became a national one. Two of the authors of the 1986 Cook County study, who were both emergency physicians at the hospital, published a 1987 piece in *JAMA* in which they estimated, based on ER studies from Chicago, Dallas, and Oakland, California, that 250,000 patients were inappropriately "dumped" every year in the United States (Ansell and Schiff 1987). Although some disputed this figure, patient advocates and their congressional sympathizers seized on this and other evidence of extensive dumping to argue for federal action against refusals of emergency care. Following several sensational dumping cases in his district, Pete Stark, the Democratic congressional representative for Alameda County, California, introduced the Emergency Medical Treatment and Active Labor Act (EMTALA) (Bedard, Yeh, and Bitterman 2000; Salisbury 1987). EMTALA stated that in any hospital receiving Medicare funds (thus virtually all U.S. hospitals),

> If any individual comes to the emergency department and a request is made on the individual's behalf for examination or treatment for a medical condition, the hospital must provide for an appropriate medical screening examination within the capability of the hospital's emergency department . . . to determine whether or not an emergency medical condition . . . exists.

The requirement also applied to women in labor. Hospitals found in violation could be fined $25,000 (later raised to $50,000) and have their Medicare status revoked. EMTALA also allowed patients to bring civil suits for violations. Stark succeeded in attaching EMTALA to the Consolidated Omnibus Budget Reconciliation Act of 1986, and it passed with no hearings and virtually no public fanfare.[7]

With little funding for EMTALA investigations under the Ronald Reagan and George H. W. Bush administrations, the law was not vigorously enforced until the mid-1990s. Since then, EMTALA has been unpopular with many providers, who resent the increased paperwork, the law's failure to define terms like "stabilize" and "emergency condition," the imposition of new liabilities, and supposed government encroachment on professional autonomy (in the words of one emergency physician, EMTALA "told hospitals how to practice medicine," Henry 2000, xiii). Some have even accused EMTALA of creating or exacerbating the overcrowding crisis in the nation's emergency rooms (Carpenter 2001; Epstein 1997), although no one has offered convincing evidence linking the two. As this chapter has shown, numerous factors led increasing numbers of people to seek care in emergency rooms well before EMTALA.

The verdict on whether EMTALA has ended the abuses it was designed to eliminate has been mixed. A former administrator of Cook County Hospital said that in her experience, the law "ended" the practice of emergency dumping in Chicago (Terrell 2003). Officials at LA County Hospital, however, were less sanguine; in 2003 they asked for state legislation to curb the still-common practice of private hospitals transferring "stabilized" patients to County for economic reasons. Six thousand such patients arrive at LA County annually (Ornstein and Weber 2003). Despite its shortcomings, and despite the George W. Bush Administration's weakening of some provisions of EMTALA in 2003, the statute will likely stand up to challenge because it reflects a public consensus on the importance and desirability of access to emergency rooms (Pear 2003).[8] Few politicians would be willing to risk the accusations of callousness that would inevitably follow from seeming to oppose their constituents' right to emergency care.

## Conclusion

This chapter has shown that there is nothing new about emergency room overcrowding, or about patients using the emergency room for nonemergency conditions. U.S. emergency rooms have been described as "in crisis" since the late 1950s. The nature and intensity of the crisis, however, has changed over time.

In the immediate post–World War II period and through the 1960s, ER utilization increased as the U.S. middle class's rising expectations of health care clashed with new types of rationing, including reduced access to private doctors, the end of house calls, and insurance limitations on payment for non-hospital care. Federal dollars from the Hill-Burton Act encouraged hospitals to construct and equip emergency facilities that far outstripped those of individual physicians, making the ER the venue of choice for patients needing or wanting a wide array of diagnostic and treatment procedures. In hospital advertising and on TV dramas, ERs were showcased as a "welcoming beacon" and an "open door" offering immediate, convenient access to the most highly trained doctors and most advanced medical technologies. ERs became crowded, but providers were, for the most part, compensated through private insurance, patient payments, and eventually Medicare and Medicaid.

By the end of the sixties and into the seventies, this began to change. White flight to the suburbs left urban pockets of largely poor minority populations drastically underserved by a dwindling number of physicians. These patients turned to the emergency room for the care they needed, but fewer were able to pay for services either directly or through insurance. Medicaid and other reimbursements were outstripped by a huge rise in medical costs, and financial pressure on hospitals led to major reductions in charity care. The overcrowding crisis also became a financial crisis for hospitals.

In the 1980s, inner-city emergency rooms faced new, huge burdens of AIDS, homelessness, drugs, and gun violence. Private hospitals responded to cuts in Medicaid and Medicare reimbursement by "dumping" emergency patients onto already-stressed county and municipal hospitals. There was now a crisis of access for the poor and uninsured who were being turned away from emergency rooms. The Emergency Medical Treatment and Active Labor Act attempted to tackle the issue of access while ignoring perennial challenges of overcrowding and unreimbursed care.

These problems persisted in the 1990s and continue today. In 2001, ninety-one percent of hospital emergency department directors "reported crowding as a problem," one that had been worsened by the closing of over a thousand emergency rooms between 1988 and 1999, mostly due to hospital mergers and consolidations (Richardson, Asplin, and Lowe 2002).[9] Despite various efforts to encourage greater use of primary-care doctors and health centers, patients' dependence on emergency rooms for routine and nonurgent care has persisted (National Center for Health Statistics 2002; Thompson and Glick 1999; Centers for Disease Control 2003). This most recent manifestation of the overcrowding crisis differs from earlier decades because of its even greater association with uncompensated care. The pressure on today's emergency rooms seems inseparable from the broader crisis of access represented by the rising ranks of the uninsured since the early 1990s, which swelled to forty-four million in 2004 (Cover the Uninsured Week 2004).

However, emergency-room crowding cannot be attributed entirely to the uninsured, since middle-class people with health insurance continue to use ERs for routine medical care; indeed, insured Americans accounted for most of the sixteen percent increase in ER visits between 1996 and 2001, according to one study (Center for Studying Health System Change 2003). Such behavior is still termed "inappropriate" and referred to as "overutilization" and even "abuse." History, however, shows that there is nothing new about middle-class demands on emergency care, and attempts to curb such utilization have always failed. The persistence of insured patients' use of ERs, from the 1950s until today, shows that emergency rooms operate as a safety net not just for the uninsured or inner-city poor, but for all types of access problems in the health system. The rise of HMOs and other forms of "managed care" since the early 1990s has led to even more pronounced forms of rationing, such as prospective and retrospective denials of reimbursement, long waits for appointments, and more cursory attention from doctors. In the current climate of cost-cutting and cost-shifting, insured patients, like their uninsured counterparts, look to the emergency room as the only place where they can't be turned away. The most recent attempt to curb ER use, in the form of retrospective denials for reimbursement by managed-care companies, led to the establishment in many states of the "prudent layperson" definition of medical urgency, which like EMTALA codified in law what patients had already been practicing: defining for themselves what constitutes an emergency or urgent condition (Guttman, Zimmerman, and Nelson 2003; Koziol-McLain et al. 2000.)

What has been perceived as an intractable crisis, then, also serves as a stabilizing force in the health-care system. Emergency rooms act as a social safety net for the problems of uninsurance, rationing, and inadequate primary and preventive care endemic to the U.S. medical system. In addition, ERs serve as a *political* safety net against demands for universal coverage. As bad as things might get, Americans and their elected officials can fall back on the comforting notion that the nation doesn't leave sick people to die in the streets—they will always be taken care of in an emergency room (Meier 2004).[10]

Many politicians and policy makers in the United States today argue for the power of market forces to solve a wide array of economic and social problems, but the open admissions policies of emergency rooms, in both law and practice, highlight a powerful strain of American resistance to market definitions of health care. Whether in the form of curbs on nonurgent visits or blatant "dumping" of the uninsured, attempts to restrict emergency-room utilization have been resoundingly rejected by the public. Emergency care has been conceived of as a right, first demanded by patients, then grudgingly accepted (and occasionally championed) by providers, and finally written into law. The current political drive to organize health care around market values will run up against a formidable barrier when it reaches the doors of the emergency room.

Due to historical circumstances rather than deliberate policy choices, emergency rooms continue to be the only part of the U.S. health system offering a statutory guarantee of access. The former director of the federal Centers for Medicare and Medicaid Services, Thomas Scully, has called EMTALA "a backdoor way to get people universal access to at least emergency room care" (Scully 2003). Scully's statement calls into question the wisdom of allowing sick people to depend on a safety net that is both unintentional and mostly unfunded. The legislators, political candidates, and Presidential administrations who have explicitly given up the fight for universal health care should, at minimum, find a way to fairly compensate the dedicated emergency room physicians, nurses, and staff who provide the nation with such an essential service. Even if they do so, it will not solve the contradictions inherent in providing emergency treatment without adequate provision for primary, preventive, long-term, and follow-up health care. As a justice of the Delaware Supreme Court mused in deciding the *Manlove* case in 1961, "[R]equir[ing] the hospital to care for emergency cases, as distinguished from others, is not logical. Why emergency cases? If the holding is sound it must apply to all the hospital services." Whether the right to emergency care will open the door to more universal rights to health care remains to be seen.

### Notes

1. Some studies distinguished between "non-emergency" conditions (which might be serious but not requiring immediate care) and "non-urgent" conditions (not requiring care within a few hours, or at all), but others did not.
2. The activist group Health PAC may have invented the term "patient dumping"; it published an article on the topic as early as 1974 (B. Roth, "Patient Dumping," *Health PAC Bulletin* [May/June 1974]: 6–10).
3. 120 Mass. 432 (1876); 229 Ala. 398 (1934). Examples of post-*Birmingham* cases include *Meiselman v. Crown Height Hospital*, 285 NY 389 (1941); *Jones v. City of New York*, 134 NYS 2d 779 (1954); *O'Neill v. Montefiore Hospital*, 202 NYS 2d 436 (1960).
4. The case is described in John Cooper, M.D., PR Institute, Princeton, N.J., July 1954, "The Liability of the Emergency Room," typescript in Emergency Hospitals and

Departments—Legal Aspects, Subject File, AHA Resource Center; undated clipping (ca. 1954), *Chicago Daily News;* "Hospital off tax free list," *Chicago American,* March 10, 1954, both in Box 8, File 6, Papers of Malcolm T. MacEachern, M.D., AHA Resource Center. The public health commissioner was Herman Bundesen.

5. For class-action lawsuits demanding hospital adherence to Hill-Burton uncompensated care requirements, see, for example, *Cook v. Ochsner Foundation Hospital,* 559 F.2d 968; 1977 U.S. App. (1977).

6. *Wilmington General Hospital v. Darius M. Manlove,* 54 Del. 15 (1961); *Guerrero v. Copper Queen Hospital,* 112 Ariz. 104; (1975).

7. 42 USC 1395dd; COBRA Section 9121; Section 1867 of the Social Security Act.

8. The Bush Administration changes narrow the definition of hospital property where patients are entitled to emergency care and ease requirements for on-call specialist coverage of ERs.

9. Apparently ER overcrowding has not been a primary factor in hospital closings. The federal Office of the Inspector General found that, for both urban and rural hospitals, closings were the result of "business related decisions or a low number of patients," while competition was also a factor for urban hospitals. Smaller hospitals were far more likely to close than the large urban hospitals with the most crowded ERs. Department of Health and Human Services, Office of the Inspector General, *Trends in Urban Hospital Closure 1990–2000,* OEI-04-02-00610 (May, 2003); *Trends in Rural Hospital Closure, 1990–2000,* OEI-04-02-0611 (May, 2003). Unfortunately, the OIG reports do not specifically address emergency departments as opposed to hospital closings.

10. This assumption was, of course, badly shaken after Hurricane Katrina.

**References**

American Hospital Association. 1963–2001. *Hospital Statistics Annual.* Chicago: American Hospital Association.

American Medical Association. 1966. *Emergency Department: A Handbook for the Medical Staff.* Chicago: American Medical Association.

Ansell, David A., MD and Robert L. Schiff, MD. 1987. Patient Dumping: Status, Implications, and Policy Recommendations. *JAMA* 257: 1500–1502.

Bedard, Larry A., Charlotte S. Yeh, and Robert A. Bitterman. 2000. The History of EMTALA. In *Providing Emergency Care Under Federal Law: EMTALA,* ed. Robert A. Bitterman. Dallas: American College of Emergency Physicians.

Berman, Joseph I., and Elizabeth Luck. 1971. Patients' Ethnic Backgrounds Affect Utilization. *Hospitals* 45: 64–68.

Blalock, William R. 1966. Emergency Care. *Hospitals* 40: 51–54.

Brown, Vernon. 1976. *The Story of Passavant Memorial Hospital, 1865–1972.* Chicago: Northwestern Memorial Hospital.

*Bulletin of the American College of Surgeons.* 1961. Editorial. March–April: 43.

Carpenter, Dave. 2001. Our Overburdened ERs. *Hospitals & Health Networks* 75: 44–47.

Center for Studying Health System Change. 2003. Insured Americans Drive Surge in Emergency Department Visits. Issue Brief No. 70, October.

Centers for Disease Control. 2003. ER Use Increased 20% Over Last 10 Years. Kaiser Daily Health Policy Report, 5 June. www.kaisernetwork.org.

CMMC Emergency Department History. 2006. Central Maine Medical Center, www.cmmc.org/pc-em-history.html.

Cover the Uninsured Week. 2004. Three Fourths of Emergency Physicians Say Number of Uninsured Patients in ERs Is Growing. Press Release, 13 May, available at cover-theuninsuredweek.org.

Curran, William J. 1997. Legal History of Emergency Medicine from Medieval Common Law to the AIDS Epidemic. *American Journal of Emergency Medicine* 18: 658–670.

Dowell, Michael A. 1984. Indigent Access to Hospital Emergency Room Services. *Clearinghouse Review* October: 483–499.

Duncan, Margaret. 1961. How to Evaluate Emergency Room Care. *Modern Hospital* 99: 168.

Eisenberg, Mickey S. 1997. *Life in the Balance: Emergency Medicine and the Quest to Reverse Sudden Death.* New York: Oxford University Press.

Epstein, Richard. 1997. *Mortal Peril: Our Inalienable Right to Health Care?* Reading, MA: Addison Wesley.

Fahey, John M. 1964. Six Ways to Deal with the Emergency Room Crisis. *Medical Economics,* 20 November.

For Urban Hospitals. 1972. File 11, Box 2, National Hospital Week Collection, AHA Resource Center.

Freidson, Eliot, and Jacob J. Feldman. 1958. *Public Attitudes toward Health Insurance.* New York: Health Information Foundation, Research Series 5.

Gee, David A. 1970. Ambulatory Care. *Hospitals* 44: 73–75, 182.

Gibson, Geoffrey. 1971. State of Urban Services—I. *Hospitals* 45: 49–54.

Goldfrank, Lewis R. 2003. Personal and Literary Experiences in the Development of an Emergency Physician. *The Journal of Emergency Medicine* 24: 73–84.

Guttman, Nurit, Deena R. Zimmerman, and Myra Schaub Nelson. 2003. The Many Faces of Access: Reasons for Medically Nonurgent Emergency Department Visits. *Journal of Health Politics, Policy, and Law* 28: 1089–1120.

Hart, Chester. 1933. A Century of Progress Hospital for Emergency Cases. *Modern Hospital* 41: 79–82.

Hayt, Emanuel, and Lillian R. Hayt. 1947. *Law of Hospital, Physician and Patient.* New York: Hospital Textbook Co.

Henry, Gregory L. 2000. Foreword. In *Providing Emergency Care under Federal Law: EMTALA,* ed. Robert A. Bitterman. Dallas: American College of Emergency Physicians.

Horgan, Patricia D. 1962. The Emergency Room Crisis: How One Hospital is Handling It. *R.N.* October: 46–57, 94.

Horty, John F. 1961a. Emergency Care—Or Lack of It—Can Make a General Hospital Liable. *Modern Hospital* 96, no. 1: 106, 159.

————. 1961b. When a Hospital Has an Emergency Room It May Be Required to Give Treatment. *Modern Hospital* 96, no. 2: 103–105.

*Hospital Topics.* 1970. Chicago Studies Emergency Services: Finds Where Improvement Is Needed. 48: 37–39.

Hoyt, Edwin P. 1970. *Your Health Insurance: A Story of Failure.* New York: The John Day Company.

Joint Commission on Accreditation of Hospitals (JCAH). 1965. Emergency Service: Standard I. *Standards for Hospital Accreditation.* Chicago: Joint Commission on Accreditation of Hospitals, July.

Koziol-McLain, Jane, David W. Price, Barbara Weiss, Agatha A. Quinn, and Benjamin Honigman. 2000. Seeking Care for Nonurgent Medical Condition in the Emergency Department: Through the Eyes of the Patient. *Journal of Emergency Nursing* 26: 554–563.

Ludmerer, Kenneth. 1999. *Time to Heal: American Medical Education from the Turn of the Century to the Era of Managed Care.* New York: Oxford University Press.

McCarroll, James R., MD and Paul A. Skudder, MD. 1960. Conflicting Concepts of Function Shown in National Survey. *Hospitals* 34: 35–38.

Meier, Conrad F. 2004. No Insurance Doesn't Mean No Healthcare. *Los Angeles Times,* 21 May. Available at www.latimes.com/news/opinion/commentary/la-oe-meier21_may21,1,187700.story?coll=la-news-comment-opinions (accessed 1 June 2004).

Michigan Blue Cross. 1965. Hospital Emergency Room Utilization Study: A Report on Emergency Room Visits in 22 Michigan Hospitals. File Drawer F-1, Hospital Emergency Units, Michael M. Davis Papers, New York Academy of Medicine.

National Center for Health Statistics. 2002. *National Ambulatory Medical Care Survey: 2000 Emergency Department Summary.* 22 April, Report No. 328. Available at www.cdc.gov/nchs/products/pubs/pubd/ad/321-330/321-330.htm#ad326.

Opdycke, Sandra 1999. *No One Was Turned Away: The Role of Public Hospitals in New York City since 1900.* New York: Oxford University Press.

Ornstein, Charles, and Tracy Weber. 2003. County May Limit Shift of Patients. *Los Angeles Times,* 11 May.

Pear, Robert. 2003. Emergency Rooms Get Eased Rules on Patient Care. *New York Times,* 3 September.

Raffensberger, John G. 1997. *The Old Lady on Harrison Street: Cook County Hospital, 1833–1995.* New York: P. Lang.

Richardson, Lynne D., MD, Brent R. Asplin, MD, MPH, and Robert A. Lowe, MD, MPH. 2002. Emergency Department Crowding as a Health Policy Issue: Past Development, Future Directions. *Annals of Emergency Medicine* 40: 388–393.

Rosenberg, Charles E. 1987. *The Care of Strangers: The Rise of America's Hospital System.* New York: Basic Books.

———. 2004. E-mail communication with the author, 28 January.

Salisbury, Lois. 1987. Testimony on Behalf of Coalition to Stop Patient Dumping, Equal Access to Health Care: Patient Dumping. Hearing Before a Subcommittee of the Committee on Government Operations, House of Representatives, One Hundredth Congress, First Session, 22 July, 257–269.

Schiff, Robert L., MD, David A. Ansell, MD, James E. Schlosser, MD, Ahamed H. Idris, MD, Ann Morrison, MD, and Steven Whitman, Ph.D. 1986. Transfers to a Public Hospital: A Prospective Study of 467 Patients. *New England Journal of Medicine* 314: 552–557

Schumer, Fern, and R. C. Longworth. 1982. County Hospital at the Brink. *Chicago Tribune,* 2 May: 33, 40.

Scully, Thomas. 2003. Interview on "All Things Considered," National Public Radio, 3 September.

Seifert, Vernon D., and J. Stanley Johnstone. 1966. Meeting the Emergency Department Crisis. *Hospitals* 40: 55–59.

Shortliffe, Ernest C., MD, Stewart Hamilton, MD, and Edward H. Noroian. 1958. The Emergency Room and the Changing Pattern of Medical Care. *The New England Journal of Medicine* 2: 20–25.

Slater, Reda R. 1970. The Triage Nurse. *Hospitals* 44: 50–52.

Smith, David Barton. 1999. *Health Care Divided: Race and Healing a Nation.* Ann Arbor: University of Michigan Press, 46–47.

Somers, Herman M., and Anne R. Somers. 1961. *Doctors, Patients, and Health Insurance.* Washington, DC: The Brookings Institution.

Stevens, Rosemary. 1989. *In Sickness and in Wealth*. New York: Basic Books.

Suggestions and Promotional Material for National Hospital Day. 1949. File 2; Sample Editorial, 1959, File 12, both in Box 1, National Hospital Week Collection, American Hospital Association Resource Center.

Terrell, Pat. 2003. Personal communication with Dr. Quentin Young, 12 June.

Thompson, Karen MacDonald, and Doris F. Glick. 1999. Cost Analysis of Emergency Room Use by Low-Income Patients. *Nursing Economics* (May/June): 42–148.

*Trustee*. 1951. The Admitting Office: Nerve Center of the Hospital. 4: 7–10.

U.S. Department of Health, Education, and Welfare (USDHEW). 1963. Hospital Emergency Service: Criteria for Organization. Washington, DC: Hospital and Medical Facilities Series under the Hill-Burton Program, Public Health Service Publication No. 930-C-3.

Webb, S. B., Jr., and R. W. Lawrence. 1972. Physician Staffing and Reimbursement Trends. *Hospitals* 46: 76.

Weinerman, E. Richard, MD, and Herbert R. Edwards, MD. 1964. 'Triage' System Shows Promise in Management of Emergency Department Load. *Hospitals* 38: 55–62.

# Policy Implications of Hospital System Failures

## The Allegheny Bankruptcy

During the late 1990s and early 2000s, the economy of the United States was rocked by a series of corporate accounting scandals and bankruptcies. Before there were Enron, Arthur Andersen, WorldCom, Tyco, and Global Crossing, however, there was Allegheny. Formally known as the Allegheny Health, Education, and Research Foundation, or more informally as AHERF, Allegheny filed for bankruptcy in U.S. Bankruptcy Court in Pittsburgh in July 1998. Filing papers cited $1.3 billion in debt owed to 65,000 creditors, making this the nation's largest nonprofit healthcare bankruptcy.

Allegheny's growth, decline, and bankruptcy caused tremendous upheaval in both Pittsburgh (where AHERF's corporate office, western Pennsylvania hospitals, and initial flagship teaching facility were located) and Philadelphia (the location of the eastern Pennsylvania hospitals directly affected by the bankruptcy filing). Hospitals repeatedly changed ownership, first among multiple nonprofit systems, and then in for-profit systems. Physician practices and medical researchers who were attracted to join Allegheny with large purchase prices and promises of new facilities and support were later jettisoned. Insurers entered into full-risk capitated contracts with Allegheny, only to have it go bankrupt without providing all of the contracted services. Suppliers and wholesalers continued to sell and deliver medical supplies after it failed to pay its bills. A handful of senior executives captured their pensions before the bankruptcy, but later repaid them—voluntarily or involuntarily. Employees of AHERF's eastern operations, on the other hand, saw their pensions wiped out after the bankruptcy and then later restored by the Pension Benefit Guaranty Corporation. Finally, months before the bankruptcy, executives tapped into the system's philanthropic funds (charitable endowments, restricted gifts) to cover operating costs.[1]

How could this have happened? The chronicle of the Allegheny bankruptcy illustrates how external policy and regulatory currents can exacerbate financial and managerial weaknesses within the firm and precipitate failure. In much of the literature about U.S. health care there is an almost romantic assumption that "regulation" and "market" are opposites—the former implying the heavy hand of government, the latter untrammeled and free. Of course, the market is not an unregulated or uninfluenced force. Both corporations and markets are regulated in numerous, complex ways, and they respond to corporate perceptions of public-policy changes. This is true, as we will show, for not-for-profit corporations such as Allegheny as well as for investor-owned firms. This chapter begins with a discussion of the causes of corporate bankruptcy and then describes how these forces led Allegheny to fail.[2] The chapter then focuses on a new and important area: the public-policy relevance of the failure of large private (nonprofit) hospital systems such as Allegheny. While the empirical literature on corporate bankruptcy argues that such failures are the result of organization-specific factors, such as the long-term decline in the firm's financial health, strategic errors, and managerial shortcomings, this chapter suggests that internal problems are strongly exacerbated by external policy and regulatory currents. The history of Allegheny is punctuated by the impacts of public-policy initiatives (at the federal, state, and municipal levels) on corporate bankruptcy, and the implications of corporate bankruptcy for public policy (at the state and municipal levels). This history illustrates the close interactions between public policy and the operation of private-sector markets and institutions.

## Causes of Corporate Bankruptcy

Beginning in the late 1960s, much of the literature on the causes of corporate bankruptcy has focused on the internal financial health of the firm. Edward Altman (1968, 1993) and John Argenti (1976) identified a series of financial ratios that correlated with bankruptcy in firms. These included the firm's cumulative profitability, return on assets, earnings stability, debt service (for example, cash flow to debt), short-term liquidity, capitalization, and total asset size. Research confirms that bankrupt hospitals are characterized by several years of negative margins, deteriorating equity positions, and low current ratios (Bazzoli and Cleverly 1994).

Additional research on bankruptcies has identified some factors associated with poor financial measures. These include extremely high and low levels of strategic initiative (that is, attempts to do too much or too little), poor accounting information or creative accounting, the strength and breadth of the top management team, and managerial incompetence (Argenti 1976; Hambrick and D'Aveni 1988; D'Aveni 1989a, 1989b; Thornhill and Amit 2003). Overall, the findings suggest that bankruptcies are a prolonged, downward spiral followed by marketing and strategic errors that seek to correct the firm's chronically weak financial position.

Only a small amount of this literature addresses the external causes of corporate bankruptcy. Researchers speak of environmental carrying capacity and entropy, industry turbulence and change, sudden environmental declines, and normal business hazards such as strikes and new legislation (Argenti 1976; Whetten 1980; Hambrick and D'Aveni 1988; Thornhill and Amit 2003). The history of AHERF reveals many of these internal financial problems. It also illustrates how external changes in the legislative and regulatory environment helped to foster these problems.

Public policy may promote conditions ripe for hospital-system bankruptcies in a number of ways:

- Federal health legislation (both proposed and enacted) may encourage the rise of consolidated and integrated health systems such as Allegheny, sometimes as an unanticipated consequence.
- Federal regulatory health policy may promote the development of an uneven balance of power in local markets between payers and providers, which places extreme financial pressure on the latter.
- Policy initiatives to deal with the poor and uninsured, undertaken by state and local government, may place additional financial pressure on the hospital industry.
- Local policy makers often endeavor to keep community hospitals open despite a history of financial distress, which only prolongs the need to close them down.
- Changes in state law regarding certificate-of-need (CON) legislation may occasion sudden market shifts that imperil hospitals.

## History of the Allegheny Health, Education, and Research Foundation (AHERF)

Allegheny was initially built around a single, large, tertiary-care facility (that is, a hospital providing high-tech services to treat specialized health conditions) in Pittsburgh called Allegheny General Hospital (AGH). AGH, a non-profit hospital established in the nineteenth century, enjoyed a strong reputation and leading market share. In 1982, perhaps in imitation of the increasingly prominent investor-owned hospital corporations, Allegheny reorganized to create a parent company, Allegheny Health Services, Inc. (AHSI), which included several subsidiaries: a foundation, a for-profit development corporation, AGH, and the Singer Research Institute. The latter two entities were separated further from the parent by an intermediary called the Allegheny Health Education and Research Corporation. Management consultants cited this complex corporate structure as too confusing and unwieldy for AHSI leaders in the mid-1980s, foreshadowing even larger and more complex structures to come later in the decade.[3]

For some time, top executives and board members of Allegheny wanted to develop a major affiliation for the residency teaching programs at AGH. As of the mid-1980s, AGH had only a limited teaching affiliation with the sole medical school in town, the University of Pittsburgh's School of Medicine. Allegheny felt quite dependent and somewhat inferior in this relationship, much in contrast to its perceived stature and competitive position in the market. It also viewed major teaching programs as a vehicle to assure a steady supply of medical students and residents and thus of the tertiary-care patients that had supported AGH in the past. The executives and board members at Allegheny feared that the limited teaching affiliation with the university posed a major competitive threat to Allegheny's survival, especially since they knew that the university and its primary teaching institution, Presbyterian-University Hospital, had considered eliminating their affiliation with AGH, and that some early proposals floated around Washington restricting approved residency programs and graduate medical education reimbursement to only those hospitals with "major" medical school affiliations. For these reasons, Allegheny acquired a financially struggling medical school in Philadelphia, the Medical College of Pennsylvania (MCP) and its hospital in 1988.

The MCP acquisition carried considerable baggage, however. MCP issued $70 million in new bond debt between 1989 and 1991 in an effort to renovate its facility.[4] Allegheny committed itself to supporting MCP with an annual subsidy paid out of the operating surplus of AGH. Allegheny also discovered that while MCP had decent basic science capabilities, it lacked strong clinical faculty in many areas, pediatrics in particular, and thus steady patient referrals to its staff from community physicians.

To deal with the problem of its new academic medical center (AMC) in Philadelphia, Allegheny pursued a second local acquisition in late 1991. United Hospitals was another struggling system poised to declare bankruptcy, with four hospitals and $137 million in outstanding debt. However, United possessed, on paper at least, certain elements that Allegheny desired: three community hospitals in the suburbs that could potentially refer to the city-based MCP Hospital. It also had a pediatric hospital, St. Christopher's Hospital for Children, that enjoyed a strong reputation but had struggled for years with an undesirable location and dilapidated facilities. Prior to the acquisition by Allegheny, United had stripped some of the operating surplus from the three community hospitals to finance the relocation and rebuilding of St. Christopher's. This move left the three community hospitals in a weakened financial position. The United acquisition marked the beginning of two AHERF customs: to cover the problems of a previous acquisition by the presumed strengths of another acquisition and to justify all of their acquisitions with arguments of expansion, greater size, and market presence. As a consequence, the mantra of expansion began to overtake prudence and due diligence (that is, close financial analysis and scrutiny).

In late 1993, Allegheny pursued yet another local acquisition—the academic health center at Hahnemann University in downtown Philadelphia. As with MCP, the Hahnemann acquisition included a medical school and a hospital. The acquisition was viewed as synergistic in several ways: Hahnemann possessed a stronger clinical program in cardiology than MCP; its hospital enjoyed a good geographic location near major expressways that patients could access in the city; it enjoyed favorable name recognition that MCP lacked; and it included a university that could further add to Allegheny's prestige. The Hahnemann acquisition also had several drawbacks. The university had no financial reserves, carried $123 million in bond debt, and was suffering deficits across its entire set of operations (for example, losses at the medical school that the hospital could no longer subsidize). Hahnemann also had major renovation needs that had long been deferred. Moreover, merging the academic departments of a second medical school with those of MCP required quite a bit of downstream effort—effort that involved time, money, and managerial attention but was never really completed.

In August 1996, Allegheny struck a deal to acquire the Graduate Health System (GHS), a sprawling empire of hospitals and physician practices in eastern Pennsylvania and New Jersey. This acquisition was, like the others, opportunistic: the system was available for purchase and increased Allegheny's share of the local market. GHS, however, was really a mixed bag of assets. It included one tertiary-care hospital in downtown Philadelphia (Graduate Hospital), a financially ailing hospital (Mount Sinai),[5] two osteopathic hospitals that had belonged to a recently bankrupt system, a hospital in Reading far to the northwest, and two hospitals in New Jersey (one of which was also struggling financially). The entire Graduate system had an accumulated deficit of $40 million and carried $174 million in bond and related debt, all of which Allegheny assumed. Moody's labeled it financially weak (Moody's Investor Service 1996).[6]

During 1996 and early 1997, Allegheny also pursued the acquisition of four more hospitals in western Pennsylvania: Forbes Metropolitan, Forbes Regional, Allegheny Valley Hospitals, and Canonsburg General Hospital. Collectively, these hospitals carried another $121 million in outstanding debt, which Allegheny assumed. These acquisitions were, in part, a competitive response to the system-building efforts of the University of Pittsburgh Medical Center (UPMC), which encompassed the university hospital and medical school and several recent hospital acquisitions.

Finally, throughout the period from 1993 to 1996, Allegheny aggressively pursued the acquisition of (mostly) primary-care physician practices across the Philadelphia and Pittsburgh metropolitan areas. These acquisitions were undertaken to achieve three goals: assure tertiary-care referrals from suburban communities to Allegheny's urban teaching hospitals; develop the primary-care capacity to complement the system's hospitals and form an integrated delivery network (IDN); and engage in full-risk, capitated contracting with local payers (that is, accept a fixed payment per year for each enrollee for agreed-upon services). Acquired practices were managed under the Allegheny Integrated Health Group, which sustained operating losses exceeding $100 million during fiscal years 1996 and 1997.

This series of acquisitions occurred quite rapidly over time and with little due diligence. Several acquisitions were quickly undertaken out of a concern that others might bid for the same assets, that the deals might fall through, or simply out of impatience. Most of the acquisitions were financial under-performers and highly leveraged. The acquisitions were also undertaken in one of the most unfavorable hospitals markets—Philadelphia—where there were multiple academic medical centers (such as the University of Pennsylvania, Thomas Jefferson University, Temple University, and Allegheny's combined MCP-Hahnemann University) and, thus, heavy competition for the same tertiary patients. More importantly, Philadelphia contained one of the most concentrated insurance markets in the country, where two major payers (Independence Blue Cross and Aetna U.S. Health Care) dominated the more fragmented hospital market (American Medical Association 2001). This resulted in multiple AMCs having little leverage in managed-care contract negotiations with two big payers and, consequently, receiving low reimbursement rates for their expensive clinical services. It is not clear that AHERF executives fully understood the Philadelphia market they were entering. At the same time that they minimized their problems, they also exaggerated their abilities to manage them.

The acquisitions undertaken to build an IDN with multiple hospitals and physicians under one corporate structure, in which the IDN is capable of assuming capitated risk, occurred at the trough of the insurance underwriting cycle. This meant that Allegheny was receiving insurance premiums that were increasing at decreasing rates while the costs of care escalated. In addition to coinciding with a poor insurance climate, Allegheny's expansion occurred just before state actions that transitioned virtually all of Philadelphia's large base of Medicaid patients to mandatory managed care (Pennsylvania's HealthChoices program of 1997), as well as just prior to federal efforts to reduce hospital reimbursement for Medicare patients (Balanced Budget Act of 1997).

All of these events crippled Allegheny's cash flow. The once-prospering hospitals in Pittsburgh (particularly AGH) that subsidized the system's expansion could no longer keep up with the costs of new acquisitions, the operating deficits of many of the system's Philadelphia holdings, and the service on the debt Allegheny had assumed, which totaled $1.2 billion by 1998. To keep its hospitals and schools operating, AHERF executives looked for any available sources of cash in its balance sheets. They found them in two different areas: funded depreciation accounts in certain AHERF hospitals and the restricted assets and charitable endowments—gifts bequeathed to the hospitals and schools over time, along with research grants and funds that supported scientists at MCP and Hahnemann.

Starting around March 1996, executives began modest transfers of monies from the funded depreciation (cash) accounts at AGH to certain eastern hospitals. The cash transfers were used for operations—that is, to compensate for a lack of operating cash in hospitals that were experiencing increases in their accounts receivable (AR). Some of the AR problems appear to have stemmed from the increased amount of AR carried by the newly acquired hospitals, physician practices, the consolidation of billing and receiving activities in the eastern region (for example, inconsistent billing systems and different AR methods for dealing with aging receivables and calculating reserves), and both inadequate collection efforts and increased uncollectible accounts. Proceeds from the 1996 Delaware Valley Obligated Group (DVOG) bond refinancing repaid these cash transfers, which then started up again in earnest in September of that year.

AHERF also executed noncash reserve transfers from other system hospitals to deal with bad-debt issues. Critics claim that AHERF made these transfers to reserve against the growing bad debt without increasing bad-debt expense. In fiscal years 1996 and 1997, Allegheny reportedly re-(mis)classified another noncash item, one of its large trust accounts (Lockhart Trust), from "temporarily restricted" to "available for use," and improperly recognized $54.7 million from these trust assets in fiscal year 1997 as income in the following year (SEC 2000a). During early 1998, AHERF reportedly tapped $78 million in cash from its restricted endowment funds, although the amount ended up being much lower.

As 1998 unfolded, Allegheny could no longer sustain itself. The system shopped for an outside buyer. Initially a new investor-owned system called Vanguard showed interest; however increasing financial troubles at AHERF and protracted due diligence by Vanguard led it to reduce its bid and ultimately back out, forcing Allegheny to declare bankruptcy in July 1998. The Bankruptcy Court judge focused on finding a buyer for Allegheny's Philadelphia assets, which were sold to Tenet Healthcare in November.

Following this, there ensued a long period of litigation by several parties to discipline Allegheny executives and recover losses incurred. The Securities and Exchange Commission (SEC) pursued four financial officers and internal accountants for misstating Allegheny's income by $114.3 million, concealing its deteriorating financial condition, issuing financial statements that were materially false, and misleading bondholders (secured creditors, since most of the bonds were insured). The Allegheny defendants settled their claims in May 2000 and paid civil monetary penalties ranging from $25,000 to $40,000 (SEC 2000b).

Simultaneously, the SEC filed a cease-and-desist order against AHERF for violating Section 10(b) of the Exchange Act and Rule 10b-5, which made it unlawful and fraudulent for any issuer of securities "to make any untrue statement of material fact or to omit to state a material fact necessary in order to make the statements made, in light of the circumstance under which they were made, not misleading." The SEC charged that in addition to overstating their consolidated net by means of inappropriate transfers, AHERF also overstated the income of DVOG by $40 million in 1996 by failing to adjust its bad-debt reserves to account for uncollectible AR; utilized transfers of approximately $99.6 million to address the bad-debt reserve shortfall not addressed in the prior year, as well as an additional shortfall in 1997; and misclassified certain restricted trust funds (SEC 2000a). The SEC order also observed that both the Obligated Group and the Corporation would have posted substantial net losses by 1997 without the fraudulent activity. This represented the first action ever undertaken by the SEC against a nonprofit healthcare firm.

The unsecured creditors sued AGH, Mellon Bank in Pittsburgh (which had received a favorable loan repayment from Allegheny just prior to the bankruptcy filing), and the insurers providing liability coverage for the directors and officers of Allegheny (D&O Insurance) to recover their losses. In January 2002, a settlement in U.S. District Court gave them $65 million, and restored $25 million to the charitable trusts of the system. The unsecured creditors ended up receiving nineteen to twenty cents on every dollar they were owed.[7]

Finally the State charged Allegheny's top three executives—CEO Sherif Abdelhak, CFO David McConnell, and Chief Counsel Nancy Wynstra—with multiple (1,500!!) felony and misdemeanor counts. The three main charges were illegal spending of restricted charitable endowment funds to support hospital operations, illegal diversion of funds for personal purposes, and illegal use of funds to make political contributions. Each executive at the time faced the possibility of seventeen to twenty-five years in jail. What happened was quite different. The CEO pleaded "no contest" to a single, consolidated misdemeanor charge of raiding the charitable endowments, was sentenced to eleven to twenty-three months in the county jail, and ended up serving only a few months due to a heart ailment. The CFO settled a lone criminal charge of receiving Allegheny money to pay for a sports stadium skybox. He was placed in an Accelerated Rehabilitation Disposition program for nonviolent first-time offenders and was sentenced to twelve months probation and 150 hours of community service, after which his slate was wiped clean. All charges were dismissed against the chief counsel, who had been undergoing treatment for breast cancer and died shortly after the proceedings.

## Public Policy and System Failure

### Legislative Proposals to Promote the Formation of IDNs

Some of Allegheny's difficulties can be traced to federal legislation and legislative proposals that encouraged the rise of large IDNs. As far back as the original Medicare legislation of 1965, Congress provided several incentives for hospitals to develop new large systems (Stevens 1989). First, hospitals were paid cost-based reimbursements (that is, reimbursements based on the hospital's reported costs to render the care) for an entirely new set of patients, the elderly. Second, hospitals were reimbursed for their capital formation efforts: for-profits received a reasonable rate of return on equity capital as part of their reimbursable costs, and, following some newly enunciated principles of the American Hospital Association, hospitals were allowed to calculate depreciation on the basis of current replacement cost instead of historical cost. These provisions prompted hospitals to spend more money, on not just technology but also new plant. They also promised enough return to induce for-profit hospital chains to form and enter the market.

Medicare also eventually encouraged many hospitals to merge for the purposes of tax savings and "Medicare recapture." Medicare's new depreciation calculations made hospitals more attractive to a potential buyer than to their current owners, since interest and depreciation could be deducted from taxes (Gray 1991). Medicare rules also specified that hospitals that changed ownership could receive an adjustment to their final allowable or reimbursable costs based on the gain (loss) on depreciated assets at the time of the sale. If the hospital's depreciable assets were purchased at higher (lower) than net book value, Medicare would share in the gain (loss), provided that Medicare's fiscal intermediary approved. In Allegheny's case, the Medicare recapture potential, often the biggest supposed savings in their hospital acquisitions, does not seem to have been approved or realized.

Following the 1965 Medicare legislation, hospitals began to form horizontal chains and systems. By the early 1990s, hospitals also began to consider vertical integration of services by formally associating with their physicians, heeding messages in the private sector (heralded by consultants and some academics) that hospitals should prepare for the future by organizing to manage capitated risk for defined patient populations. Vertically integrated IDNs that combined doctors and hospitals were viewed as *the* vehicle to do so.

In 1993, the Clinton Health Plan (formally known as the Health Security Act) spurred on both horizontal and vertical system building on a widespread scale. Ironically, while the Clinton plan was never passed (or even really debated) in Congress, it exerted an enormous impact on the hospital industry. The proposed plan encouraged the formation of accountable health plans (AHPs), which were coalitions of various providers (physicians, hospitals) and payers in local markets that might then contract with proposed state-based health insurance purchasing cooperatives (HIPCs), later renamed Regional Health Alliances. The plan envisioned that three or four AHPs might exist in a local market to contract with the state HIPCs. Hospital providers, especially those in fragmented markets, saw this as the beginning of a "survival of the biggest" struggle: the hospitals that would be left standing to contract with the HIPC would be those that belonged to large hospital systems with large market share. AHERF's executives cited the Clinton Health Plan in the strategy documents that produced their version of an IDN.

The Clinton plan exerted other effects as well. First, the plan suggested the advent of greater federal regulation of health care. Providers scrambled to align with one another to deal with the increased uncertainty and potential threat. Second, the plan added to the growing fears of hospital executives, who were already witnessing the penetration of HMOs and other forms of managed care into their markets; they responded with a lemming-like instinct of follow the leader. Even three years after the plan's demise in 1994 hospital merger activity skyrocketed, likely encouraged by the plan's embrace of managed care, which became even more prominently perceived as "the wave of the future." During 1994–1996, UPMC became very active in building a large hospital system in Pittsburgh through acquisitions. UPMC's emergence prompted AHERF to commence its own system-building efforts in Pittsburgh during 1996–1997—and thus to construct systems and compete in two different markets.

There is additional evidence for these (largely unanticipated) consequences of federal legislative activity. The Clinton Health Plan, and its analyses, concentrated heavily on the regulatory and demand-side aspects of the program, and neglected to think about the provider organizations necessary to contract with large state purchasers (the supply side). An entire volume devoted to the plan, published in 1994, made little mention of large hospital systems or hospital-physician or hospital–health-plan alliances (Jolt and Leibovici 1994). This neglect may be due to the plan's decentralization of authority to the states to certify the quality of the proposed AHPs and decide with which of them to contract.

Hence, both Medicare and the Clinton Health Plan encouraged hospitals to form large systems. To date, the evidence has shown the performance of these systems to be lackluster (Burns and Pauly 2002). There is no firm evidence that such systems enjoy economies of scale in their operations, and some evidence that they take years to learn how to operate. There is also some evidence that hospitals that invested more of their operating surplus in systems development during the 1990s suffered proportionately greater losses in their operating margins and declines in the return on their assets than those that invested less of their operating surplus (Burns, Gimm, and Nicholson 2005).

Concurrent with the Clinton Health Plan, some states also passed legislation encouraging the rise of IDNs. In 1993 the state of Minnesota passed "MinnesotaCare" that encouraged providers to develop "Integrated Service Networks," or ISNs: "organizations that were accountable for the costs and outcomes associated with delivering a full continuum of health-care services to a defined population" (Laws of Minnesota 1993, Chapter 345, House File 1178). The ISNs were networks of physicians, hospitals, and other providers that would furnish all needed services in exchange for a fixed payment (Kralewski et al. 1995). The Allina Health System, the largest ISN in the Twin Cities, formed the following year as an outgrowth of this legislation and other congruent initiatives. The state of Washington passed similar legislation at the same time.

What were the outcomes of these developments? For the most part, what these ISNs and IDNs belatedly achieved was countervailing power in dealing with large managed-care insurers in local markets. By the end of the decade, there were increasing reports of large hospital systems like Allina successfully pushing managed-care firms to the bargaining table to renegotiate discounts. Honest system executives began publicly admitting that this bargaining power over insurers served as the main (but undisclosed) rationale for their system's formation. Researchers countered that it had negative welfare effects, such as increased hospital prices (Feldman and Wholey 2001). The Federal Trade Commission (FTC) and the Department of Justice (DOJ) began a series of hearings and investigations to reexamine the antitrust issues posed by large hospital providers (FTC 2002, 2004).

To be sure, Allegheny was an extreme case; few other hospital systems in the IDN movement actually went bankrupt during the 1990s. Some of the unique aspects about the AHERF case were its high dependence on Medicaid funding, the absence of any state government bailout, the consolidation of its billing activities, the dispersion of its operations in two cities, and the lack of concern on the part of board members at corporate headquarters in Pittsburgh for what was occurring several hundred miles away in Philadelphia. Detroit Medical Center, however, has come quite close to bankruptcy, even with a $50 million bailout from the state of Michigan; many other hospitals have suffered double-notch downgrades in their bond ratings and some have seen their systems disintegrate.

This history suggests that federal and state policy initiatives, taken together, may have both intended effects and, more important, sometimes massive unintended effects. The advent of consolidation in the hospital industry can be traced back to Medicare's reimbursement provisions. Hospital consolidation was clearly an unanticipated consequence. The rise of the for-profit hospital chains just after Medicare's enactment led to similar system formations in the nonprofit hospital sector. The Clinton initiative served as the major impetus to hospital executives in forming IDNs in the 1990s, according to their own recollections. But even after the plan was scuttled, IDNs formed at an increasing rate for the next several years. Clearly, some hospital executives interpreted the plan as the harbinger of further federal health reforms to which the IDN model was suited. Other executives undoubtedly copied the example of their peers and conformed to the IDN trend. The plan also scared the industry into a protective, defensive strategy that failed to serve consumers. Hospitals played this defensive role for the rest of the decade and managed to blunt the efforts of managed care (Goldsmith 2003).

One might argue from this history that policy makers should stop trying to reengineer changes in the provider system from the top down. One might instead argue that system reform should be attempted from the bottom up by encouraging (but not mandating) local-level experiments and adaptations in service delivery. In 2002, Secretary of Health and Human Services Tommy Thompson challenged the National Academy of Science "to identify bold ideas that might change conventional thinking about the most serious problems facing the health care system." One of the academies, the Institute of Medicine, responded the following year by proposing five areas of local experimentation to craft solutions to these difficult problems: chronic care, primary care, information and communications technology infrastructure, state health insurance, and liability (IOM 2003).[8] Such an approach is consistent with emerging research on organizational change (Burns, Bazzoli, and Dynan 2003). In contrast, top-down legislative initiatives have fostered a host of unintended consequences that led to the further corporatization of the hospital industry, the rise of a countervailing power against managed care, and increased health-care costs.

## Regulatory Policies Promoting the Power of Payers in Local Markets

At the same time that policy makers were encouraging the rise of large hospital systems, they were also utilizing managed care as their favorite vehicle to hold down the rate of increase in health-care spending. Managed care thus increasingly penetrated not only the private insurance market but also the Medicaid market and, to a lesser extent, the Medicare market. Between 1991 and 1998, the percentage of Medicaid beneficiaries enrolled in managed-care plans skyrocketed from 9.5 to 53.6 percent; between 1995 and 1998 the number of Medicare beneficiaries in Medicare+Choice plans doubled from eight percent to sixteen percent. In the private insurance market, the managed-care plans' (HMO, PPO, and POS) share of employee coverage among employers with two hundred or more workers jumped from fifty-six to eighty-six percent between 1992 and 1998. HMO enrollment rose from twenty-two to thirty percent; PPO enrollment rose from twenty-six to thirty-four percent, and POS enrollment rose from eight to twenty-two percent. Overall enrollment in managed care nationwide grew from thirty-two million in 1989 to forty-two million in 1993 to nearly seventy-nine million by 1998.

The spread of managed care in Philadelphia was even more remarkable. By July 1997, eighty-seven percent of Medicaid recipients and thirty percent of Medicare beneficiaries were enrolled in managed care (Wigglesworth 1997). Between 1994 and 1997, managed care penetration across all market segments rose from forty-three to fifty-seven percent in southeastern Pennsylvania. The Philadelphia metropolitan area became one of the most concentrated insurance markets among large cities in the country, with two payers accounting for ninety percent of market share (American Medical Association 2001).

These developments meant that an increasing percentage of the hospital's total patient mix was now being reimbursed by managed-care plans rather than indemnity (fee-for-service) plans. Managed-care plans sought to reduce hospital utilization and the rates paid for that utilization.[9] This exerted a double effect: a decrease in inpatient days and reduced payment for those fewer days. Moreover, now that an increasing number of both Medicare and Medicaid patients were covered by managed care, hospitals found there were fewer places to shift costs—that is, to cover losses in one activity with profits from another. More importantly, at least in the Philadelphia market, they found that the two powerful insurers in the private sector gained increasingly more bargaining clout as they also provided coverage in the public sector. Thus, a concentrated payer market became even more concentrated across all types of insurance coverage.

Insurer actions to delay and/or deny hospital claims compounded the problem of insurer concentration. Hospital executives in Philadelphia complained that insurers utilized their market power to make unilateral changes in provider contracts, denied payment for services retrospectively, arbitrarily changed levels of care, and took months to pay medically necessary claims. Perhaps reflecting these actions, a survey of hospital AR projections found that on any given day hospitals had outstanding bills of two billion dollars, of which one billion was sixty days old and eight hundred million was more than ninety days old (Wigglesworth 1999). To help alleviate this situation, the state of Pennsylvania passed Act 68 (the Quality Health Care Accountability and Protection Act) in 1998. Act 68 included a provision requiring prompt payment from managed care to providers within forty-five days for undisputed clean claims. However, the act failed to require insurers to notify providers of claim status or deficiencies. Providers claimed that managed care payers used this loophole to deny or delay claims payment due to uncertain dollar amounts, the patient's failure to complete a coordination-of-benefits questionnaire, or the insurer's assertion the claim was never received.

Federal regulators (that is the FTC and DOJ) intervened very infrequently as insurers engaged in their own merger and acquisition activity to boost their local market power (Feldman, Wholey, and Christianson 1999). One may assume that the federal government's lack of antitrust enforcement during the 1990s reflected their belief and desire that managed care would exert its market power to hold down provider price increases and utilization, thereby saving money for the purchasers of health care (government, employers, and individual consumers). By contrast, federal regulators' attempts to prevent the formation of provider cartels were nearly always unsuccessful. Between 1995 and 2000, the FTC/DOJ challenged seven hospital mergers that were all consummated (Greaney 2002). Judges may have been convinced that managed care was a good thing and that hospital consolidation contributed to its ends.

Thus, during the 1990s policy makers at different levels of government pursued agendas that simultaneously promoted the development of large hospital systems and sought to limit their bargaining power by encouraging the spread of managed care organizations (MCOs). The mix of intended and unintended effects of governmental policies ultimately produced a marketplace of large, powerful buyers and suppliers. Ironically, the implicit strategy of utilizing MCOs to dampen hospital costs served as one of the most important spurs to hospital consolidation. In Philadelphia, AHERF and other systems sought to amass capacity to match the market shares achieved by the two big commercial payers. A lack of market concentration and capital limited just how much success they could achieve. In the end, AHERF spent a lot of money on system building and achieved little leverage over the payers.

This strategy of utilizing managed care to hold down provider spending impacted hospital revenues in several ways during the mid-1990s, especially in Philadelphia. First, hospitals saw their reimbursement rates drop anywhere from twenty to forty percent, according to statements by former system executives. Second, hospitals saw an increase in the time taken by MCOs to reimburse them. Third, hospitals saw a substantial percentage of their emergency room visits and inpatient days denied for coverage by MCOs. Such measures contributed to deteriorating cash flow and margins at area hospitals. The weakened financial health made it difficult for large systems like AHERF to support all of the capacity they had acquired in building their IDN models.

### Health Policy Initiatives to Deal with the Poor and Uninsured

During the 1990s, Pennsylvania had a large Medicaid population of 1.75 million (1996–1998), ranking sixth in the nation. Not surprisingly, state and local policy initiatives to control public spending on health care exerted a major impact on hospital providers. In 1977, for example, the city of Philadelphia closed down its municipal hospital (Philadelphia General) and expanded existing services at its District Health (ambulatory care) Centers. National evidence shows that urban public hospitals account for one-third of the care of the uninsured (Cunningham and Tu 1997; Mann et al. 1997). With no public hospital, Medicaid recipients and the uninsured poor naturally migrated to the nearest private hospital—oftentimes AMCs based at Temple University, Hahnemann University, MCP, and the University of Pennsylvania. The result was a larger census of Medicaid patients in those AMCs and greater AMC dependence on state Medicaid funding (and adequate funding levels). Philadelphia stands out as the largest U.S. city without a public hospital.

In addition, national evidence shows that hospitals serving a large share of Medicaid patients also absorb a disproportionate share of the uncompensated burden of treating the uninsured (Mann et al. 1997). Acute-care hospitals in southeastern Pennsylvania provided $335 million in uncompensated care in 1998, up seventeen percent over 1997.[10] Of this amount, $75 million was rendered to individuals who were denied eligibility due to Welfare Reform in the State (Act 35); this represented half of the state total (Wigglesworth 1997). Within the city of Philadelphia, AMCs experienced high increases in the number of uninsured seeking treatment in their emergency rooms (twenty-seven to forty-nine percent) and their levels of uncompensated care (one to eight million dollars). Even the district health centers experienced a twenty percent increase in the number of uninsured patients they treated between 1996 and 1998. Before the tobacco settlement monies made available after 2000, Pennsylvania had no comprehensive funding mechanism, such as an uncompensated care pool, to reimburse hospitals for the care of these patients.

This dependence on Medicaid became painfully obvious to hospital providers as the state Medicaid program cut reimbursement rates during the 1980s, reduced the number of medically needy from General Assistance programs during the 1990s by over 56,000 people (9.6 percent) in southeastern Pennsylvania (Act 35), and then transitioned eighty-seven percent of the city's Medicaid beneficiaries (half a million people) to mandatory managed care programs in 1997 (HealthChoices). According to the Delaware Valley Hospital Council, rates paid to hospitals under HealthChoices fell as much as twenty percent. Removal of patients from general assistance rolls shifted the costs of care for these patients from the state to the hospitals. The impact was the familiar "low pay, slow pay, and no pay" refrain echoed by providers in other Medicaid programs. The resulting financial pressure on providers led 145 hospitals to file suit in U.S. District Court against the Pennsylvania Department of Public Welfare in 1988 for higher disproportionate share payments and revised diagnosis-related group rates (that is, inpatient hospital payment rates), to lobby state legislators for fiscal relief for their own institutions (for example, Temple University), and/or to establish Medicaid HMOs in the late 1990s (which suffered losses in their first years of operation).

### Policymakers' Efforts to Keep Hospitals Open

One peculiarity of the Philadelphia hospital market has been the incidence of bankruptcy over time; another, the reluctance to let hospitals close. Hospital bankruptcies over just a six-year period are itemized in Table 12-1.

Indeed, the same financially distressed hospitals filed for bankruptcy at multiple points in time during the last twenty years of the twentieth century. Sometimes the struggling hospitals were rescued by private individuals or organizations; at other times, they were rescued through public-policy initiatives to ensure access to care.

In the private sector, for example, the Central Division of Metropolitan Hospitals went bankrupt in 1989, was acquired by new owners and renamed Franklin Square Hospital, faced payroll and finance problems by 1991, was subsequently purchased by the Cooper Health System in New Jersey and renamed Cooper Hospital–Center City, before finally closing in 1993. In the public sector, Girard Medical Center and St. Joseph's Hospital defaulted on their bond payments in both 1979 and 1990, filed for bankruptcy in 1990, and

Table 12-1  **Hospital Bankruptcies, 1988–1993**

| Hospital/System | Year of Bankruptcy |
|---|---|
| St. Mary's Hospital | 1988 |
| University Medical Center | 1988 |
| St. Joseph's Hospital | 1988 |
| Metropolitan Hospital System | 1989 |
| Central Division | |
| Springfield Division | |
| Parkview Division | |
| Franklin Square Hospital | 1990 |
| Girard Medical Center | 1990 |
| Sacred Heart Medical Center | 1992 |
| Neumann Medical Center | 1993 |
| Cooper Hospital | 1993 |

were subsequently reorganized with federal financing as the North Philadelphia Health System.

During the Allegheny bankruptcy, the city of Philadelphia faced the prospect of several local hospitals closing if a buyer was not located. Allegheny was reported to be the city's largest employer and, not surprisingly, state and local government officials stepped in to ensure these jobs were not lost. The mayor of Philadelphia (who lived in MCP's neighborhood) and the governor of Pennsylvania worked together to develop a package that would attract Tenet Healthcare to purchase the hospital assets and Drexel University to manage the combined Hahnemann/Medical College of Pennsylvania University.

These actions bespeak a public interest in maintaining hospital jobs in a market that is heavily dependent on health-care employment and looks to the health-care sector for whatever little job creation exists. In Philadelphia, for example, health care accounted for thirteen percent of private-sector jobs. Between 1982 and 1995—a period during which the regional employment base shrank—the sector added 82,000 jobs. Moreover, the city possessed five AMCs, and boasted that roughly twenty to twenty-five percent of the nation's physicians received some portion of their medical training in the city. The Pennsylvania governor at the time declared that job creation was the essence of his administration. It is, thus, not surprising that public officials secured Tenet's commitment not to shutter any of the hospitals it acquired, at least initially. By 2004 (six years after the bankruptcy), however, Tenet had decided to close one of Allegheny's hospitals (City Avenue Hospital) and sell another (Elkins Park). Tenet tried to close a third (MCP Hospital) but was persuaded by the new governor (and former mayor of Philadelphia) to sell it for $1 to the hospital's medical staff in order to try (unsuccessfully) to keep it open.

The experience of the last twenty years suggests that local policy makers often intervene in the local hospital market to ensure the survival of distressed institutions. This occurs despite downward trends in local hospital utilization and occupancy rates and calls for downsizing of local capacity. Such actions may only serve to delay the inevitable closure of these institutions that repeatedly file for bankruptcy. Indeed, bankruptcy may be viewed as the market's way of "getting rid of the deadwood"—a process in which politics interferes. Political interference to prop up troubled hospitals may actually create a moral hazard problem, since hospital executives may engage in more risky behavior and strategies if they expect a bailout. Given the state's reluctance to let hospitals close, closure may only come through the managerial actions of investor-owned systems like Tenet, which have a bent toward rationalizing capacity and are accountable to shareholders.

The city of Philadelphia and the state of Pennsylvania generally lacked any investor-owned community hospitals (medical-surgical facilities). Investor-owned entry was hampered by the existence of state certificate-of-need (CON) laws (which required prior state-level approval for new hospital construction and major capital equipment purchases) and the requirement for review of any hospital ownership conversions from nonprofit to investor-owned by the state attorney general. In the absence of the investor-owned, the nonprofits may have lacked the motivation to compete on cost. Indeed, recent research has found that the presence of a handful of investor-owned hospitals in a local market may induce more imitative (that is, both revenue increasing and cost-competitive) behavior on the part of nonprofit hospitals (Cutler and Horwitz 1999; Kessler and McClellan 2001; Silverman and Skinner 2001; Duggan 2002). It is telling that the executives in charge of the Philadelphia nonprofit hospitals and AMCs greatly feared the entrance of large investor-owned chains like Tenet and their impact on local competition. Taken together, these findings suggest that the entry of investor-owned hospitals into local markets can not only induce greater profitability and efficiency but also rationalize excess hospital capacity. Some states, however, prohibit such entry by law (for example, Minnesota) or feature strong provider resistance (for example, Massachusetts).

## Certificates of Need

One of the interesting episodes in the Allegheny saga was the sunset of Pennsylvania's CON legislation in late 1996. Opponents included some community hospitals in northeast Philadelphia (Abington and Frankford) that wanted to develop their own open-heart surgery programs to keep these lucrative patients in-house rather than transfer them to AMCs downtown. These hospitals found some sympathetic ears among state legislators who believed that CON cost the state money, represented merely a more expensive way to build plant, and did not really retard the approval of projects. Other legislators grew tired of being caught between competing hospitals in their districts over new construction projects. Both groups of legislators were happy to allow CON to go away.

Within days of CON's demise, Abington Hospital opened its open-heart program. Two more hospitals followed over the ensuing two years. A study of the Philadelphia market for open-heart surgeries reveals some dramatic changes in the competitive market. Between 1996 and 1999, the market experienced a twenty-five percent increase in the number of open-heart programs, but no significant change in the number of other heart procedures (for example, coronary artery bypass with graft, or CABG). Instead, volume shifted from the older established programs (such as those at the AMCs, especially Hahnemann) to the new programs in outlying community hospitals (Crawford et al. 2002). The loss of CON and the entrance of new competitors siphoned off some of AHERF's most profitable patients and further hurt its cash flow.

This volume shift was accompanied by some very expensive duplication of capacity in the city. Each of the three new heart programs cost between twelve and fourteen million dollars to set up. This expansion of specialized programs—and the rise of single-specialty hospitals nationally—illustrates what researchers have recently observed and referred to as a new medical arms race (Devers, Brewster, and Casalino 2003). Researchers have suggested that CON may have served as a mechanism to resist the development of expensive and duplicative facilities (Hackey 1993; Robinson et al. 2001). Indeed, there is some evidence that Detroit's automakers incur lower health-care costs per employee and lower hospital inpatient and outpatient costs per one thousand members in CON states (Piper 2003). There is also some case-study evidence that single-specialty hospitals are most prevalent in states without CON.

The wider body of evidence on CON's impact on hospital costs, how-ever, is inconclusive (Conover and Sloan 1998; Morrisey 2003). One expla-nation for this may be the reluctance or inability of investor-owned hospitals to enter and gain share in CON markets, and thus to exert competitive effects on nonprofits (Marketing and Planning Leadership Council 2003a).[11] Policy analysts also suggest that the rise of single-specialty hospitals is not so much due to the lack of CON as it is to Medicare's overpricing of surgi-cal procedures.[12]

Nationwide, CON laws remain in place in thirty-six states. One rationale for leaving them in place (and perhaps even making them tougher) is to pro-vide a "check and balance" on community-hospital investments that do not serve rising demand but rather add duplicative capacity. During 2002 lawmak-ers in twenty states considered a variety of legislative proposals ranging from repeal to reinstatement of CON (Romano 2003). The overall trend, however, appears to be deregulation: most states have moved to dismantle portions of their CON laws. Since the majority of CON projects get approved anyway, its demise may allow for greater long-term efficiency as competition determines which programs (like open-heart surgery) will survive. In the shorter term, however, such deregulation will subject general medical-surgical hospitals to greater competitive pressures, further reduce their already slim operating mar-gins, and nudge a handful toward bankruptcy.

## State Oversight of Nonprofit, Charitable Institutions

### Protection of Charitable Endowments

Pennsylvania Attorney General Mike Fisher originally sought to recover $78.5 million in endowments that Allegheny allegedly misused (Hensley 2000). This amount roughly corresponds to the amount that the CEO directed one of his subordinates to spend out of endowed funds in February 1998 to cover the system's outstanding bills. In March 2000, Fisher revised the figure downward to $52.4 million. This lower amount represented what the subordinate's staff reportedly told Abdelhak was the amount that was restricted and could not be used; it may also reflect the lower bound of what the forensic accountant hired by the state determined was illegally used. When Abdelhak pleaded no contest to a single misdemeanor account of misusing funds, however, the figure mentioned was only about $35 million. Why did the figure drop so much? Why was the charge reduced from a criminal charge to a misdemeanor? And why did the number of charges drop from 1,500 to just one?

The answers to these questions are intertwined. The preliminary hearing into these issues lasted thirty-seven weeks, on and off, over a calendar year—the longest such hearing in the state's history. One reason for the hearing's length was the complexity of the case (which itself lasted two-and-a-half years). Another was the hundreds of endowments involved, which explains the number of charges filed. For each endowment, there were two charges: theft by failure to make required disposition of funds received (18 Pa. C.S.A. Section 3927[a], a third-degree felony), and misapplication of entrusted property (18 Pa. C.S.A. Section 4113[a], a second-degree misdemeanor). A demographic analysis of Allegheny's endowments reveals that the hundreds of endowments were of varying amounts (ranging from as little as ten dollars to as much as $4.6 million), given by various donors at various times in history, with a variety of restrictions on their use. Some contained no restrictions on the hospital's borrowing the money (for example, to pay hospital bills). Other endowments were tapped by medical school deans and department heads on a regular basis as a discretionary fund—further suggesting there were no apparent restrictions on their use. Moreover, these donations accumulated over a lengthy period in disparate hospitals that came to be acquired by Allegheny. Allegheny consolidated the accounts in written summaries of who gave how much and for what purpose. The written source documents (originals) were not centrally maintained and may have been discarded or lost as the hospitals and medical schools were acquired.

In court, the defense argued successfully that without the original bequests, the attorney general could not prove the original donor's will. The AG could not rely on Allegheny's or its hospital's summarization of what those bequests contained. In addition, the court judge ruled that the prosecution had to group all of its charges into one consolidated count, rather than pursue multiple instances of criminal and civil wrongdoing. In a plea-bargaining agreement, Abdelhak pled no contest to a single misdemeanor but received more jail time than was stipulated for such an offense.

The defense also argued that Abdelhak (mis)used the endowments for a laudable cause: to save the hospitals and the jobs of its employees. Abdelhak himself stated that, "My intent was to keep the hospital in operation for the patients and the 20,000 persons employed there" (Becker 2002, 6). According to an editorial in the *Pittsburgh Post-Gazette,* "Sherif Abdelhak was a defeated general. He was burning the furniture belonging to someone else, but he was doing it so that the defenders of his fortress wouldn't freeze to death" (*Pittsburgh Post-Gazette,* 2002). Newspaper accounts at the time of the hearing suggest the court judge may have felt similarly.

This chronicle suggests that states might consider requiring better record-keeping of charitable endowments among their nonprofit organizations. States might also consider what their laws and statutes say about the use of endowment funds. Officials in the Attorney General's office in Pennsylvania suggest that the current laws on the books may be adequate for prosecuting misuse of these funds. What is lacking, however, is enforcement. This may be partly a function of the small size of the attorney general's office responsible for regulating nonprofits (fifteen attorneys). Indeed, an earlier analysis of the Allegheny bankruptcy argued that the AG's office may also be underfunded and underequipped (in terms of statutory authority) to review transactions such as acquisitions of one nonprofit organization by another (Burns et al. 2000). The lack of state regulatory oversight places an even greater burden on the nonprofit's board of trustees, who may also be hampered in this role.

### Governance Oversight in Nonprofit Organizations

Various features of AHERF's operation led to management's domination over the board. Among other things, the board was enormous: AHERF had a network of ten boards responsible for its various operations with little membership overlap. Perhaps only a handful of top executives really understood the entire financial picture. Strategic decisions were made without board oversight; for example, AHERF corporate bylaws did not prohibit movement of monies without the knowledge of, or approval by, the trustees.

After AHERF's demise, it became clear that the weak board would be held to a low legal standard. None of the board members were prosecuted under criminal statutes. Several board members were sued for gross negligence and mismanagement, breach of fiduciary duty, and corporate waste. Because the trustees had served on the board without compensation, a little-known statute which provided for a level of trustee protection from liability now partially applied. The "Little League Statute," 42 Pa.C.S.A § 8332.2, states that where trustees of nonprofit organizations serve without compensation, they are not liable for any civil damages as a result of any acts or omissions relating to their performance as trustees unless they knew, or had reason to know, that the act or omission created a substantial risk of actual harm to the person or property of another. Liability by the trustees is thus established only if their behavior was "substantially below" the ordinary standards practiced in like circumstances by similar persons performing similar duties.

The Little League Statute was not the basis for any of the litigation against AHERF's directors. It was nevertheless relevant in the litigation for several reasons. First, the statute applies to cases of negligence and breach of fiduciary duty. Second, as uncompensated volunteers, the statute granted AHERF's directors limited immunity from liability, allowing for recovery only upon showing that their performance fell substantially below expectations. The statute is not clear on precisely how far below the norm the performance must fall (perhaps gross negligence), but a showing of simple negligence would be insufficient to impose liability. Third, the Committee of Unsecured Creditors which brought the civil suit concluded that the directors' breach of fiduciary duty fell substantially below general standards. Fourth, the directors could utilize the statute as an affirmative defense.

As the moniker implies, the Little League Statute was intended to promote volunteerism by protecting individuals who volunteer on the myriad of nonprofit organizations that enrich every community. The statute made it difficult to sue volunteer board members of a baseball or soccer team because, for example, two players collided and were injured. The rationale for the legislation was, of course, that these organizations do not have the wherewithal to buy the kind of insurance required. Did the statute apply to an organization like AHERF, with assets exceeding a billion dollars? There is discussion in the legislative history as to whether the statute should be limited to Little League–type entities or whether the statute should extend to the boards of organizations like AHERF or the University of Pennsylvania. The legislative intent ultimately was to apply this statute to organizations like AHERF.

Since the Little League Statute was enacted, there have been no other cases like AHERF in Pennsylvania. That no AHERF directors were criminally prosecuted in the case, despite a pretty compelling argument for misconduct on their part, argues for the need of new legislation to deal with corporate governance misconduct. It also raises the question whether a Little League Statute is the correct legislative guard against misuse of assets held in the public interest.[13] The heightened standard for proving misconduct is especially troubling in light of AHERF's by-laws, which like those of almost every other nonprofit, provided for protection from individual liability for directors and officers. Even as provider malpractice premiums went unpaid, director and officer insurance from individual liability was increased fourfold from fifty to two hundred million dollars. In addition, the absence of shareholders in nonprofit institutions made it even easier for the AHERF boards to remain insulated from scrutiny and prosecution.

The size, complexity, and indispensability of big hospital systems and other nonprofit organizations like AHERF place them in a different league from a soccer team or Boy Scout troop. So much more is at stake with large organizations like these, not the least of which are donations of both time and money (often considerable sums) made by many individuals for the community good, for example, the governor and the mayor's efforts to marshal the monies needed to keep the hospitals going after AHERF went bankrupt. Many jobs were at stake. All this would not have happened for a Little League team.

Legislators and the public must deal differently with big-league nonprofit organizations like AHERF. As with for-profit corporations, there is a tension between persuading qualified individuals to serve on nonprofit boards and requiring them to exhibit a high standard in their oversight. Individuals sitting on boards of nonprofits of a certain size should perhaps be paid, thus disqualifying them from the group envisioned by the statute. Alternately, if a nonprofit organization is providing protection from individual liability for its board, there is no rationale for the law to give these individuals the special consideration reserved for small organizations without the same wherewithal. The legislature should pay close attention to the standards by which directors and officers of large firms like AHERF, by virtue of being nonprofit, steward funds entrusted to them.

## Application of Corporate Governance Reforms
## to the Nonprofit Sector

AHERF occurred just prior to several major bankruptcies in the corporate sector. Congress responded to the growing number of corporate scandals at Enron, WorldCom, and Tyco by passing the Sarbanes-Oxley Act of 2002. Among the act's reforms:

- CEO and CFO responsibility for financial reports (for example, certification that the firm's financial statements contain no misstatements or omissions)
- A code of ethics/conduct for the CEO and CFO
- Independent directors on the board's Audit Committee (that is, no compensation beyond director's fees)
- The presence of a financial expert on the Audit Committee (for example, someone with prior experience in auditing and accounting and an understanding of generally accepted accounting principles)
- A requirement that the full Audit Committee review financial statements every quarter
- The avoidance of improper company influence on corporate audits

The overall thrust of Sarbanes-Oxley was to increase transparency of financial results, responsibility, and independence of the board; accountability of the top executives; and diffusion of best practices in corporate governance. There is no guarantee that such reforms will prevent future financial scandals among the Fortune 500 firms. Indeed, some claim that the act was hastily passed with several inconsistencies and unresolved issues (for example, should the board chairman be separate from the CEO? Should a majority of board members be independent of the firm, that is, unaffiliated with the company in any way?). Nevertheless, Sarbanes-Oxley may be a good first step to improve corporate governance.

In light of the problems at Allegheny, one might ask if Sarbanes-Oxley reforms are relevant and appropriate remedies for governance problems in the nonprofit sector. At a minimum, the issues addressed by the act constitute relevant questions for outside agencies that deal with hospitals. These agencies include bond-rating companies such as Moody's Investors and Standard & Poors, banks that issue credit, and municipal authorities that issue bonds. The analysis that follows considers the applicability and feasibility of certain portions of Sarbanes-Oxley as they might be applied to nonprofit hospital systems such as Allegheny.

The first two elements of Sarbanes-Oxley—certification of financial statements and a code of ethics/conduct—seem fairly straightforward. The CEO and CFO at Allegheny were the people most knowledgeable about the system's financial status and covered up its deteriorating performance. They released critical fiscal-year results six months after the deadline, and then later retracted them because of the errors they contained. This violated SEC requirements, which led to the prosecution of the top executives. If Sarbanes-Oxley were in place, the penalties would have been more substantial (for example, one million dollars and/or up to ten years' imprisonment for "knowing" violation, and five million dollars and/or twenty years' imprisonment for "willing" violation).[14]

Some observers believe that national legislation like Sarbanes-Oxley that bolsters the standards of accountability for publicly-owned corporations will invite states to increase their regulation of nonprofits and charities. There are reports that some states have increased their nonprofit oversight in the light of bankruptcies and asset sales (Jaklevic 2002). Attorney General Mike Hatch of Minnesota, for example, gained visibility through his efforts to dismantle portions of the Allina Health System due to its excessive spending (Reilly 2003).

Indeed, New York Attorney General Eliot Spitzer introduced legislation during the 2003–2004 legislative session (Senate Bill 4836) to amend the state's not-for-profit corporation law and the religious corporations' law along the lines of Sarbanes-Oxley (New York State Assembly 2003).[15] In addition to guidelines for nonprofit board members regarding their responsibilities (Office of the Attorney General of the State of New York 2000), the sales and dispositions of assets involving nonprofit and religious corporations (State of New York Department of Law 2002), and the appropriation of endowment fund appreciation (State of New York Department of Law, 2003), the legislation called for the following:

- Certification of annual reports by the CEO, CFO, and Treasurer (for example, "the financial information contained therein fairly represents in all material aspects the financial condition and results of operations of the corporation")
- More stringent provisions for filing of accurate financial reports, with violations resulting in lawsuits and board member removal
- Creation of a board audit committee (with three or more board members) for corporations whose financial statements are audited by a public accountant or has at least three million dollars in assets
- Oversight of the public accountant or auditing firm by the audit committee
- Prohibition of corporate compensation for any member of the audit committee other than board membership fees
- Prohibition of business activities between the corporation and its board members

The New York AG's action appears to be the first of its kind in the United States. By spring 2003, twenty other states were reportedly considering the implementation of similar rules, and some expect all states to follow New

York's example due to the prominence and reputation of its AG (Sandler 2003). Some state legislative proposals also seek to increase the fines imposed on CPAs who violate the Security and Exchange Act (Connecticut), impose professional rules of conduct promulgated by state boards of accountancy (Washington), and increase state enforcement of corporate fraud (Texas) (American Institute of Certified Public Accountants 2003).

Reliance on offices of the state attorneys general to regulate nonprofit organizations may be insufficient to prevent bankruptcies such as Allegheny. One reason is the limited size of the AG's office staff. Compared to some other states, the AG's office in Pennsylvania had a relatively large number of attorneys overseeing nonprofit organizations, reflecting the tens of thousands of charities that operate in the state—a legacy of philanthropic efforts and lots of small liberal arts colleges. Yet, even this large staff was inadequate to regulate nonprofits, according to a spokesman for the Pennsylvania AG (Stark and Goldstein 2002).

Other elements of Sarbanes-Oxley are more problematic. The stipulation of independent directors, for example, requires board members to have no material relationship to the hospital corporation, for example, no prior employment, no receipt of money from the corporation, and no business relationship (consultants or suppliers to hospital administration). This requirement becomes more difficult to maintain as hospitals develop into far-ranging geographic systems with multiple business subsidiaries and employment relationships with physicians. Business relationships between board members (or, just as important, members of their families) and hospitals become more enmeshed as the systems become geographically and financially more complex.

Another problem is that nonprofit hospitals typically do not compensate their board members for their participation while for-profit firms do. This may retard the recruitment of talented executives to sit on nonprofit boards. Some analysts feel that compensation is a device to get board members to confront corporate issues seriously. Compensation might also be tied to board members' performance and the length of time they commit to board duties.

Even more difficult is the need to have a financial expert on the audit committee of the board. IRS stipulations for 501(C)(3) corporations have led hospital boards to be primarily composed of "community representatives." Given the presence of roughly five thousand hospitals, there may be an insufficient supply of financial experts willing to sit on their boards, especially those willing to work without pay. Recent corporate scandals and fears of liability may also be shrinking the pool of potential board members.

This situation leaves the hospital with the need to train some of its current board members in finance rather than recruit financial experts from the outside to serve on the board. Alternatively, the hospital may need to hire outsiders to advise the board in the areas of finance and auditing. The hospital may also need to provide staff assistance to their audit committees to help them analyze and interpret financial statements from complex hospital systems.

What complicates this entire process of oversight is the different nature of health-care finance compared to that of private industry. Health-care involves a mix of public and private payers, third-party reimbursement, and different accounting rules—features that financial experts from outside the industry probably do not understand. Even if the hospital is successful in recruiting a financial expert to sit on its board, the expert may also need to be trained in health-care finance. Such complexity has become even more apparent recently with the problems at Tenet Healthcare involving Medicare "fraud and abuse" and "outlier billing" for admissions with unusually large expenses. Nevertheless, it should be noted that a large share of Medicaid patients is a major contributor to hospital financial distress. No level of financial acumen on the board will solve this problem.

Another complicating factor is that at some nonprofit organizations, management, not the board of directors, has historically assumed responsibility and oversight of the auditing process. Corporate boards in the nonprofit arena are going to have to assume much more responsibility for corporate oversight than ever before. This can entail having their own separate counsel for the audit committee, more meetings in "executive session" without the CEO present, and more critical review of CEO and corporate strategy. Such reviews will be difficult for board members who are drawn from community organizations that lack health-care experience and who rely on the CEO for guidance and assistance in their deliberations.

To be sure, the application of Sarbanes-Oxley reforms to nonprofits is not the only avenue to improving nonprofit governance. Eliot Spitzer himself has stated that these reforms may actually go too far by requiring "too much ministerial activity" in areas of compliance (Leynse 2003, 132). Other avenues of reform involve improvements in board structure and the information and financial tools at their disposal. Various lawyers and consultants have advocated for better selection and training of new board members, evaluation and assessment of board members, reductions in the size of large nonprofit boards, and imposition of term limits (Marketing and Planning Leadership Council 2003b; McDermott, Will and Emery and American Governance and Leadership Group 2003).

Others have argued that structural changes will be ineffective without changes in board process. What is needed, they argue, is the board's ability to: engage in constructive conflict, especially with the CEO; avoid destructive conflict among board members; work together as a team and avoid board dominance by a small number of members; know the appropriate level of strategic involvement, and go beyond merely monitoring the CEO; and address decisions comprehensively, in depth, with outside expert help when needed, and in view of the alternatives (Finkelstein and Mooney 2003). Few of these processes were at work in the AHERF board room.

Finally, others have stressed the importance of information (for example, qualitative and quantitative data, leading and lagging indicators) and financial models to represent the discounted value of the firm's future cash flows (Kocourek, Burger, and Birchard 2003). Such models would help board members evaluate how value is created by the organization's various divisions, detect areas of operation where management has failed to execute its plans, and understand management's view of the long-term implications of current day issues (Cornell 2003).

## Conclusion

The empirical literature on corporate bankruptcy identifies the causes of failure in the long-term financial health of the organization. The firm's financial health is influenced primarily by other internal factors: corporate strategy, accounting, and management. To be sure, AHERF's bankruptcy can be explained using the empirical literature's focus on internal causes. AHERF suffered a long-term financial decline, as evidenced by poor financial ratios (profitability, liquidity, solvency). This decline itself was occasioned by poor strategic decision making such as the acquisition of poorly performing hospitals and hundreds of physician practices—all as part of its IDN development plan. The decline was also hastened by collection problems (for example, consolidated billing systems) and a lack of information on which to base sound decisions (for example, entrance into new markets such as Philadelphia or new business lines such as risk contracting). The decline was also furthered by classic managerial mistakes: preoccupation with large size and growth, trying to do too much too quickly, exaggerating management's ability to administer a complex enterprise, pursuing conflicting goals (for example, develop university and AMC affiliations and increase profitability), and succumbing to corporate fads such as IDNs.

Yet, despite all of these internal difficulties and errors, AHERF might have survived and even attained a dominant position in the Philadelphia marketplace if not for a series of external changes in the policy and regulatory environment that exploited the internal weaknesses and vulnerabilities of the system. These changes included the private-sector transition from fee-for-service payment to managed care, the nearly simultaneous spread of managed care to the public sector, the decline in reimbursement rates, welfare reform, and the demise of CON.

This chapter has highlighted some of these external forces at work in the AHERF bankruptcy and broadly outlined some of the interactions between public policy and the operation of private-sector markets and institutions that can lead to bankruptcy. Public-policy initiatives undertaken at multiple governmental levels have had enormous impacts on hospital markets and strategies. These effects were both intended and unintended. At the same time, we believe the behavior of hospital markets in response to these initiatives can lead to extreme financial difficulties (such as bankruptcy) which have enormous implications for future public policy.

Given the largely decentralized and pluralistic system of financing and delivering health care in this country, we believe that policy efforts to re-engineer the system from the top down will either fail or lead to serious and unanticipated side effects. Reengineering efforts, including system building and consolidation (both vertical and horizontal), have achieved very dubious results in our health-care system. If they are to be pursued, they should be led by providers in local markets in response to local incentives and opportunities—not governmental mandates.

But market forces have not really been allowed to operate here. One local incentive for system building was the growing purchasing power of managed-care plans. Hospital systems were developed to respond to both legislative proposals and market forces. Policy efforts to promote hospital systems ran counter to other policy initiatives to foster greater bargaining power in the hands of local payers who reimbursed hospitals for services. By allowing managed-care plans to amass large market shares but forbidding hospital systems to develop anywhere near such shares, policy makers created an imbalance of power in some markets—an imbalance which some professional organizations believe is growing (American Medical Association 2001).

System-building efforts by providers in local markets have also been retarded by state and local health policies dealing with Medicaid funding, welfare reform and coverage of indigent-care costs, support of chronically failing hospitals, and hospital capacity (for example, CON). In each case, states have pursued strategies that have shifted costs of treating the poor to hospitals, inhibited the closure of hospitals in over-bedded markets, and fostered an oversupply of duplicative technology. All of these efforts have placed hospitals under severe financial pressure.

One area where policy initiatives may be welcome is state oversight of charitable institutions. States should consider beefing up their scrutiny of non-profit organizations, their strategic initiatives (for example, mergers and acquisitions), and their charitable estates. There may be thousands of such organizations within a given state, making it impossible for the small staff of the public charities division of the AG's office to monitor. Some possible remedies include the enlargement of these staffs or at least the appropriations for their enforcement activities; the promulgation of new legislation regarding the recording and disposition of endowment funds; and the adaptation of federal legislation dealing with publicly owned corporations to the nonprofit sector. Where relevant, states should also examine the growing size of their nonprofit organizations and reconsider whether they are still Little League players or should be held to major-league standards of accountability.

## Notes

The authors wish to thank Mark Pauly, Rosemary Stevens, and Mark Pacella for their helpful comments on an earlier draft of this chapter.

1. Only a small amount of philanthropic funds was spent on personal items such as a skybox at Three Rivers Stadium in Pittsburgh and a gift for athletic locker room improvements at the high school attended by the CEO's son (later returned). The absence of widespread use of corporate funds for personal purposes and self-aggrandizement distinguishes the AHERF bankruptcy from recent bankruptcies in the corporate sector.
2. For a more detailed discussion of the AHERF bankruptcy see Burns et al. 2000.
3. Jeff Goldsmith, personal communication.
4. The reader may ask why MCP issued the bonds rather than the corporate parent, AHERF. The reason is that hospital bonds are typically guaranteed by the revenues of the facility issuing them.
5. Mount Sinai Hospital had been sold to GHS in 1987 by its former owner for less than $11 million, after having undergone a $30 million renovation; it was losing a reported $2.5–3.5 million per year.
6. These figures for the Graduate debt may pertain only to its Pennsylvania hospital operations. Graduate also operated a two-hospital system in New Jersey, Zurbrugg, whose debt may not be included in the $174 million amount. If this is true, the total debt may have reached as high as $200 million.
7. Figures as of January 2004.
8. Skeptics of the challenge issued by Tommy Thompson and the IOM proposal suggest these "local experiments" are still top-down proposals that providers are allowed to implement more gradually.
9. Policy analysts suggest that insurers pursued strategies like these because employers wanted them to. Employers may never have embraced the value of integrated delivery networks, perhaps due to their expensive imitation of one another's system-building efforts and their failure to contain costs.

10. Data supplied by Pennsylvania Health Care Cost Containment Council and the Delaware Valley Hospital Council. We should note that the percentage of uninsured adults under the age of sixty-five in Philadelphia and in the state of Pennsylvania is lower than the national average: 14.6 percent in the city versus 17.7 percent in municipalities nationwide, 1994–96 and 11.6 percent in the state versus 18.2 percent in states nationwide, 1996–98.

11. Some researchers have raised concerns about the falling procedure volumes at AMCs and their potential impact on quality outcomes; however, in the short-term at least (one-year window from 1998 to 1999), there was no difference in risk-adjusted inpatient mortality rates between hospitals with cardiac programs established before and after CON termination (Robinson et al. 2001). The researchers attribute these findings to the sharing of heart surgeons among open-heart programs established before and after CON termination. This may have been facilitated by the relatively close geographic proximity of the older and newer heart programs. Of course, these results are based on only one year of observations in one market. Longer-term studies across multiple states suggest that risk-adjusted mortality rates for Medicare beneficiaries undergoing CABG surgery are substantially lower in states with CON in place (Rosenthal and Sarrazin 2002).

12. Mark Pauly, personal communication.

13. Members of AHERF's executive committee, for example, had ties to Mellon Bank which, as a creditor of AHERF, had inside information regarding AHERF's financial situations and debt compliance.

14. The Sarbanes-Oxley Act was recently applied in the federal prosecution of Health-South Corporation and its chairman who, the SEC alleged, committed massive accounting fraud and overstated the corporation's earnings by at least $1.4 billion since 1999 (Solomon, Charns, and Terhune 2003). The CEO and CFO at HealthSouth were also charged by the DOJ with securities fraud, wire fraud, and certification of false financial records. Both executives swore in two separate public filings during 2002 that the firm's financial statements were accurate. The CFO pleaded guilty to DOJ charges and has described how executives allegedly falsified financial statements to inflate the firm's revenues and earnings to meet Wall Street analysts' expectations and keep up the stock price. The CEO was recently acquitted of all thirty-six criminal counts he faced. Analysts suggest the government may have difficulty prosecuting large, complex accounting-fraud cases.

15. This legislation has since been scaled back (for example, the bill now encourages but does not require nonprofit-board audit committees) and reintroduced in 2005.

## References

Altman, Edward. 1968. Financial Ratios, Discriminant Analysis and the Prediction of Corporate Bankruptcy. *Journal of Finance* 23, no. 4: 589–609.

———. 1993. *Corporate Financial Distress and Bankruptcy* Second ed. New York: Wiley.

American Institute of Certified Public Accountants. 2003. *The State Cascade: An Overview of the State Issues Related to the Sarbanes-Oxley Act.* www.aicpa.org/statelegis/index.asp (accessed 7 October 2003).

American Medical Association. 2001. *Competition in Health Insurance: A Comprehensive Study of US Markets.* Chicago: AMA.

Argenti, John. 1976. *Corporate Collapse.* New York: Wiley.

Bazzoli, Gloria, and William Cleverly. 1994. Hospital Bankruptcies: An Exploration of Potential Causes and Consequences. *Health Care Management Review* 19, no. 3: 41–51.

Becker, Cinda. 2002. No Contest for Ex-AHERF Chief. *Modern Healthcare* 32, no. 5: 6–7.

Burns, Lawton, Gloria Bazzoli, and Linda Dynan. 2003. Considerations and Conclusions Regarding Organizational Change. Unpublished manuscript. Wharton School, University of Pennsylvania.

Burns, Lawton, John Cacciamani, James Clement, and Welman Aquino. 2000. The Fall of the House of AHERF: The Allegheny Bankruptcy. *Health Affairs* 19, no. 1: 7–41.

Burns, Lawton, Gilbert Gimm, and Sean Nicholson. 2005. The Financial Performance of Integrated Health Networks. *Journal of Healthcare Management* 50, no. 3: 191–212.

Burns, Lawton, and Mark Pauly. 2002. Integrated Delivery Networks (IDNs): A Detour on the Road to Integrated Healthcare? *Health Affairs* 21, no. 4: 128–143.

Conover, Christopher, and Frank Sloan. 1998. Does Removing Certificate of Need Regulations Lead to a Surge in Health Care Spending? *Journal of Health Politics, Policy and Law* 23, no. 3: 455–481.

Cornell, Bradford. 2003. The Information that Boards *Really* Need. *MIT Sloan Management Review* 44, no. 3: 71–76.

Crawford, Albert, Neil Goldfarb, Reuel May, Kerry Moyer, Jayne Jones, and David Nash. 2002. Hospital Organizational Change and Financial Status: Costs and Outcomes of Care in Philadelphia. *American Journal of Medical Quality* 17, no. 6: 236–241.

Cunningham, Peter, and Ha Tu. 1997. A Changing Picture of Uncompensated Care. *Health Affairs* 16, no. 4: 167–175.

Cutler, David, and Jill Horwitz. 1999. Converting Hospitals from Not-For-Profit to For-Profit Status: Why and What Effects? In *The Changing Hospital Industry: Comparing Not-For-Profit and For-Profit Institutions,* ed. D. Cutler. Chicago: University of Chicago Press.

D'Aveni, Richard. 1989a. Dependability and Organizational Bankruptcy: An Application of Agency and Prospect Theory. *Management Science* 35: 1120–1138.

———. 1989b. The Aftermath of Organizational Decline: A Longitudinal Study of the Strategic and Managerial Characteristics of Declining Firms. *Academy of Management Journal* 32: 577–605.

Devers, Kelly, Linda Brewster, and Lawrence Casalino. 2003. Changes in Hospital Competitive Strategy: A New Medical Arms Race? *Health Services Research* 38, no. 1: 447–469.

Devers, Kelly, Linda Brewster, and Paul Ginsburg. 2003. Specialty Hospitals: Focused Factories or Cream Skimmers? *Issue Brief No. 62.* Washington, DC: Center for Studying Health System Change. April. Available at http://hschange.com/CONTENT/552/ (accessed 29 June 2005).

Duggan, Mark. 2002. Hospital Market Structure and the Behavior of Not-For-Profit Hospitals. *Rand Journal of Economics* 33, no. 3: 433–446.

Federal Trade Commission (FTC). 2002. *Workshop on Health Care and Competition Law and Policy.* 9 September. www.ftc.gov/ogc/healthcareagenda.htm (accessed 9 October 2003).

———. 2004. *Improving Health Care: A Dose of Competition.* July. www.ftc.gov/reports/healthcare/040723healthcarerpt.pdf (accessed 20 September 2004).

Feldman, Roger, and Douglas Wholey. 2001. Do HMOs have Monopoly Power? *International Journal of Health Care Finance and Economics* 1, no. 1: 7–22.

Feldman, Roger, Douglas Wholey, and Jon Christianson. 1999. HMO Consolidations: How National Mergers Affect Local Markets. *Health Affairs* 18, no. 4: 96–104.

Finkelstein, Sydney, and Ann Mooney. 2003. Not the Usual Suspects: How to Use Board Process to Make Boards Better. *Academy of Management Executive* 17, no. 2: 101–113.

Goldsmith, Jeff. 2003. Is the Past Prologue? Presentation at Federation of American Hospitals Conference. *The American Hospital: What Does the Future Hold?* 21 April. Washington, DC.

Gray, Bradford. 1991. *The Profit Motive and Patient Care.* Cambridge, MA: Harvard University Press.

Greaney, Thomas. 2002. Whither Antitrust? The Uncertain Future of Competition Law in Health Care. *Health Affairs* March/April: 185–196.

Hackey, R. 1993. New Wine in Old Bottles: Certificate of Need Enters the 1990s. *Journal of Health Politics, Policy and Law* 18: 927–935.

Hambrick, Donald, and Richard D'Aveni. 1988. Large Corporate Failures as Downward Spirals. *Administrative Science Quarterly* 33, no. 1: 1–23.

Hensley, Scott. 2000. AHERF Executives Arrested: PA Attorney General Says Three Stole Endowment Funds. *Modern Healthcare* 30, no. 12: 2–3.

Institute of Medicine (IOM). 2003. *Fostering Rapid Advances in Health Care: Learning From System Demonstrations.* Washington, DC: National Academies Press.

Jaklevic, Mary Chris. 2002. Echoing Down From Wall Street. *Modern Healthcare* 32, no. 12: 8–9, 16.

Jolt, Harvey, and Martin Leibovici, eds. 1994. *U.S. Health Care in Transition: Reforming America's Health System—Analysis, Reactions, and Alternatives.* Philadelphia: Hanley & Belfus.

Kessler, Daniel, and Mark McClellan. 2001. The Effects of Hospital Ownership on Medical Productivity. National Bureau of Economic Research, Working Paper 8537. http://www.nber.org/papers/w8537 (accessed 20 May 2003).

Kocourek, Paul, Christian Burger, and Bill Birchard. 2003. Corporate Governance: Hard Facts about Soft Behaviors. *Strategy+Business* 30: 59–69.

Kralewski, John E., Andrea de Vries, Bryan Dowd, and Sandra Pothoff. 1995. The Development of Integrated Service Networks in Minnesota. *Health Care Management Review* 20, no. 4: 42–56.

Leynse, James. 2003. Straight Talk from Eliot Spitzer. *Business Week,* 6 October: 129–132.

Mann, Joyce, Glenn Melnick, Anil Bamezai, and Jack Zwanziger. 1997. A Profile of Uncompensated Hospital Care, 1983–1995. *Health Affairs* 16, no. 4: 223–232.

Marketing and Planning Leadership Council. 2003a. *Impact of CON Laws on Hospital Costs and For-Profit Competition* (March 24). Washington, DC: Advisory Board. http://www.advisory.com/members/default.asp?contentID=34187&collection ID=682&program=11&filename=34187_50_11_03–25–2003_0.pdf (accessed 29 June 2005).

———. 2003b. *Effective Board Structure and Development* (19 March). Advisory Board: Washington, DC. http://www.advisory.com/members/default.asp?contentID=34260 &collectionID=682&program=11&filename=34260_50_11_03–27–2003_0.pdf (accessed 29 June 2005).

McDermott, Will and Emery and The American Governance Leadership Group. 2003. *Sarbanes-Oxley Reforms for Nonprofit Boards.* Audio Teleconference, 6 May.

Moody's Investor Service. 1996. Moody's Downgrades Philadelphia Hospitals and Higher Education Facilities Authority Graduate Health System's Debt to Ba From Baa. *Rating News,* 26 August.

Morrisey, Michael. 2003. Certificate of Need, Any Willing Provider and Health Care Markets. *Federal Trade Commission and Department of Justice Hearings on Health Care Competition: Quality and Consumer Protection/Market Entry.* 10 June. Washington, DC. http://www.ftc.gov/ogc/healthcarehearings/docs/030610morrisey.pdf (accessed 30 June 2005).

New York State Assembly. 2003. 226th Annual Legislative Session. Bill Summary-S04836. http://assembly.state.ny.us/leg/?bn=S04836 (accessed 26 September 2003).

Office of the Attorney General of the State of New York. 2000. *Right From the Start: Guidelines for Not-for-Profit Board Members.* http://www.oag.state.ny.us/charities/ charities.html (accessed 25 September 2003).

Piper, Thomas. 2003. Certificate of Need: Protecting Consumer Interests. *Federal Trade Commission and Department of Justice Hearings on Health Care Competition: Quality and Consumer Protection/Market Entry.* Washington, DC, 10 June. http://www2.ftc .gov/ogc/healthcarehearings/docs/030610piper.pdf (accessed 30 June 2005).

*Pittsburgh Post-Gazette.* 2002. AHERF Whimper–Its Former CEO is Sentenced on a Single Count. 8 September: B-2.

Reilly, Patrick. 2003. Power of Attorneys. *Modern Healthcare* 33, no. 34: 20.

Robinson, Jamie L., David Nash, Elizabeth Moxey, and John O'Connor. 2001. Certificate of Need and the Quality of Cardiac Surgery. *American Journal of Medical Quality* 16, no. 5: 155–160.

Romano, Michael. 2003. Pros and Cons of Certificates. *Modern Healthcare* 33, no. 16: 4–5.

Rosenthal, Gary, and Mary Sarrazin. 2002. Impact of State Certificate of Need Programs on Outcomes of Care for Patients Undergoing Coronary Artery Bypass Surgery. Unpublished manuscript. Iowa City, IA: University of Iowa College of Medicine.

Sandler, Susan. 2003. SEC Rules & Actions Send CPA Firms Mixed Messages. *Accounting Office Management & Administration Report* March, no. 1: 14–15. Institute of Management & Administration. Available at www.ioma.com.

Securities and Exchange Commission (SEC). 2000a. *Securities Exchange Act of 1934 Release No. 42992 (June 30th), Accounting and Auditing Enforcement Release No. 1283 (June 30th): Administrative Proceeding File No. 3–10245.* http://www.nabl.org /library/securities/misc/secenf/3–10245.html (accessed on 9 September 2002).

———. 2000b. *Litigation Release No. 16534 (May 2nd), Accounting and Auditing Enforcement Release No. 1254 (May 2nd): SEC v. David W. McConnell and Charles P. Morrison.* (United States District Court for the Eastern District of Pennsylvania, Civil Action No. 00 CV 2261).

Silverman, Elaine, and Jonathan Skinner. 2001. Are For-Profit Hospitals Really Different? Medicare Upcoding and Market Structure. Working Paper # 8133. National Business of Economic Research. www.nber.org/papers/w8133 (accessed 4 October 2003).

Solomon, Deborah, Ann Charns, and Chad Terhune. 2003. Health South Faked Profits, SEC Charges–A $1.4 Billion Overstatement Cited as CEO is Accused of Ordering "Massive Accounting Fraud." *Wall Street Journal,* 20 March: C1.

Stark, Karl, and Josh Goldstein. 2002. Former Employers, Health Care Analysts Absorb Lessons of Allegheny's Downfall. *Philadelphia Inquirer,* 1 September.

State of New York Department of Law. 2002. *A Guide to Sales and Other Disposition of Assets Pursuant to Not-For-Profit Corporation Law 510–511 and Religious Corporations Law 12.* http://www.oag.state.ny.us/charities/charities.html (accessed 25 September 2003).

———. 2003. *New York State Attorney General Eliot Spitzer Advises Not-for-Profit Corporations on the Appropriation of Endowment Fund Appreciation.* http://www.oag .state.ny.us/press/reports (accessed 25 September 2003).

Stevens, Rosemary. 1989. *In Sickness and In Wealth.* New York: Basic Books.

Thornhill, Stewart, and Rafi Amit. 2003. Learning about Failure: Bankruptcy, Firm Age, and the Resource-Based View. *Organization Science* 14, no. 5: 497–509.

Whetten, David. 1980. Sources, Responses, and Effects of Organizational Decline. In *The Organizational Life Cycle,* eds. John Kimberly and Robert Miles, 342–374. San Francisco: Jossey-Bass.

Wigglesworth, Andrew. 1997. *Testimony Before the State House Health and Human Services Committee on the Impact of Act 35.* 28 August. www.dvhc.org/rr/housetest3.htm (accessed 18 December 2002).

———. 1999. *Statement Before the Pennsylvania House Insurance Committee.* 16 December. www.dvhc.org/rr/awtest12_16.htm (accessed 18 December 2002).

# The Rise and Decline of the HMO

## A Chapter in U.S. Health-Policy History

Health maintenance organizations or HMOs were the object of many of the most bitter criticisms of American health care at the end of the twentieth century. Media accounts drew on experiences of doctors and patients to depict HMOs as impersonal, bureaucratic entities that were primarily interested in controlling costs (or generating profits) rather than enabling doctors and hospitals to meet the needs of patients.[1] A national Harris poll in 1998 found that a solid majority (fifty-eight percent) of the American people believed that the quality of medical care that people receive would be harmed rather than improved by "the trend toward more managed care—with more people belonging to HMOs, PPOs, and other managed care plans" (Jacobs and Shapiro 1999, 1025). In response to managed care, serious efforts were made at the national level in the late 1990s to pass a patients' "bill of rights," even though health insurance and health-care organizations are regulated primarily at the state level. Notably, between 1995 and 2001, forty-seven states passed laws to regulate HMOs and other forms of managed care (Sloan and Hall 2002). In 1999, in introducing a special issue of the *Journal of Health Politics, Policy and Law*, editor Mark Peterson called the "managed care backlash," the issue's topic, "the most significant health policy issue since Congress pulled the plug on health reform" (874). By the beginning of the twenty-first century, HMOs had become a powerful symbol of a health-care system gone awry.

Their power, however, was much more than symbolic. In 2000, more than eighty million Americans were enrolled in HMOs, and two-thirds were in plans affiliated with ten national managed-care organizations (InterStudy

2000). This concentration of control is especially significant because HMOs are involved in both the financing of care and the provision of services.

How did these powerful organizations come to be? The answer lies in the interaction of public policy and the market. The HMO is itself an invention of American public policy, the HMO Act of 1973. Early champions depicted HMOs' combination of prepayment and group practice as an organizational form with self-regulatory mechanisms that could simultaneously enhance access, improve quality, and contain costs without creating the undesirable tradeoffs that were characteristic of the existing fee-for-service payment system of indemnity insurance.[2]

Since passage of the 1973 legislation, HMOs have moved from the periphery to the center of the American health-care system and from depiction as policy solution to policy problem. Many changes occurred among HMOs over this period. The most rapid and dramatic organizational changes took place in the 1980s. The typical HMO in 1980 was a locally controlled nonprofit plan whose salaried physicians served the plan's enrollees on a full-time basis. By the middle of the decade, the typical HMO was a for-profit plan that was part of a national firm and that contracted with office-based physicians who saw other patients as well as the HMO's patients. InterStudy, a research organization that had tracked HMOs for the federal government since the mid-1970s, aptly characterized this fundamental change in the title of its 1987 report "From HMO Movement to Managed Care Industry" (Hale and Hunter 1988). Ensuing developments led to the public-policy backlash against managed care in the 1990s.

This chapter examines the origins and evolution of HMOs—from periphery to center, from solution to problem, from movement to industry. What are HMOs? How did they become important? How could they have become so willing to act in ways that would generate broad and vocal opposition—what came to be called the managed care backlash (Peterson 1999)? I will show that this was not the result of one "health policy." Rather, many disparate but interweaving factors accounted for both the success and the ultimate problems of HMOs. These included

- Key decisions built into the HMO Act of 1973 and its subsequent amendments
- The Reagan Administration's decision to end financial support of HMOs and to encourage private investment in them
- Specific tax-policy decisions
- Provisions of the Employee Retirement Income Security Act (ERISA) of 1974
- The operation of the health-care market at different periods

## Major Organizational Trends, 1970 to the Present

The organizational history of HMOs can be described in terms of trends in enrollment, numbers of HMOs, HMO models, ownership form, and local versus national control. On each of these dimensions, HMOs have undergone remarkable change over the past thirty years.

The number of HMOs grew from about 30 or 40 (estimates vary) in 1970 to more than 650 in the mid-1980s and, after a period of consolidation, grew again in the mid-1990s (Figure 13.1). During that time enrollment increased steadily from an estimated three million to more than eighty million (Figure 13.2). The 175 HMOs that existed in 1976 (the first year a comprehensive census was conducted) averaged enrollment of fewer than 35,000 people; the average enrollment in 2000 was more than 125,000 people. HMOs had become an industry.

Considerable volatility accompanied the growth of the industry. After the number of plans peaked at 679 during 1987, consolidations and failures ensued, with the number of plans falling to fewer than 540 in 1993.[3] HMOs operated in an intensely competitive arena. During the 1980s, some 473 HMOs failed, merged, or were acquired by another plan; such transactions increased in frequency as the decade progressed (Christianson, Wholey, and Sanchez 1991).[4] Enrollment growth slowed at the decade's end. When it picked up

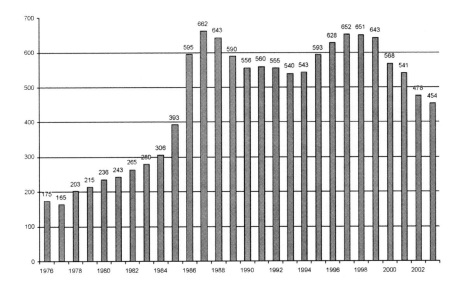

**Figure 13.1**  Number of HMO Plans, 1976–2003

Source: InterStudy

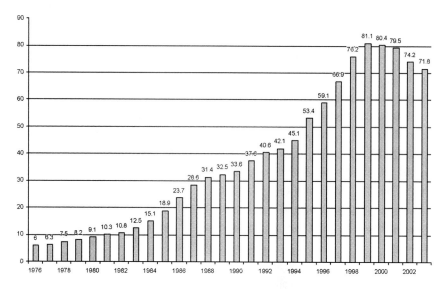

**Figure 13.2**   Number of HMO Enrollees, 1976–2003
Source: InterStudy

sharply in the mid-1990s, the number of plans began to increase again, peak-
ing in 1998. After that, the number of plans declined sharply and for the first
time the number of HMO enrollees began to decline, dropping from 80.4 million in 2000 to 71.8 million in 2002 (InterStudy 2002).

   Important organizational characteristics of the HMOs also changed over
time. The number of recognized types of HMOs grew (Figure 13.3), as did the
distribution of enrollment among the types (Figure 13.4). In 1980, InterStudy

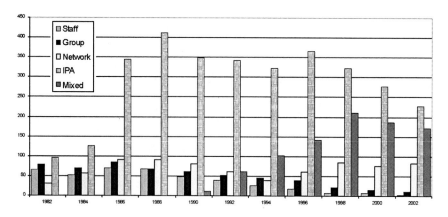

**Figure 13.3**   Number of HMOs by Type
Source: InterStudy

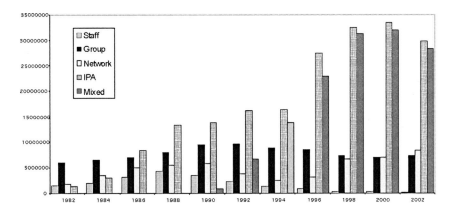

**Figure 13.4** Number of HMO Enrollees by Type
Source: InterStudy

classified HMOs into three types. In two of these, the *staff model* and the *group model,* the physicians served the HMO's enrollees exclusively. In the staff model, these physicians were the plan's employees. In the group model, the physicians were in a separately incorporated multi-specialty group practice that contracted with the HMO. Staff- and group-model plans were both variants of the older prepaid group practice (such as Kaiser). *Independent practice association* plans (IPAs) provided physician services through contracts with

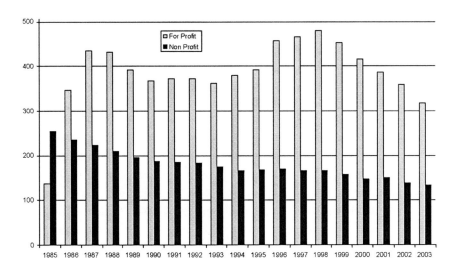

**Figure 13.5** Number of HMOs by Profit Status
Source: InterStudy

individual physicians who had their own practices or with associations of physicians in independent practices.[5] In IPAs, unlike staff- and group-model plans, an HMO's physicians were able to see patients other than the HMO's enrollees. Indeed, in many IPAs, a given HMO's enrollees were only a small share of a physician's patient population. In IPAs, physicians were commonly paid on a fee-for-service basis, as in ordinary indemnity insurance.

In 1981, InterStudy added the *network* model to their taxonomy to reflect the fact that some HMOs were contracting with two or more independent group practices. The *mixed* category was added to the taxonomy in 1990 because a growing number of HMOs had multiple types of arrangements (for example, some staff physicians but also contracts with independent practitioners).

The staff and group models declined from eighty-one percent of HMO enrollment in 1980 to twenty-eight percent in 1993, although number of enrollees in staff and group models increased over this period, from 7.4 to 11.7 million. Other models—the network model in the early 1980s and the IPA model in the late 1980s and early 1990s—grew much faster. The market share of network models peaked at twenty-seven percent of enrollment in 1985, while the IPA model continued to grow—from 18.6 percent of enrollment in 1980 to more than forty-three percent by 1996. By the end of the century the group and staff models accounted for less than ten percent of enrollment. In the early 1980s, when InterStudy began to track model types, they identified some 147 group- and staff-model plans; there were 112 in 1990 and only 17 in 2002.

The shift toward plans built on the insurance-carrier model (Enthoven and Tollen 2004) changed the character and operating methods of HMOs. IPAs had as many similarities to non-HMOs (insurance companies or preferred-provider organizations) that administered corporate health-benefit plans as to group- or staff-model HMOs. Group- and staff-model plans can use collegial, peer-oriented processes for managing utilization and quality, have policies and procedures developed by medical staff, and make internal referrals across specialties (Freidson 1975). IPAs and networks rely heavily on utilization-management methods (for example, pre-hospital certification) to control costs (Gray and Field 1989; Welch, Hillman and Pauly 1990; Gold 1995). These methods entail little collegial contact at the practice-setting level and lend themselves to centralization of cost containment activities across multiple plans. The changes in the prevailing forms of organization affected how HMOs came to influence health care (Pauly, Hillman and Kerstein 1990). The decentralized models' use of utilization management methods and gatekeeping contributed to an adversarial relationship between plans and physicians, and became controversial because the organization, not just the doctor and patient, was shaping care.

Group- or staff-model plans also had significant advantages regarding systems of accountability. It is much more feasible to develop uniform procedures, records systems, and informational technology systems when the medical staff serves only the HMOs' patients than when physicians see patients from six or eight plans, each of which may have its own set of policies and practices. When purchasers began to demand information about plan performance in the early 1990s, HMO industry leadership in the development of performance measures came from the group- and staff-model plans, then in the minority. These plans tended to perform best on the plan-performance measures adopted by the National Committee on Quality Assurance (Himmelstein et al. 1999).

Because the physicians in the IPA model worked in their own offices, new IPAs could be established with smaller capital outlays than if facilities were built for care of thousands of enrollees. Creating networks of established physicians' practices had other advantages as well, easing entry of new plans into markets by building on existing doctor-patient relationships. As demand for HMO services increased in the 1980s, most capital flowed to IPAs.

Simultaneously with the organizational changes, HMOs became increasingly for-profit, rather than nonprofit, corporations. The earliest reported ownership data reported by InterStudy are for 1981, when only eighteen percent of plans, containing twelve percent of enrollees, were for-profit (InterStudy 1985). Another study of the sixty largest HMOs in 1981 found that twenty percent (with twelve percent of enrollees) were for-profit (Touche Ross & Co. 1982).[6] By 1986, sixty percent of plans were for-profit (InterStudy 1990). The for-profit share continued to grow. Although most of the for-profit growth came from new plans, a substantial minority were plans that had once been nonprofit. The transformation of the field away from the nonprofit form is important because most research (published after the for-profit transformation had occurred) found nonprofits perform better than for-profits with regard to quality (Consumer's Union 1999; Greene 1998; Ha and Reschovsky 2002; Himmelstein et al. 1999; Landon et al., 2001; Landon and Epstein, 2001; Palmiter 1998; Patterson 1997; ProPAC 1994; Riley et al. 1997; Rossiter et al. 1989).[7] It is likely that this difference reflects the predominance of group and staff models among nonprofits and the IPA and network models among for-profits.

A further major trend was the move to multi-plan firms. Most early HMOs and their precursors were locally controlled; as recently as 1983, only twenty-five percent of plans belonged to organizations that operated more than one plan (National Industry Council for HMO Development 1983).[8] By 1986, however, sixty-two percent of HMOs (and 73.5 percent of enrollees) were in the forty-three organizations that InterStudy called "national managed care firms" (InterStudy 1987).[9] This pattern of predominant control by national firms has persisted ever since. National firms now control about sixty percent of plans and about three-quarters of enrollees. The largest such organization has been a nonprofit organization, Kaiser Foundation Health Plan, with eight plans and 8,355,495 enrollees in 2002, but most national firms are for-profit.

I interviewed senior executives of several leading national firms in the late 1990s, asking about the reasons for, and significance of, the operation by a single organization of plans in multiple locations.[10] They mentioned eight advantages of such horizontal integration.[11]

1. The ability to exploit intellectual capital by replicating successful models and methods
2. Greater access to capital
3. Cost advantages in purchasing (especially drugs and computer systems)
4. Scale economies in expertise and in transaction processing
5. Protection against adverse local conditions (economic slumps, competitive changes) provided by geographic diversity
6. The marketing advantage of a single brand
7. The ability to market to and serve national accounts
8. The ability to reduce irrational practice variations by generating data on large numbers of patients, and by having economies of scale in technology assessment and in the development and dissemination of practice guidelines and clinical pathways

In a 1999 article, Berkeley economist James Robinson mentioned a similar list of factors in his analysis of economies of scale underlying the transformation of health plans into "national, full-service corporations" that offered multiple "products," reached purchasers through multiple "distribution channels," and offered multiple networks of providers (Robinson 1999, 8).

The national firms in the late 1990s were quite variable in their degree of centralization. At one extreme was the Blue Cross system, where plan- or state-level boards had full responsibility for all plan operations and the national organization was comprised of representatives from each plan. At Kaiser, plan-level boards were largely responsible for plan operations, but capital plans and operating budgets were approved at the national level, which also provided strategic direction and quality assurance. Most of the

Blues, like Kaiser, were nonprofits. But United Health Care, a for-profit firm, was also quite decentralized, with each plan a wholly owned subsidiary with its own board and CEO. At the other extreme were firms such as Humana, Wellpoint, and PacifiCare, which had only nominal local governance structures to the extent required by law. In most of the national firms, many areas of policy were set nationally, as were many functions, such as finance, monitoring, underwriting, and information technology. Network management was generally a local function.

## The Policy History of HMOs

The HMO Act of 1973 provides a natural starting point in considering how public policy has contributed to the evolving contours of the HMO field, but the ideas behind the HMO concept can be traced to the prepaid group practices of the 1930s and earlier. Working models of the plans for which the act provided support existed long before it was passed (Starr 1982). Between the late nineteenth century and 1970, at least 120 HMO precursors existed in the form of prepaid group practices, or "foundations for medical care," the IPA-precursor that had been developed in California as a form of prepaid care using practice-based physicians (Durso 1992). Some ancestor organizations were instruments of reform-oriented visionaries; others were practical ways for unions to provide medical coverage for members or for corporations to provide medical care to workers on large enterprises in remote areas. The combination of prepaid financing and physicians' group practice had strong advocates among scholars and New Deal politicians going back to the landmark Committee on the Costs of Medical Care (1927–1932). However, no national movement was ever launched on behalf of the prepaid group practice (PGP) model because its advocates had a higher priority—national health insurance—that pitted them against opposition that was also strongly set against prepaid group practice, most notably the American Medical Association, which represented the fee-for-service practitioners who predominated in American medicine (Brown 1983).

After the passage of the legislation establishing Medicare in 1965, the politics of prepaid group practice changed, even though the legislation had included the famous provision stating that "nothing in this title shall . . . authorize any Federal officer . . . to exercise any supervision or control over the practice of medicine or the manner in which medical services are provided" (Brown 1983). Medicare paid physicians on the traditional fee-for-service basis. The small percentage of the elderly population enrolled in that era's prepaid group practices (mainly Kaiser) presented a practical problem for

Medicare's payment system and could have offered an opportunity to lend federal support to the PGP concept. There were strong advocates of PGP in the Social Security Administration that was implementing Medicare, but they avoided actions that might trigger opposition from organized medicine during Medicare's fragile early years.

Medicare's costs increased much more rapidly than expected, and by 1971, a Republican president (Richard Nixon) called for legislation to provide federal support to build a network of PGPs, now called health maintenance organizations. The idea proved to have bipartisan appeal. As Lawrence Brown (1983) notes, liberals saw the PGP model as a corrective to the fragmented nature of the benefits provided by the Medicare law; the model also addressed conservatives' concerns about the fiscal implications of the open-ended re-imbursement methods that were built into the Medicare law (199). As PGPs were described, they "offered comprehensive preventive, ambulatory, and inpatient care; faced incentives to serve patients before illnesses developed; and operated with budgets fixed in advance each year." Brown characterized President Nixon's HMO initiative as relying "almost entirely on the literal theory of prepaid group practice" (196).

The HMO concept was first suggested to senior officials in the U.S. Depart-ment of Health, Education, and Welfare in February 1970 by Paul Ellwood, M.D., who was then the executive director of the American Rehabilitation Foundation. It was Ellwood who coined the term *health maintenance organi-zation*.[12] The USDHEW officials, who included Under Secretary John Veneman and Lewis Butler, the assistant secretary for planning and development, were considering how the Nixon Administration might respond to two problems—rapidly rising costs in the Medicare and Medicaid programs and the growing congressional pressure for a national health insurance program.

Ellwood, an evangelistic and inspirational speaker, argued that fee-for-service created problematic incentives. He suggested a major public-policy ini-tiative be undertaken to develop HMOs that would encourage prevention, timely primary care, and economical use of resources. The policy makers were Californians who knew and admired Kaiser's PGPs that used full-time salaried physicians to serve an enrolled population. Ellwood saw Kaiser as a prototype but believed it would not be feasible to try to create Kaiser-like plans through-out the nation because of cost, certain resistance from organized medicine, and the lack of a track record in most parts of the country. Thus he suggested that the organization-building effort should include other models, such as the San Joaquin County Medical Foundation, which included Kaiser's prepayment fea-ture but that did not use full-time salaried physicians (Brown 1983). Thus, from their earliest origins as a Nixon Administration initiative, HMOs included IPAs as well as prepaid group practices.

For a relatively conservative administration, the inclusion of IPAs within the definition of HMOs served important purposes regarding cost, scale, and potential opposition. IPAs were relatively inexpensive to establish and did not require physicians to give up either their office practices or fee-for-service medicine. They thus generated much less resistance from physicians; indeed local medical societies became the major early sponsors of IPAs.

The HMO program, which was announced in a major health speech by President Nixon, was initially discussed in grand terms by its advocates within the administration. In a 1971 USDHEW White Paper described the administration's expectations for the development of HMOs: 450 by the end of 1973; 1,700 by the end of fiscal-year 1976 (enough to serve forty million people); and sufficient capacity to enroll ninety percent of the population by the end of the decade. However, the legislative parameters that emerged from the White House and its Office of Management and Budget called for a modest investment: $23 million for planning grants for HMOs, $22 million for grants and loans to launch HMOs in medically underserved areas, and $300 million in loan guarantees to enable fledgling HMOs to borrow money (Brown 1983). Although the vision was grand, the provision for HMO funding was appropriate only for a limited demonstration program. The modesty not only reflected the administration's desire to minimize the program's cost and the federal government's role, but also its expressed hope that the organizations created under the HMO program would be able to attract investor capital.

The HMO Act was the compromise of several powerful individual and institutional players who had very different views about HMOs and what their role should be. Although fault lines changed to some extent in the three years of struggle over this legislation,[13] the ultimate conflict involved the Nixon Administration and three key Democratic congressional figures—Senator Edward Kennedy (MA), chair of the health subcommittee of the Committee on Labor and Public Welfare; Representative Paul Rogers (FL), chair of the Subcommittee on Health and the Environment; and physician/attorney Representative William Roy (KS), a junior member who took an intense interest in the topic. The administration may have proposed a demonstration program, but the congressional drafters of the legislation envisioned HMOs as a path toward larger change in the health system. The Senate in 1972 passed a Kennedy bill that authorized more than five billion dollars over three years, and Roy had one billion dollars in his first bill.

As passed in 1973, the HMO Act authorized only $375 million to be spent over five years. It provided for grants and loans for planning and developing new HMOs; however, it did not include operating subsidies. Thus, the organizations that had been designed in the give-and-take of the legislative process would have to succeed in a marketplace in competition with existing organizations. Furthermore, the legislation included several potentially expensive provisions (from the Kennedy and Roy-Rogers proposals) requiring, for example, that HMOs would have to provide treatment for alcohol and drug abuse, aid in mental health crises, and offer preventive dental care for children. HMOs thus would have costs that their competitors would not necessarily bear, giving them a disadvantage in competition with established insurers. HMOs were also required (thanks to Kennedy) to accept all applicants ("open enrollment") and to charge a uniform price to all enrollees ("community rating"). Not surprisingly, these provisions had been strongly opposed by the Group Health Association of America, the trade association of the prepaid group practices, on the grounds that open enrollment would attract people who already had expensive conditions, which would require the HMO to charge rates that would not be competitive in the marketplace (Brown 1983). Dubbed the "anti-HMO" Act of 1973 by academics, the legislation's combination of provisions was unworkable from the beginning.

Not all of the act's provisions, however, were negative. One of its most important components was a "dual choice" provision that required employers who offered health benefits to twenty-five or more employees to provide an HMO option if a federally qualified HMO was available. Since most large employers offered health benefits, the dual choice provision opened many markets to HMOs (provided, of course, that they could compete on price). The "federal qualification" process meant that the federal Office of Health Maintenance Organizations (OHMO) was not only responsible for trying to stimulate HMOs, it was also in the business of regulating them.

Implementation would have been difficult under any circumstances, but the HMO Act was put into operation by an administration that objected to several of its provisions. Congress had included features that did not comport with the modest demonstration program the Nixon Administration had envisioned, such as ongoing regulation of HMOs, provisions to override obstructive state laws, and a revolving loan fund that could make the program difficult to terminate (Brown 1983). Opinion was divided about whether genuine difficulties or deliberate bureaucratic sloth characterized the early implementation of the HMO Act.

Whatever the cause, most of the appropriated funds were returned unspent to the treasury during the program's initial years. Only a handful of plans managed to qualify for federal funding in the first few years, fewer, actually, than the department had been quietly supporting without explicit legislative authorization in the years prior to the passage of the act.[14] Seen from this perspective, the act initially slowed the development of HMOs.

Amendments to the act in 1976 relaxed most of the provisions that were allegedly making it impossible for HMOs to meet the requirements of federal qualification (open enrollment, community rating, generous benefit packages) while also successfully competing with insurers who were not subject to these requirements. The 1976 legislation and additional amendments in 1978 changed the demonstration-program orientation that had persisted through the Ford Administration, increasing the authorization and extending the program into the future. Administrative changes during the Carter Administration corrected many implementation problems that had plagued the program during its early years.[15]

Notwithstanding its early problems, the HMO Act had profound effects on the future trajectory of the HMO field. In establishing a grant and loan program to support the development of HMOs, the act defined and legitimized HMOs and codified important basic concepts, including capitation, community rating, a structure that included enrolled members and participating providers, and comprehensive benefits that promoted health by covering routine physicals and that minimized copayments and deductibles. The basic architecture created by the act gave a federal imprimatur to an HMO concept that included for-profits as well as nonprofits and IPAs as well as PGPs. This was important because both for-profit ownership and the IPA had been matters of controversy when the HMO Act was being drafted.

Because the initial Nixon Administration approach for HMOs aimed at providing the maximum stimulus for HMOs with a minimum amount of federal spending, its proposal emphasized loans and loan guarantees, with minimal regulation or restriction on what could be called an HMO, and with hopes for stimulating private investment. This is why Nixon's plan included both IPAs, the preferred vehicle of organized medicine (which was influential in the Nixon White House) and for-profit HMOs. Initially, Congressman Roy was against both for-profit ownership and IPAs, and Senator Kennedy adamantly opposed IPAs. Kennedy, who was pushing strongly for major health reform at the time, saw the proposed use of federal funds to create IPAs as retreading "the same old ways of delivering health services under different names." Kennedy viewed IPAs as mere associations of fee-for-service practitioners and saw no justification for federal subsidies. His bill, which passed the Senate in 1972 and his committee in 1973, restricted support to the PGP model.[16] During the highly contested floor debate on the 1973 legislation, however, Kennedy unexpectedly offered a compromise substitute bill that broadened the definition of eligible HMOs to include IPAs (Brown 1983, 227, 163). Thus, in the HMO Act, IPAs met the federal definition of an HMO.

While the original Nixon strategy of HMO development envisioned the encouragement of private investment and for-profit plans, investor ownership was viewed negatively by both Kennedy and Roy. As a result, with narrow exceptions, federal support for HMO planning and development under the act was limited to nonprofits. The act did not permit either grant or loan support for for-profit HMOs, though there was a loan guarantee provision for for-profits located in medically underserved areas.

The reasons for not offering support for for-profits can be inferred from congressional hearings and statements. First there were worries that for-profit HMOs would take the money but provide little or poor-quality care—in short, that commercial plans would be less trustworthy than supposedly more stable, community-oriented nonprofit plans. Second, there were concerns that for-profit ownership was inconsistent with the reformers' social goals and ideals, as reflected in provisions such as the requirements for open enrollment and community rating. Some legislators also believed that it would be inappropriate for the federal government to provide venture capital to for-profit entrepreneurs in health care. Thus, although the act provided for support of for-profit HMOs only under very limited conditions, it did not preclude the creation and federal qualification of for-profit HMOs.

By the time the federal government ended its grant program to HMOs in fiscal 1981,[17] it had provided a total of "$145 million for 657 grants and $185 million for eighty-five loans and loan guarantees" and "over one hundred plans had received Federal support for initial development."[18] The Federal Office of HMOs noted that during the life of the program, the total number of HMOs in the country had increased from "about thirty in 1971 to nearly 250 in 1981 and membership had tripled to over ten million" (Touche Ross & Co. 1982, 9). The federal HMO program could not claim credit for all of this growth, however. As of mid-1981, only about forty percent of the functioning HMOs (with twenty-three percent of HMO enrollment) had received support under the HMO Act, and less than one-third of the organizations that had received support had an operational HMO (Harrison and Kimberly 1982).

In retrospect the 1973 act not only provided a starting point from which more effective efforts could build, but also legitimated the term *HMO* as a vehicle for both public and private policy making. The use of legislation to create an alternative form of health-care delivery had succeeded to a substantial extent, even if not exactly along the path that the legislative sponsors envisioned.

## The Transformation of the HMO Field

The election of Ronald Reagan marked a dramatic turning point in the history of HMOs. The program faced reauthorization in 1981, and the new legislation fundamentally changed the nature of the HMO program. Federal support for the development of HMOs was halted, and the OHMO assumed a new role—the active promotion of HMOs as an opportunity for investors. Activities included publications such as data-filled "investor's guides" and sponsorship of conferences for the investor community (Touche Ross & Co. 1982; 1983). The field as it existed at the beginning of the 1980s reflected the act's influence.

The HMO Act of 1973 had primarily been a source of capital for nonprofit HMOs, and fewer than twenty percent of the plans that existed in 1982 were for-profit. However, the act also provided structure when the Reagan Administration decided to halt federal support of HMOs and promote them as an investment opportunity. Some for-profit HMOs were federally qualified (and thus benefited from the dual-choice requirement), and the IPA model provided an ideal vehicle for entry into local markets. It was flexible, posed no difficulties with state laws restricting the hiring of physicians (because physicians in an IPA maintained their own practices), generated little resistance from the medical establishment, and required minimal capital. So, despite the original intentions of its congressional sponsors, the HMO Act provided the structure that facilitated the transformation of HMOs into for-profit IPAs.

The 1982 *Investors' Guide,* which was prepared under contract by the accounting firm Touche Ross & Co., presented a detailed analysis of thirty-nine HMOs and reported that sixteen had been profitable in 1979 and 1980, with a median return-on-equity of more than thirty percent. Four had returns of more than forty-five percent. James Turnock, an author of the report, was quoted in *Business Week* as observing that, for investors, HMOs "were like any business. If you can pick a winner, you can make a lot of money." In the same article, Paul Ellwood observed that a well-run HMO meets the needs of both clients and investors. The article reported that Citicorp Venture Capital was pursuing investments in HMOs ("an area of great potential that we are actively pursuing," reported an executive), as were Merrill Lynch, Kidder Peabody, Hartford Insurance, Nationwide Insurance, and Humana, which was then a hospital company. It went on to note that Warburg Paribas Becker had invested one million dollars in Health Group International of Ventura County, California, and was predicting that the "year-old plan could earn $3 million to $4 million after taxes by 1986. . . . Some HMO experts," believed that "$1.8 billion in investment would be needed to meet potential demand for HMOs" (*Business Week* 1982).

Additional stimulus was provided by changes in the Medicare law. In 1982 a payment method was adopted whereby HMOs that enrolled Medicare beneficiaries would receive Medicare premiums based on ninety-five percent of the average cost of Medicare services in the fee-for-service system (Langwell and Hadley 1986). Since HMOs should be able to eliminate much waste and reduce unnecessary services, this premium was attractive, particularly in geographic areas where existing Medicare costs were unusually high.

The investment world responded quickly to the signals sent by the federal government. The first stock offering by an HMO company (U.S. Health Care Systems) was issued early in 1983. Initially priced at $20, the stock tripled in price in the first few months and split twice. Two other companies (Maxicare Health Plans and HealthAmerica) quickly followed suit in going public, and by the middle of 1984 they had been joined by four others (Inter-Study 1984). During this period, insurance companies rapidly entered or expanded their involvement in the HMO field; by 1986 some ten insurers owned multiple HMOs, led by Cigna (with more than 900,000 enrollees in twenty-four plans) and Prudential (600,000 enrollees in twenty-two plans) (InterStudy 1987).[19]

When the federal government's role changed from supporting non-profit HMOs to encouraging private investment, there were approximately 240 HMOs with about ten million enrollees. As previously described, the typical HMO was a group- or staff-model plan, and most plans were nonprofit and locally controlled.[20] Within five years, the industry had been transformed. There were some twenty-four million enrollees in some 600 HMOs. The majority of HMOs were for-profit. IPAs far outnumbered group- and staff-model plans. And more than sixty percent of enrollees were in plans affiliated with organizations that operated in multiple states (so-called national firms). The shift toward for-profit HMOs, IPAs, and national firms, though conceptually distinct, were, in fact, all part of one change.

The efforts of the OHMO to encourage private investment and the changed Medicare policies were not the only factors that led to the transformation of the HMO field into the managed-care industry.[21] Several other policy actions also contributed in important ways. The role of each should be understood.

## ERISA

Much of the growth in demand for HMO services in the 1980s came from companies that had employees in multiple states. HMOs' access to this market was enhanced not only by the HMO Act's dual-choice provision but also by legislation that had been passed for other purposes in the previous decade. The Employee Retirement Income Security Act of 1974 (ERISA) helped to create the market conditions that led to the transformed structure of the managed-care industry in the 1980s (Fox and Schaffer 1989).

The main rationales for ERISA were the desirability of uniform national standards for corporate pension and benefit plans, and the argument that diverse and conflicting state and local requirements made it more difficult for companies that operated in multiple states to offer benefit plans. Health insurance was (and continues to be) regulated by the states. Employers and insurance companies chafed under ever-proliferating requirements passed by state legislatures that increased the cost of providing health insurance, such as mandating that particular types of services or providers be covered. Under standards created pursuant to ERISA, corporations could *self*-insure (thereby escaping state regulation that applied to insurance companies) and purchase administrative services for their plan from newly formed "third-party administrator" companies, as well as from insurance companies or HMOs. This enabled national employers to offer uniform health benefits throughout the country and to escape costly state regulatory requirements. By the early 1980s, after ERISA had survived important legal challenges, awareness spread in the corporate sector about the potential savings of self-insuring, "administrative services only" contracts, and the "ERISA preemption" of state regulation. A market opportunity was created for organizations that could administer corporate health-benefit programs on a multi-state or national basis.

When health-care costs became a major concern for large corporate employers in the early 1980s, HMOs were an attractive option because they cost less than conventional health insurance. If HMO companies were able to administer health-benefit programs in multiple states in which a self-insuring company had employees, that employer could save money in several ways— by self-insuring (and thus not compensating insurers for risk-taking), escaping the costs of state mandates and regulations because of ERISA, and purchasing from fewer rather than more "vendors."[22] Administering benefit plans for self-insuring employers proved to be particularly compatible with IPAs' mode of doing business, as did establishing (or purchasing) plans quickly in multiple states.

ERISA's preemption of state laws that "relate to" employee benefit plans had an additional effect that contributed to the growth of HMO enrollment in self-insuring companies. ERISA was generally interpreted by the courts not only to preclude coverage of enrollees by state-enacted consumer-protection legislation but also to prevent patients from bringing malpractice actions against organizations (including HMOs) that administered the benefit programs of self-insuring companies. ERISA became one of the battle grounds of health policy in the 1990s, and, although there was some slippage at the margins, it has been successfully defended by the corporate and managed-care industries. It was estimated in the late 1990s that more than one-third of the 150 million insured Americans were in a self-insured plan (Noble and Brennan 2001).

## Policy by Taxation

Two other areas of regulatory activity—one federal and one state—also contributed to the transformation of HMOs. Federal tax policies discouraged the organization of HMOs on a nonprofit basis. Internal Revenue Service policy actions that were hostile to tax exemptions for nonprofit HMOs began, ironically, in 1974, almost immediately after passage of the HMO Act, whose intent was to stimulate the creation of such organizations. Though the details are somewhat arcane, the IRS raised three issues about the legitimacy of tax exemption for HMOs: whether HMOs, because they served only enrolled populations, provided a sufficiently broad *community* benefit to justify exemptions; the extent to which HMOs operated for the private benefit of affiliated physicians; and the similarity of some HMOs to commercial (tax-paying) health insurers. The latter two issues were particularly salient for IPAs.

A key event was a 1974 case in which the Internal Revenue Service denied the application for a 501(c)(3) tax exemption from a new HMO named Sound Health. Applying the reasoning it had developed in making tax policy for hospitals, the IRS reasoned that because Sound Health was to be supported by premiums and provide service only to subscribers, it lacked the "broad public benefit" needed for exemption as a charitable organization. Under this reasoning no HMO could qualify for exemption.

A 1978 Tax Court decision reversed the IRS decision regarding Sound Health, finding community benefit in many of the plan's characteristics,[23] but by that time, the IRS had developed reservations about two features that were particularly conspicuous in IPAs. In the early 1980s, IRS general counsel memoranda indicated that IPAs could not qualify for tax exemption because their primary activity was conducting a business—the business of insurance—that was similar to businesses operated for profit, and the organizations' primary beneficiaries were the physicians associated with the plan. By the mid-1980s, when demand for and enrollment in HMOs was surging and new IPAs were being created in large numbers, tax experts were advising that the IRS would make it difficult for such plans to qualify for tax exemptions.[24] Although the IRS did not reject large numbers of applications for exemptions from HMOs, its actions and policy pronouncements created uncertainty in the minds of groups that might have considered starting new nonprofit plans in the 1980s.[25] The ending of federal support under the HMO Act in 1982 only compounded the effect.

In 1986, congressional concern about reports of increasingly commercial practices among Blue Cross and Blue Shield plans led to legislation that made it difficult for nonprofit insurers to keep their tax exemption unless they adopted specific practices subsidizing low-income beneficiaries (Schlesinger, Gray, and Bradley 1996). This legislation also legitimized IRS hostility toward tax exemptions for IPAs because they retained risk and therefore assumed an important attribute of an insurance plan. This legislation set the stage for a wave of for-profit conversions of Blues plans in the 1990s.

## Conversions from Nonprofit Status

Contributing to the for-profit transformation of the HMO field in the 1980s was the failure of state regulators to provide oversight in an obscure corner of the law of charities—the for-profit conversion of nonprofit organizations. It was often possible for entrepreneurs to acquire the assets of nonprofit plans for a fraction of their true value. These entrepreneurs were commonly insiders.

In the late 1970s, with almost no discussion in either the health-policy or legal worlds, a few nonprofit HMOs converted to for-profit ownership. Some forty-six plans converted before 1985 (Ginsberg and Buchholtz 1990), and at least another sixty converted before 1997. The total amounts to perhaps one-third of the nonprofit plans that existed in the early 1980s (Bailey 1994). HMO conversions often took the form of leveraged buyouts by groups composed of the HMO's management, key physicians, and board members. Access to capital for expansion was commonly cited as the rationale for conversion. Lax state regulation and uncertainty about how HMOs should be valued allowed insiders to determine the price by which the assets of nonprofit HMOs would be acquired. It became apparent that conversion prices had often been set much too low when some of the converted HMOs were subsequently sold, enriching those who had engineered the conversion. For example, California's Inland Health Plan was converted in 1985 for a "fair market price" of $562,000, of which most went to charity; the new owners sold the company a year later for $37.5 million.[26]

The Health Net and Blue Cross of California cases of the 1990s finally alerted all parties to the amount of wealth represented by an HMO's assets; negotiations between the state of California and Blue Cross of California resulted in a conversion price of $3.2 billion, which was used to create three foundations (Bell 1996; Fox and Isenberg 1996; Hamburger et al. 1995). In the late 1990s, many states passed legislation to regulate the for-profit conversion of nonprofit health-care organizations, but the pace of HMO conversions had actually peaked in the mid-1980s (thirty-nine plans converted between 1985 and 1987).[27]

### The Loss of HMO Distinctiveness

The thirty HMOs and three million enrollees of 1970 became almost seven hundred HMOs and eighty million enrollees thirty years later. But what became of the logic behind the federal stimulus of the HMO as an alternative to indemnity insurance in which physicians and hospitals were paid on a fee-for-service basis? This too was dramatically changed by the transformation in the 1980s.

Early research showed that use of services (and therefore cost) was substantially less in HMOs than under indemnity insurance (Luft 1981). The cost difference was generally attributed to the effects of the contrasting incentive structures—fee-for-service rewarded the provision of more services—although there was uncertainty about how HMOs actually affected services. Notably, most of the early evidence about HMO performance was collected from group- or staff-model plans where physicians were salaried and not subject to the economic incentives of fee-for-service medical care. However, the rapid enrollment growth in the 1980s took place primarily in plans, such as IPAs, in which physicians were paid on a fee-for-service basis.

These plans needed cost containment methods to discourage unnecessary utilization of services, a problem they shared with conventional forms of health insurance. During the 1970s and early 1980s, as health-care cost increases became a major concern for all purchasers of health care, new cost-containment approaches were developed and new organizational forms emerged to make use of them.

One new organizational form exerted market power to control costs. *Preferred provider organizations* (PPOs) were invented in the early 1980s around the simple idea of offering to steer enrolled patients toward hospitals that would offer discounts. A plan that included incentives to patients for use of the hospitals that offered discounts could be offered to purchasers (e.g., employers) at a reduced price. PPOs occupied a hazy middle ground between traditional fee-for-service indemnity insurance, in which insured individuals had free choice of providers, and HMOs in which enrollees' coverage applied only to providers in the network. That distinctive feature of HMOs blurred in the 1990s as many plans begin offering an option called *point of service,* which allowed enrollees to receive partial coverage for services provided outside the HMO's network. By the mid-1990s, about ten percent of HMO enrollment was in point-of-service or "open" plans (InterStudy 1996).

The proliferation of organizational forms was facilitated by the florescence in the 1980s of a family of cost-containment methods, known collectively as utilization management, that responded to the incentives created by fee-for-service payment (Gray and Field 1989). Utilization *review* had been a cost-containment staple of Medicare and the indemnity insurance world. It was based on retrospective review of records to assess whether services that had been provided to patients were necessary and appropriate. Utilization *management* was also carried out by parties who were accountable to purchasers, but its review processes occurred *prior to* the provision of services so that coverage could be denied for services deemed unnecessary or inappropriate. Utilization-management methods included second-opinion programs (soon abandoned as cost ineffective), mandatory prior authorization of elective hospitalization and certain surgical and diagnostic procedures, prior authorization of specialty referrals, and concurrent review of ongoing hospitalizations. Use of these methods eventually helped trigger the public backlash against managed care.

Utilization review and management activities were carried out by several kinds of organizations, including IPA-model HMOs (Hale and Hunter 1988; Gray and Field 1989). Specialized utilization-management firms sprung up that could be hired by insurance companies, HMOs, PPOs, or third-party administrators. Many insurance companies and third-party administrators developed their own utilization-management programs. The use of utilization management came to be known as managed care, and the various kinds of organizations that carried out utilization management—including HMOs—became known, without clear definition or clear lines being drawn, as *managed-care organizations.* By the early 1990s, hybrid terms such as *managed fee-for-service* began to appear in the literature.

Except for the prepaid group practices, distinctions between HMOs and other kinds of health-care services became increasingly difficult to discern. People who were paid to notice (health-services researchers, regulators, trade association officials) could perhaps do so, but there was research evidence that enrollees often were not certain of whether or not they were enrolled in an HMO (Reschovsky, Hargraves, and Smith 2002).

The emergence of the various organizational permutations meant that an array of options existed in addition to prepaid group practices, whose physicians served only enrolled members, and traditional indemnity insurance, in which beneficiaries had freedom of choice in selection of providers. A large employer in the 1990s could offer, for example, an IPA, an IPA with a point-of-service option, and a PPO. Typically, there would be an inverse relationship between the degree of openness or freedom of choice in a plan and its price.

Single insurance companies began offering a similar choice of plans. "HMO" no longer necessarily referred to an organization; it could be, instead, one of several "products" offered by an organization. Customers of a single managed-care organization might choose from options ranging from a plan in which all services were provided by members of a network to a plan in which enrollees had broad freedom of choice. There was not necessarily a one-to-one match between the name of an organization and the name of an HMO (or HMO product) that it might operate. Organizations could even "rent" one another's provider networks, further attenuating the relationship between physicians and the managed-care organizations with which they had contracts.

Increasingly, beginning in the 1980s the term *health plan* came into use, lumping HMOs together with other kinds of organizations. In the 1990s, the unit of analysis for plan performance in some parts of the country, particularly California, became the medical group (which might contract with multiple health plans) rather than health plans themselves. Many HMOs were essentially virtual organizations. As a new century began, HMOs had largely ceased to exist as distinctive organizations.

The history of the American Association of Health Plans provides a nice capsule of the evolving loss of HMO distinctiveness. AAHP was formed in 1995 by the merger of the Group Health Association of America (staff- and group-model HMOs) and the American Managed Care and Review Association (IPAs and utilization-review organizations). Other associations subsequently merged into it. In 2003, its web site said that the more than one thousand member plans (providing coverage to 170 million Americans) included "health maintenance organizations (HMOs), preferred provider organizations (PPOs), other similar health plans and utilization-review organizations (UROs)." In this organizational sense, HMOs, PPOs, UROs, and "others" are all "health plans." In late 2003, the AAHP merged with the Health Insurance Institute of America, the trade association of the commercial health-insurance industry, eliminating a line between conventional health insurance and the HMOs that had been invented as the alternative. The new organization was called America's Health Insurance Plans. Its web site describes it as the voice of America's health insurers, representing "nearly 1,300 member companies providing health insurance coverage to more than 200 million Americans."[28] The word *HMO* does not appear in the web site.

## Conclusion

Many years ago, the political scientist Robert Alford used the term *dynamics without change* to describe health care in the United States (Alford 1972). Surveying the HMO field, one can legitimately ask what has been accomplished in the thirty years since Paul Ellwood pointed to the advantages of the prepaid group practice as a model of health reform that a Republican administration could adopt as an alternative to centralized regulation. It had attractive attributes (a budget, peer control, etc.) and corrected well-known deficits of the existing fee-for-service indemnity model. To make widespread adoption feasible, however, it was necessary to graft some key features of the prepaid group practice onto models that paid fee-for-service. To minimize the federal role, it was desirable to allow (and in the Reagan Administration, to actively seek) investment from the private sector.

I have described how the resulting growth of the HMO types that paid physicians on a fee-for-service basis led first to the development of utilization management methods ("managed care") and then to the emergence of (and blurring of boundaries with) non-HMO forms of managed care. Managed-care organizations were able to halt the growth of health-care costs for a few years in the mid-1990s—no small accomplishment (Fronstin 2001). But there soon followed the virulent and effective anti–managed-care backlash of the late 1990s, which led organizations that used utilization management methods to abandon them and to increase the size of their provider networks. In the wake of these changes the world of managed care came to look very much like the indemnity insurance system that HMOs had supposedly replaced, with insurers using their size to negotiate discounts in the amount they paid to providers. The number of prepaid group practices counted in the most recent InterStudy survey—seventeen—is about the same as existed in 1970 when Paul Ellwood first proposed to policy makers that a national program be created to stimulate the growth of new entities that would be called health maintenance organizations.

The ultimate question raised by this chapter is whether the HMO as a policy invention has been a success. Two answers can be given. The positive answer would emphasize the extent to which concepts associated with HMOs have permeated the health-care system—notably the growth of thinking in terms of the health of populations (rather than solely of individuals) and the development of methods to measure the performance of individuals and organizations in the health-care system. The negative answer would emphasize the very limited extent to which plans that embody the pure features of an HMO have survived and grown. Paradoxically, the same factors account both for the growth and fading of HMOs as a policy invention.

Could this story have been different? Of course. As I've shown, a series of decisions made by policy makers led first to the enormous growth of the organizational entities called HMOs and then to their organizational transformation from local nonprofit entities into national mostly for-profit firms, which in turn led both to the aggressive use of cost-containment methods that made "managed care" the villain of American health care and to the loss of organizational distinctiveness for HMOs. The inclusion of IPAs in the original definition of HMOs contributed substantially to all of this. However, had they not been so included, it seems unlikely that prepaid group practices could have grown to fill the space that later came to be occupied by other organizational forms.

Might the rapid growth of IPAs (and the associated utilization management methods) have occurred in the 1980s if the model had not undergone a decade of development and legitimization under the shaping influence of federal qualification as HMOs? Perhaps. The pressures that health-care costs exerted on government and corporate purchasers of care in the late 1970s and early 1980s would probably have led to the growth of organizations that had some capacity for influencing health-care costs. The IPA as an organizational form might well have become an attractive option at that time, even in the absence of successful federally qualified examples. Without question, however, the HMO Act made that development both more feasible and, therefore, more likely.

The most interesting aspect of HMOs as an instrument of federal health policy was that they were designed in a political process but had to compete with other organizations in the health-care marketplace. Once the most burdensome of the original federal requirements were lightened or removed, HMOs did compete effectively, with significant price advantages over conventional unmanaged health insurance. In the 1980s and 1990s, indemnity insurance was largely replaced not only by HMOs but also by other organizational forms that used the methods of managed care. The competitive arena shifted from HMO versus conventional insurance to competition among different types of managed-care arrangements, including preferred-provider organizations. In this competition, the prepaid group practices that had provided the original inspiration for the act were progressively supplanted by other types of organizations.

The economist James Robinson has analyzed the eclipse of the prepaid group practice—the pure form of the HMO—in terms of economic factors that favored other models (Robinson 2004). In Robinson's analysis, PGPs as an organizational model faced challenges that are common to all enterprises that share certain key characteristics—vertical integration, prospective payment, and employee ownership. The PGPs' exclusive linkages between insurers and providers run into diseconomies that are generally found in vertical integration arrangements between suppliers and customers. Customers (the insurer half of the HMO) can usually benefit economically by purchasing from specialized firms that serve many customers rather than owning their own exclusive source of supply. Capitated payments reward recipients for reducing costs in both legitimate and illegitimate ways, and salaried physicians have attenuated incentives for productivity. Multispecialty groups run into a host of problems that arise in large organizations and employee-owned firms. Robinson mentions "bureaucratic lethargy, internal factionalism, a widening chasm between individual initiative and group performance, incentives for each participant to ride on the coattails of others, and ever-growing difficulty in maintaining [necessary] coordination and cooperation." Where different specialties are involved, an additional list of diseconomies of scope may emerge: "loss of managerial focus," the difficulty of competing in multiple markets involving different technologies and consumers," the "difficulty in assigning rights and responsibilities," and politicization of decisions about who should be paid how much (202–210). Notwithstanding these disadvantages, there is evidence that group- and staff- model plans performed better on quality measures. However, few purchasers proved willing to make the investments required to engage in sophisticated purchasing in which quality as well as price would be considered, as in the market framework of "managed competition" in which PPGs could compete effectively (Robinson 2004).[29]

If there is an irony in the story told in this chapter, however, it is not that PGPs—the model that inspired the HMO Act—fell prey to problems that come with the territory of their organizational form. It is that their replacement as the dominant form of managed care in the 1980s came at the hands of organizations that were also creations of the HMO Act—IPAs, which evolved in the 1990s under pressure of the anti–managed-care legislation and the demands of corporate purchasers into organizations that were similar in many respects to the conventional insurance that HMOs had been designed to replace. The ability of these organizations (whether called HMOs or PPOs) to control cost came to rely heavily on size. Their ability to influence quality and target inappropriate services was largely lost with the abandonment of utilization management and tight networks of providers. With multiple health plans having contractual arrangements with most providers in their market, the ability of plans to influence care patterns (for example, by providing practice guidelines or providing feedback based on retrospective utilization review) was weak. And with services increasingly being provided outside the plan because of point-of-service options, the plan performance measures that had been developed by the National Committee on Quality Assurance became less and less meaningful.

This chapter has illustrated both the power and limitations of public-policy decisions to stimulate change in the health care system. In the HMO example, an interaction between policy decisions and market forces shaped the trajectory of an organizational field that moved from peripheral ideal to mainstream villain. The roots of this trajectory lay in compromises made in securing passage of the original HMO Act, although many other subsequent policy decisions—in administrative agencies, the courts, and succeeding Congresses and presidential administrations—all played a shaping role. The many influential policy decisions—regarding governmental versus private sources of capital, the ERISA exemption from state regulation, tax-exempt status, and others—had intended and unintended consequences, as well as foreseen and unforeseeable effects.

But policy decisions are only half of the story, because HMOs were asked to succeed in a competitive marketplace where they were subject to powerful economic and institutional forces. It is probably impossible to design organizations in a public-policy process that will function as anticipated once they are required to attract private capital and succeed in a competitive marketplace. In a health-care system that is deeply resistant to change, the grand policy idea that was HMO was weathered away by thirty years of public policy and market forces.

## Notes

This work was supported in part by an Investigator Award in Health Policy Research from The Robert Wood Johnson Foundation and by the Atlantic Philanthropies. The views expressed are those of the author and do not imply endorsement by The Robert Wood Johnson Foundation. I am grateful for suggestions by Larry Brown, Dan Fox, Mark Schlesinger, and Rosemary Stevens.

1. Reflecting this, my search on the Google search engine in September 2003 using the combination of "HMO" and "greed" produced 4,560 hits, and the combination of "HMO" and "horror" produced 12,000.

2. As a crude measure of the interest generated by HMOs, between 1971 and late 2003 almost 2,600 articles appeared in the literature covered by the National Library of

Medicine's MedLine system that had either "HMO" or "health maintenance organization" in the title. (More than 5,300 articles had those words in either the title or abstract.)

3. This is the number of HMOs that was reported operational in June 1987. The number shown in Figure 13-1 is InterStudy's year-end number.

4. For example, of the 178 HMOs that failed during the 1980s, 131 failures occurred between 1986 and 1990. There were 124 mergers between 1986 and 1990 (there had been 20 in the previous five years), and 88 HMOs were acquired by national firms in the same period (up from 46 in the previous five years).

5. Some IPAs also contract with multi-specialty group practices, but InterStudy defined a plan as an IPA if it was predominantly organized around solo, single specialty practices.

6. Though the sixty represented only one-fourth of all HMOs, they included eighty percent of enrollment.

7. One study did not find a quality difference (Born and Simon 2001).

8. *The 1983 Investor's Guide to Health Maintenance Organizations,* published by the Federal Office of Health Maintenance Organizations in 1983, identified thirty-one for-profit HMOs owned by organizations that controlled multiple plans. This represented approximately twelve percent of plans then in existence.

9. In this report, InterStudy listed Blue Cross plans separately from the forty-two "National HMO Firms." In subsequent reports, they were combined. In 1986, the Blues plans accounted for 13.5 percent of plans and 13 percent of enrollment.

10. The organizations included Kaiser Foundation Health Plans, Blue Cross Blue Shield Association, United Healthcare Corporation, Humana, Inc., Foundation Health Corporation, CIGNA Corporation, NYLCare Health Plans, WellPoint Health Network, Pacificare Health Systems, and Prudential Health Care.

11. This discussion is based on a paper originally presented at the annual meeting of the American Sociological Association in 1998.

12. According to Falkson's history of those events (1980, 32), Ellwood first used the term *health maintenance organization* at that initial February 5, 1969 meeting with the Nixon Administration officials, though he had been "toying with" the term *health maintenance* in preparation for the meeting. In response to my own query about the policy history of HMOs, Ellwood pointed me to Falkson's book. Falkson also notes that the concept of health maintenance was discussed earlier by Richard Weinerman (1968).

13. See Brown's detailed account.

14. Brown (276) indicates that only four HMOs had received support as of the summer of 1976 when Paul Rogers held a hearing and that about one hundred HMOs had received development grants in the years prior to the passage of the Act (278).

15. See Brown, Chapter 6 for a detailed account.

16. The Group Health Association of America, the trade association of the prepaid group practices, which had been frustrated by PGPs' inability to participate in Medicare because of its fee-for-service payment system and which would otherwise have been delighted by the Nixon discovery of the virtues of prepayment, opposed the inclusion of IPAs within the definition of HMO.

17. The loan program ended a bit later.

18. It is not clear how many HMOs are actually referred to in these numbers.

19. Two insurers were part of joint ventures with hospital companies, Equicor and Partners National Health Plans.

20. According to the March 1982 *Investor's Guide*, 99 of the 250 plans were "affiliated" with larger organizations. 48 of these were Blue Cross plans, which are connected by a service mark but are not under a single corporate governance structure. Four for-profit organizations owned 26 plans: INA/Connecticut General (10 plans), Prudential (7), Wausau (7), and CNA (2).

21. This phrase is borrowed from Hale and Hunter.

22. For example, a cost-saving program implemented by Xerox in the mid-1990s involved a company-wide effort to reduce the number of suppliers by ninety percent. This approach was also applied to its health benefits program. See, Gray 1982, 258.

23. The Court noted that Sound Health operated an open emergency room, had research and educational programs, had established a fund for subsidizing premiums for the poor, had a community-based board, facilitated membership of Medicare and Medicaid patients, and showed no evidence of inappropriate insider benefit. Because any member of the community could enroll in the plan, the Tax Court also rejected the original IRS view that the plan served only the private interests of its members. Sound Health Association v. Commissioner of Internal Revenue Service (13 November 1978).

24. The 1986 legislation that ended the federal tax exemptions for nonprofit health insurers created further complexities for establishing new tax-exempt plans that assumed risks and did not employ physicians. The IRS considered such organizations to be insurers of the sort that lost their exemptions in 1986.

25. By the mid-1980s, the comments of "experts" about the problems that the IRS posed for IPAs have a taken-for-granted quality—as if everyone who knew the rules of the game already understood. For example, a matter-of-fact comment that most new physician-controlled IPAs are starting out as for-profit plans to avoid problems with the IRS is attributed to attorney Jeffrey Kraft, a partner in Gardner, Carlton, and Douglas in Chicago in a 1989 news account about nonprofit HMO conversions in a trade publication in 1989 (Larkin 1989).

26. For other examples see Bailey 1994 and Hamburger, Finberg, and Alcantar 1995.

27. These data are based partly on InterStudy reports and partly on data reported to state insurance commissioners. A research team at the New York Academy of Medicine confirmed most of these conversions by telephone in 1999.

28. www.ahip.org. (accessed 1 July 2004).

29. The terminology of managed competition bears explanation. The idea is that plan sponsors (corporations or governmental programs such as Medicare) would offer beneficiaries a choice among multiple health plans ("multiple choice") and contribute a fixed amount of premium pegged to the least expensive option ("defined benefit"). Premiums would be adjusted so that plans would receive more if sicker beneficiaries enrolled; this was to assure that plans would compete on price and quality, not on enrolling comparatively healthy individuals. Sponsors would also measure quality in different plans and report this information to beneficiaries so that the beneficiaries could choose among plans based on both cost and quality. The leading advocate of managed competition is Alain Enthoven. See Enthoven 1980.

## References

Alford, Robert. 1972. The Political Economy of Health Care: Dynamics without Change. *Politics and Society* 2: 127–164.

Bailey, Anne L. 1994. Charities Win, Lose in Health Shuffle. *Chronicle of Philanthropy* 14.

Bell, Judith E. 1996. Saving Their Assets: How To Stop Plunder at Blue Cross and Other Nonprofits. *The American Prospect,* May–June, 60–66.

Born, Patricia H., and Carol J. Simon. 2001. Patients and Profits: The Relationship between HMO Financial Performance and Quality of Care. *Health Affairs* 20: 167–174.

Brown, Lawrence D. 1983. *Politics and Health Care Organization: HMOs as Federal Policy.* Washington, DC: Brookings Institution.

*Business Week.* 1982. Investors are Eying HMOs. June 14, 114.

Christianson, Jon B., Douglas R. Wholey, and Susan M. Sanchez. 1991. State Responses to HMO Failures. *Health Affairs* 10: 78–92.

Consumer's Union. 1999. How Does Your HMO Stack Up? *Consumer Reports* 64: 23–29.

Durso, K. A. 1992. Profit Status in the Early History of Health Maintenance Organizations. Ph.D. dissertation, Yale University.

Enthoven, Alain. 1980. *Health Plan: The Practical Solution to the Soaring Cost of Medicare.* Reading, MA: Addison-Wesley.

Enthoven, Alain C., and Laura A. Tollen, eds. 2004. *Toward a 21ˢᵗ Century Health System: The Contributions and Promise of Prepaid Group Practice.* San Francisco: Jossey-Bass.

Falkson, Joseph L. 1980. *HMOs and the Politics of Health System Reform.* Chicago: American Hospital Association and Bowie, MD: Robert J. Brady.

Fox, D. M., and P. Isenberg. 1996. Anticipating the Magic Moment: The Public Interest in Health Plan Conversions in California. *Health Affairs* 15: 1.

Fox, D., and D. Schaffer. 1989. Health Policy and ERISA: Interest Groups and Semi-preemption. *Journal of Health Politics, Policy & Law* 14.

Freidson, E. 1975. *Doctoring Together: A Study of Professional Social Control.* New York: Elsevier.

Fronstin, Paul. 2001. The History of Employment-based Health Insurance: The Role of Managed Care. *Benefits Quarterly*: Second Quarter; 17, 2; ABI/INFORM Global.

Ginsberg, A., and A. Buchholtz. 1990. Converting to For-Profit Status: Corporate Responsiveness to Radical Change. *Academy of Management Journal* 33: 445–447.

Gold, M. 1995. *Arrangements between Managed Care Plans and Physicians.* Washington, DC: Prospective Payment Review Commission.

Gray, Bradford H. 1982. *The Profit Motive and Patient Care.* Cambridge, MA: Harvard University Press.

Gray, Bradford H., and Marilyn J. Field, eds. 1989. *Controlling Costs and Changing Patient Care? The Role of Utilization Management.* An Institute of Medicine Report. Washington, DC: National Academy Press.

Greene, J. 1998. Blue Skies or Black Eyes? HEDIS Puts Not-for-Profit Plans on Top. *Hospitals and Hospital Networks* 72: 26–30

Ha, T. Tu, and James D. Reschovsky. 2002. Assessments of Medical Care by Enrollees in For-Profit and Nonprofit Health Maintenance Organizations. *The New England Journal of Medicine* 346: 1288–1293.

Hale, Judith A., and Mary M. Hunter. 1988. *From HMO Movement to Managed Care Industry.* Excelsior, MN: InterStudy.

Hamburger, E., J. Finberg, and L. Alcantar. 1995. The Pot of Gold: Monitoring Health Care Conversions Can Yield Billions of Dollars for Health Care. *Clearinghouse Review,* August–September: 473–504.

Harrison, Deborah H., and John R. Kimberly. 1982. Private and Public Initiatives in Health Maintenance Organizations. *Journal of Health Politics, Policy and Law* 7: 80–95.

Himmelstein, David U., Steffie Woolhandler, Ida Hellander, and Sidney M. Wolfe. 1999. Quality of Care in Investor-Owned vs. Not-for-Profit HMOs. *Journal of the American Medical Association* 282: 159–163.

InterStudy. 1984. *HMO Status Report 1982–1983.* Excelsior, MN: Decision Resources, Inc.

———. 1985. The InterStudy 7. *HMO Summary: June 1985.* Excelsior, MN: Decision Resources, Inc.

———. 1987. *National HMO Firms. 1986. A Report on Companies that Own or Operate HMOs in Two or More States.* Excelsior, MN: Decision Resources, Inc.

———. 1990. *The InterStudy Edge. Managed Care: A Decade in Review 1980–1990.* Excelsior, MN: Decision Resources, Inc.

———. 1993. *The InterStudy Competitive Edge 3.2.* Excelsior, MN: Decision Resources, Inc.

———. 1996. *The InterStudy Competitive Edge 6.1. Part II: HMO Industry Report.* Minneapolis: Decision Resources, Inc.

———. 2000. *The InterStudy Competitive Edge 10.1 Part II: HMO Industry Report.* Minneapolis: Decision Resources, Inc.

———. 2002. *The InterStudy Competitive Edge 12.1 Part II: HMO Industry Report.* Minneapolis, MN: Decision Resources, Inc.

Jacobs, Lawrence R., and Robert Y. Shapiro. 1999. The American Public's Pragmatic Liberalism Meets Its Philosophical Conservatism. *Journal of Health Politics, Policy, and Law* 24: 1021–1031.

Landon, Bruce, and Arnold M. Epstein. 2001. For-Profit and Not-for-Profit Health Plans Participating in Medicaid. *Health Affairs* 20: 162–171.

Landon, Bruce E., Alan M. Zaslavsky, Nancy D. Beaulieu, James A. Shaul, and Paul D. Cleary. 2001. Health Plan Characteristics and Consumers: Assessments of Quality. *Health Affairs* 20: 274–286.

Langwell, Kathryn M., and James P. Hadley. 1986. Capitation and the Medicare Program: History, Issues, and Evidence. *Health Care Financing Review* Annual Supplement: 9–20.

Larkin, H. 1989. Law and Money Spur HMO Profit Status Changes. *Hospitals* 63: 68–69.

Luft, Harold S. 1981. *Health Maintenance Organizations: Dimensions of Performance.* New York: Wiley.

National Industry Council for HMO Development. 1983. *The Health Maintenance Organization Industry: Ten Year Report 1973–1983.* Washington, DC: Washington Industry Council for HMO Development.

Noble, Alice A., and Troyen A. Brennan. 2001. The States of Managed-Care Regulation: Developing Better Rules. In *The Challenge of Regulating Managed Care,* eds. John E. Billi and Gail B. Agrawal, 29–57. Ann Arbor: University of Michigan Press.

Palmiter, Sharon. 1998. Factors Associated with HEDIS Scores for Selected Preventive Services in HMOs. Ph.D. dissertation, University of Rochester.

Patterson, Carol. 1997. For-Profit Versus Nonprofit Health Maintenance Organizations: Efficiency and Efficacy. Ph.D. dissertation, University of California, Berkeley.

Pauly, M. V., A. L. Hillman, and J. Kerstein. 1990. Managing Physician Incentives in Managed Care: The Role of For-Profit Ownership. *Medical Care* 28, no. 11: 1013–1024.

Peterson, Mark. 1999. Introduction: Politics, Misperception, or Apropos? *Journal of Health Politics, Policy and Law* 24: 873–886.

———. ed. 1999. *Journal of Health Politics, Policy and Law* 24 (5). Special issue on the managed care backlash.

Prospective Payment Assessment Commission (PROPAC). 1994. *Enrollment and Disenrollment Experience in the Medicare Risk Program*. Washington, DC: PROPAC.

Reschovsky J. D., J. L. Hargraves, and A. F. Smith. 2002. Consumer Beliefs and Health Plan Performance: It's Not Whether You Are in an HMO but Whether You Think You Are. *Journal of Health Politics, Policy, and Law* 27, no. 3: 353–377.

Riley, G. F., M. J. Ingber, and C. G. Tudor. 1997. Disenrollment of Medicare Beneficiaries from HMOs. *Health Affairs* 16: 117–124.

Robinson, James C. 1999. The Future of Managed Care Organization. *Health Affairs* 18: 7–24.

———. 2004. The Limits of Prepaid Group Practice. In *Toward a 21th Century Health System: The Contributions and Promise of Prepaid Group Practice*. eds. Alain C. Enthoven and Laura A. Tollen. San Francisco: Jossey Bass.

Rossiter, L. F., K. Langwell, T. T. Wan, and M. Rivnyak. 1989. Patient Satisfaction among Elderly Enrollees and Disenrollees in Medicare Health Maintenance Organizations: Results from the National Medicare Competition Evaluation. *Journal of the American Medical Association* 262: 57–63.

Schlesinger, M., B. Gray, and E. Bradley. 1996. Charity and Community: The Role of Nonprofit Ownership in a Managed Health Care System. *Journal of Health Politics, Policy, and Law* 21, no. 4: 697–751.

Sloan, Frank A., and Mark A. Hall. 2002. Market Failures and the Evolution of State Regulation of Managed Care. *Law and Contemporary Problems* 65: 169–206.

Starr, P. 1982. *The Social Transformation of American Medicine*. New York: Basic Books.

Touche Ross & Co. 1982. *Investor's Guide to Health Maintenance Organizations*. Washington, DC: U.S. Government Printing Office.

———. 1983. *Investor's Guide to Health Maintenance Organization*. Washington, DC: Office of Health Maintenance Organizations, U.S. Department of Health and Human Services.

Weinerman, Richard E. 1968. Problems and Perspectives of Group Practice. *Bulletin of the New York Academy of Medicine* 44: 1423–1434.

Welch, W. P., A. L. Hillman, and M. V. Pauly. 1990. Toward New Typologies for HMOs. *The Milbank Quarterly* 68, no. 2: 221–243.

# Contributors

**Robert A. Aronowitz, MD,** is an associate professor of history and sociology of science and family practice and community medicine at the University of Pennsylvania. His research interests are in the history of twentieth-century disease, epidemiology, and population health. He is the author of *Making Sense of Illness: Science, Society, and Disease* (1998) and is currently completing a book on the history of breast cancer.

**Lawrence Brown,** a political scientist, is a professor of health policy and management at Columbia University. His research interests include health-policy analysis and formation and the politics of health care. In recent years his research has focused on health-care reform, including Medicaid and Medicare policies and managed care. He has also studied the provision of medical care for the uninsured.

**Alexandra P. Burns, JD,** is an attorney in private practice. Her interests include the intersections between state responsibility and private duty.

**Lawton Robert Burns, Ph.D., MBA,** is the James Joo-Jin Kim Professor and a professor in the Departments of Health Care Systems and Management at the Wharton School at the University of Pennsylvania. He is also the director of the Wharton Center for Health Management and Economics. He is the author of *The Health Care Value Chain* (2002) and *The Business of Health Care Innovation* (2005).

**Robert Cook-Deegan** is a former physician and molecular biologist who turned to health policy and research policy in 1982 when he joined the congressional Office of Technology Assessment as a science fellow. After six years at OTA, he joined the staff of the National Institutes of Health for one year as its Human Genome Project was beginning. He then worked for eleven years at the Institute of Medicine and the National Research Council before joining the faculty of Duke University in 2002, as the director of the Center for Genome Ethics, Law, and Policy, Institute for Genome Sciences and Policy.

**Amy L. Fairchild** is an assistant professor in the Department of Sociomedical Sciences at Columbia University's Mailman School of Public Health. She is the author of *Science at the Borders: Immigrant Medical Inspection and the Shaping of the Modern Industrial Labor Force* (2003). Her work at the intersection of history, ethics, and politics has appeared in *Science, American Journal of Public Health, Bulletin of the History of Medicine,* and *Journal of the American Medical Association.*

**Bradford H. Gray** is the editor of *The Milbank Quarterly*. He is also a principal research associate at the Urban Institute's Health Policy Center. He formerly was the director of the Division of Health and Science Policy at the New York Academy of Medicine. He is author of *Human Subjects in Medical Experimentation: A Sociological Study of the Conduct and Regulation of Clinical Research* and *the Profit Motive and Patient Care: The Changing Accountability of Doctors and Hospitals*. He is a member of the Institute of Medicine of the National Academy of Sciences.

**Gerald N. Grob** is the Henry E. Sigerist Professor of the History of Medicine (Emeritus), and a member of the Institute for Health, Health Care Policy, and Aging Research at Rutgers University. He is a historian of mental health policy and medicine. His many books include *The State and the Mentally Ill, Mental Institutions in America, Mental Illness and American Society, From Asylum to Community: Mental Health Policy in Modern America, The Mad among Us: A History of the Care of American's Mentally Ill, Interpretations of American History: Patterns and Perspectives,* and *The Deadly Truth: A History of Disease in America.*

**Colleen M. Grogan** is an associate professor in the School of Social Service Administration at the University of Chicago. Her areas of research include health policy, health politics, and the American welfare state. She is currently working on two book manuscripts; one, with Michael Gusmano, explores efforts to include representatives of the poor in health-policy decision making; the other, based on research from her Robert Wood Johnson Health Policy Research Investigator Award, examines the political history of the U.S. Medicaid program from its roots in the nineteenth century to the present.

**Beatrix Hoffman** is an associate professor of history at Northern Illinois University. Her research on emergency rooms is part of her larger project, "A History of the Right to Health Care in the United States," which has received support from the Robert Wood Johnson Foundation and the National Endowment for the Humanities.

**Michael McGeary** is a senior program officer at the Institute of Medicine, Washington, DC. A political scientist, his research interests include the development of the U.S. science and technology enterprise after World War II. At the IOM, he has directed a number of studies of NIH research priorities and programs.

**Gerald Markowitz** is a Distinguished Professor of History at John Jay College of Criminal Justice and the Graduate Center, City University of New York. He is the recipient of numerous grants from private and federal agencies, including the Milbank Memorial Fund, National Endowment for the Humanities, and the National Science Foundation. Together with David Rosner he has authored and edited books and articles on environmental health and occupational safety and health, including, most recently, *Deceit and Denial: The Deadly Politics of Industrial Pollution* (2002).

**David Mechanic** is the René Dubos University Professor of Behavioral Sciences and the director of the Institute of Health, Health Care Policy, and Aging Research at Rutgers University. He also directs the Robert Wood Johnson's Investigator Awards in Health Policy Research Program. His research and publications deal with the social aspects of health and health care.

**Charles E. Rosenberg** is a professor of the history of science and Ernest E. Monrad Professor in the Social Sciences at Harvard University. He has written widely on the history of medicine and science and is currently at work on a history of conceptions of disease during the past two centuries.

**David Rosner** is a professor of history and public health at Columbia University and the director of the Center for the History of Public Health at Columbia's Mailman School of Public Health. He is author of nine books and over eighty articles and review essays. His most recent book is *Deceit and Denial: The Deadly Politics of Industrial Pollution* (2002).

**Rosemary A. Stevens** is a DeWitt Wallace Distinguished Scholar in social medicine and public policy at Weill Cornell Medical College, and the Stanley I. Sheerr Professor Emeritus in the history and sociology of science at the University of Pennsylvania. She has a longtime scholarly and applied interest in public and private responsibilities in American medicine, with many related publications, and is currently focusing on medical specialization from both a historical and policy perspective.

**Nancy Tomes** is a professor of history at the State University of New York at Stony Brook. She is the author of three books, most recently *The Gospel of Germs: Men, Women, and the Microbe in American Life* (1998). With support from the National Humanities Center and the Robert Wood Johnson Foundation, she is completing a book on changing conceptions of the patient-consumer's role in the evolution of modern American medicine.

# Index

AAHP (American Association of Health Plans), 330–331

AARP (American Association of Retired Persons), 221

Abdelhak, Sherif, 281, 293–294

ABIM (American Board of Internal Medicine), 63–64, 66, 69, 70

Abington Hospital (Philadelphia), 291

ABMS. *See* American Board of Medical Specialties

abortion, 26, 27. *See also* reproductive rights

academic-industrial complex. *See* "medical-industrial complex"

academic medical centers (AMCs) (teaching hospitals): commercial exploitation of research at, 19, 146–147, 154, 192–195; competition between hospitals for, 276–278; defined, 184; description of, 51, 53; emergency rooms of, 252, 253, 288; managed care contracts in, 278, 279; Medicaid and Medicare in, 40, 45, 288; medical specialties in, 65; as NIH constituents, 176, 183–185, 190–195; in Philadelphia, 290, 291–292; research in, 34, 179–184, 186; and voluntary national professional service, 72. *See also* education (medical); hospitals; "medical-industrial complex"; *specific institutions*

accessibility (to health care), 8; emergency room as rational response to general lack of elsewhere, 251, 255–256, 267, 268; of HMOs, 310; poor vs. wealthy gap in, 100, 102; as a right, 15, 24, 28, 85, 87, 91; urban vs. rural gap in, 91–92. *See also* coverage; deflection; insurance (health)

accountability. *See* responsibility

accountable health plans (AHPs), 282, 283

accreditation (of hospitals), 53. *See also* hospitals: standards for

Accreditation Council for Graduate Medical Education (ACGME), 61, 72

ACGME (Accreditation Council for Graduate Medical Education), 61, 72

ACSH (American Council on Science and Health), 135–136

acupuncture, 34

ADC (Aid to Dependent Children), 206

adenoidectomies, 52, 55

adolescent medicine specialty, 70

advertising (marketing; public relations), 181; deceptive corporate, 93, 131, 132–137, 153; direct, of prescription drugs, 101, 153, 163, 165–166, 245; emergency-room-related, 252–254, 258, 266; as mirror of society, 28; through physician detailing, 163; regulation of, 94

Advisory Board for Medical Specialties, 56. *See also* American Board of Medical Specialties

Advisory Committee on Genetic Testing, 140

Aetna U.S. Health Care, 278, 286

African Americans, 144–146

Agency for Health Care Policy and Research (AHCPR), 36, 37. *See also* Agency for Healthcare Research and Quality (AHRQ)

Agency for Healthcare Research and Quality (AHRQ), 36–39, 196

agent orange, 136

AGH (Allegheny General Hospital), 275–276, 279, 281

aging population: drugs taken by, 153; expensive choices facing, 104, 216; impoverishing of, to become eligible for Medicaid, 213, 217–219; lack of insurance for, 95; long-term care for, 202–225, 237–238; medicalization of, 153, 161–167; as Medicare and Medicaid beneficiaries, 40, 202, 214, 215, 281; as pressure group, 22, 28; women in, 166; younger generations pitted against, 213, 214–217, 220. *See also* pensions

Agriculture Department (U.S.), 177, 187

AHA. *See* American Hospital Association

AHCPR (Agency for Health Care Policy and Research), 36, 37

AHERF (Allegheny Health, Education, and Research Foundation), 273–308

AHPs (accountable health plans), 282, 283

AHRQ (Agency for Healthcare Research and Quality), 36–39, 196

AIDS, 19, 22, 28, 266; lay advocacy about, 170n. 5; reporting of, 124–125; research protocols on, 99

Aid to Dependent Children (ADC), 206

Aid to Dependent Families, 205

Aid to the Blind, 205

Air Force Office of Scientific Research, 186

alcoholism, 15, 132; and mental illness, 240, 242, 245. *See also* fetal alcohol syndrome; substance abuse

Alford, Robert, 331

Allegheny General Hospital (AGH), 275–276, 279, 281

Allegheny Health, Education, and Research Foundation (AHERF), 273–308; bankruptcy scandal, 8, 273–308

CPSIA information can be obtained at www.ICGtesting.com
Printed in the USA
BVOW03s2356270813

329736BV00008B/42/P